Complications in Knee and Shoulder Surgery

Robert J. Meislin • Jeffrey Halbrecht
Editors

Complications in Knee and Shoulder Surgery

Management and Treatment Options for the Sports Medicine Orthopedist

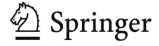

Editors
Robert J. Meislin, MD
Orthopedic Surgery
NYU Hospital for Joint Diseases
New York, NY
USA

Jeffrey Halbrecht, MD
The Institute for Arthroscopy and Sports Medicine
San Fancisco, CA
USA

ISBN: 978-1-84882-202-3   e-ISBN: 978-1-84882-203-0
DOI: 10.1007/978-1-84882-203-0

British Library Cataloguing in Publication Data
A catalogue record for this book is available from the British Library

Library of Congress Control Number: 2009926046

© Springer-Verlag London Limited 2009
Apart from any fair dealing for the purposes of research or private study, or criticism or review, as permitted under the Copyright, Designs and Patents Act 1988, this publication may only be reproduced, stored or transmitted, in any form or by any means, with the prior permission in writing of the publishers, or in the case of reprographic reproduction in accordance with the terms of licenses issued by the Copyright Licensing Agency. Enquiries concerning reproduction outside those terms should be sent to the publishers.
The use of registered names, trademarks, etc., in this publication does not imply, even in the absence of a specific statement, that such names are exempt from the relevant laws and regulations and therefore free for general use.
Product liability: The publisher can give no guarantee for information about drug dosage and application thereof contained in this book. In every individual case the respective user must check its accuracy by consulting other pharmaceutical literature.

Printed on acid-free paper

Springer is part of Springer Science+Business Media (www.springer.com)

"Learn from the mistakes of others—you can never live long enough to make them all yourself."

– John Luther

In dedication to our mentors, Victor Frankel, MD, and Joseph Zuckerman, MD—orthopedic surgeons who taught us about leadership, hard work, and dedication to detail ... and most importantly—how to stay out of trouble!

In appreciation,

– Robert J. Meislin, MD
Jeff Halbrecht, MD

Preface

"To Err is Human..." Alexander Pope

Any surgical intervention has potential risks and complications. This book is designed as a reference tool and a roadmap for the sports medicine orthopedist to minimize the complications in knee and shoulder surgery. Some complications are avoidable; some are not. By understanding the functional anatomy at risk, proper surgical setup, proper equipment, and proper patient selection, a preventative approach to complications can be instituted.

The authors of these chapters represent leaders in orthopedic sports medicine and have provided novel methods for dealing with intraoperative complications and situations that can occur in the midst of a "routine" arthroscopic reconstruction. In discussing these issues, we hope to raise the surgeon's awareness of potential complications and to provide wisdom and advice to properly avoid and treat these problems should they arise.

How one deals with complications truly tests the mettle of the surgeon. Keeping one's "cool" in the midst of an intraoperative complication will be facilitated by having an algorithmic approach. We hope that this book will improve your outcome should these problems occur.

Some complications are unavoidable. Arthrofibrosis or stiffness may take place in the best of hands. Infection may surface postoperatively in the most sterile OR. We provide you with the background to confront these challenges. A list of ten "Pearls" are offered at the beginning of most chapters as a quick reference card.

Because revision surgery automatically has inherent complications, the authors have provided their respective experience with these more complex cases. Techniques are described and pictures are included. We hope that this collective experience will provide confidence and solutions in these trying moments. And from that both the surgeon and the patient will surely benefit.

Robert J. Meislin, MD
New York, NY

Jeffrey Halbrecht, MD
San Francisco, CA

Contents

1 **Avoiding and Managing Complications in Meniscus Repair**........ 1
   Trong B. Nguyen and Peter R. Kurzweil

2 **Avoiding and Managing Complications in Meniscus Transplantation**..................................... 19
   Benjamin Shaffer and J.R. Rudzki

3 **Avoiding and Managing Complications in Cartilage Restoration Surgery**..................................... 37
   Bert R. Mandelbaum, Joshua A. Johnston, and Jason M. Scoop

4 **Avoiding and Managing Complications in ACL Reconstruction**.... 53
   Don Johnson and Olufemi Ayeni

5 **Avoiding and Managing Complications in PCL Reconstruction**..... 75
   Shane T. Seroyer and Christopher D. Harner

6 **Avoiding and Managing Complications of Collateral Ligament Surgery of the Knee**..................... 91
   Leon E. Paulos and Kirk Mendez

7 **Avoiding and Managing Complications in Osteotomies of the Knee**................................... 115
   David A. Vasconcellos, J. Robert Giffin, and Annunziato Amendola

8 **Avoiding and Managing Complications in Patella Surgery**........ 133
   Michael V. Elman, Scott Zimmer, and Anthony A. Schepsis

9 **Avoiding and Managing Complications Associated with Arthroscopic Knee Surgery: Miscellaneous Knee Conditions**... 165
   Eric J. Strauss and Robert J. Meislin

10 **Avoiding and Managing Complications in Shoulder Labral Repair**..................................... 175
    Jeffrey S. Abrams

11 **Avoiding and Managing Complications for Shoulder Superior Labrum (SLAP) Repair**........................... 189
    Michael S. Bahk and Stephen J. Snyder

12 **Avoiding and Managing Complications of Arthroscopic Biceps Tenodesis**... 207
Michael S. Bahk, Joseph P. Burns, and Stephen J. Snyder

13 **Avoiding and Managing Complications of Arthroscopic Rotator Cuff Repair**... 225
John Trantalis and Ian K.Y. Lo

14 **Avoiding and Managing Complications of Surgery of the Acromioclavicular Joint**................................ 245
Matthew T. Provencher, Lance LeClere, Anthony A. Romeo, and Augustus A. Mazzocca

15 **Complications of Arthroscopic Shoulder Surgery: Miscellaneous Shoulder Conditions**........................ 265
Alexander Golant and Young W. Kwon

Index... 273

Contributors

Jeffrey S. Abrams, MD
Orthopedic Surgery, Princeton Orthopedic Associates and Sports Medicine, Princeton, NJ, USA

Annunziato Amendola, MD
Department of Orthopedics and Rehabilitation, University of Iowa Hospitals and Clinics, Iowa City, IA, USA

Olufemi Ayeni, MD, FRCSC
Sports Medicine Clinic, Carleton University, Ottawa, ON, Canada

Michael S. Bahk, BA, MD
Southern California Orthopedic Institute, Van Nuys, CA, USA

Joseph P. Burns, BA, MD
Southern California Orthopedic Institute, Van Nuys, CA, USA

Michael V. Elman, MD
Orthopedic Surgery, Boston University Medical Center, Boston, MA, USA

J. Robert Giffin, MD
Department of Orthopedic Surgery, University of Western Ontario, London, ON, Canada

Alexander Golant, MD
Orthopedic Surgery, NYU Hospital for Joint Diseases, New York, NY, USA

Christopher D. Harner, MD
Department of Orthopedics, University of Pittsburgh Medical Center, Pittsburgh, Allegheny County, PA, USA

Donald H. Johnson, MD, FRCSC
Sports Medicine Clinic, Carleton University, Ottawa, ON, Canada

Joshua A. Johnston, MD
Orthopedic Surgery, Santa Monica Orthopedic and Sports Medicine Group, Santa Monica, CA, USA

Peter R. Kurzweil, MD
Department of Sports Medicine, Southern California Center for Sports Medicine, Long Beach, Los Angeles, CA, USA

Young W. Kwon, MD, PhD
Department of Orthopedic Surgery, NYU Hospital for Joint Diseases,
New York, NY, USA

Lance LeClere, MD, LT, MC, USN
Orthopedic Surgery, Naval Medical Center San Diego, San Diego, CA, USA

Ian K.Y. Lo, MD, FRCSC
Surgery, University of Calgary, Calgary, AB, Canada

Bert R. Mandelbaum, MD
Orthopedic Surgery, Santa Monica Orthopedic and Sports Medicine Group,
Santa Monica, CA, USA

Augustus A. Mazzocca, MD
Orthopaedic Surgery, University of Connecticut Health Center, Farmington,
CT, USA

Robert J. Meislin, MD
Orthopedic Surgery, NYU Hospital for Joint Diseases, New York, NY, USA

Kirk Mendez, MD
Private Practice, Orthopedic Specialist of Nevada, Las Vegas, NV, USA

Trong B. Nguyen, MD
Orthopedic Surgery, Southern California Center for Sports Medicine,
Long Beach, Los Angeles, CA, USA

Leon E. Paulos, MD
Department of Orthopedic Surgery, Baylor College of Medicine,
Houston, TX, USA

Matthew T. Provencher, MD, LCDR, MC, USN
Department of Orthopedic Surgery, Naval Medical Center San Diego,
San Diego, CA, USA

Anthony A. Romeo, MD
Department of Orthopedics, Rush University Medical Center, Chicago, IL, USA

J.R. Rudzki, MD
Department of Orthopedic Surgery, The George Washington University
School of Medicine, Washington, Washington, DC, USA

Anthony A. Schepsis, MD
Orthopedic Surgery, Boston University Medical Center, Boston, MA, USA

Jason M. Scopp, MD
Peninsula Orthopedic Associates, Salisbury, MD, USA

Shane T. Seroyer, MD
Department of Orthopedic Surgery, University of Pittsburgh Medical Center,
Pittsburgh, PA, USA

Benjamin S. Shaffer, MD
Department of Orthopedic Surgery, The George Washington University School of Medicine, Washington, Washington, DC, USA

Stephen J. Snyder, MD
Southern California Orthopedic Institute, Van Nuys, CA, USA

Eric J. Strauss, MD
Orthopedic Surgery, NYU Hospital for Joint Diseases, New York, NY, USA

John N. Trantalis, MBBS
Orthopedics, University of Calgary, Calgary, AB, Canada

David A. Vasconcellos, MD
Department of Orthopedics and Rehabilitation, University of Iowa Hospitals and Clinics, Iowa City, IA, USA

Scott Zimmer
Sports Medicine, Boston University School of Medicine, Boston, MA, USA

Chapter 1
Avoiding and Managing Complications in Meniscus Repair

Trong B. Nguyen and Peter R. Kurzweil

Top 10 Pearls

- Patient selection is vital to a successful repair.
- Treat a Meniscus Repair like a bony nonunion.
- Reduce the tear and hold reduction with temporary fixation.
- Create a stable repair that can withstand flexion and extension of the knee. Test it!
- Insert fixator perpendicular to tear to provide compression at the meniscal repair site.
- Avoid fixator threads or barbs crossing the repair site – they prevent compression.
- Medial distraction, through use of a femoral distractor or pie-hole incisions of the medial collateral ligament (MCL), is sometimes necessary, especially in tight knees, to avoid scuffing the articular surface.
- Consider the use of adjunctive healing factors, such as, "fibrin" platelets, or newer platelet-rich plasma (PRP) concentrates.
- Revision repairs for failures often require more "formal" suture repair techniques.
- Adherence to the postoperative protocol is crucial to the success of the procedure.

T.B. Nguyen (✉)
Southern California Center for Sports Medicine,
Long Beach, CA, USA
e-mail: trong.nguyen.md@gmail.com

P.R. Kurzweil
Department of Sports Medicine, Southern California Center for Sports Medicine, Long Beach, Los Angeles, California, USA

Introduction and Background

Preventing complications in meniscal repairs begin with a thorough understanding of the anatomy and function of the meniscus. Over the last 25 years, our awareness of meniscal properties and behavior has grown, resulting in a desire to restore the anatomy of the meniscus, casting aside the once common, reflexively performed menisectomies. From meniscal repairs and partial menisectomies to entire meniscal allograft transplantation, the range of treatment options subsequently developed has paralleled the expansion of our knowledge.

This chapter will focus on the various techniques employed in meniscal repairs. In addition, we will emphasize the procedural steps that we believe the community orthopedists will need to undertake and the concepts that need to be understood to minimize the risk of complications. As with any surgery, reducing the rate of complications and failures begins as soon as the orthopedic surgeon meets the patient in the office. A thorough history and physical examination, as well as appropriate imaging studies are needed to help make the diagnosis and identify associated pathology. Finally, an in-depth conversation with the patient is needed regarding the treatment options, risks, and benefits of the different surgical procedures available. Moreover, a preoperative discussion with the patient regarding postoperative rehabilitation, restrictions, and expectations will be necessary to avoid confusion and promote compliance with physical therapy protocols. In select patients, particularly, highly competitive or scholarship athletes, this step is crucial because it could mean the difference between a quick return to sport or a season-ending operation. Some individuals may also need a quick return to their job for financial reasons.

Functional Anatomy at Risk

Our basic understanding of the microvascular anatomy of the meniscus stems from Arnoczky and Warren's classic study where cadaveric specimens of the medial and lateral menisci of the human knee were analyzed by histology and tissue clearing (Spalteholz) techniques.[1] It was found that the menisci are supplied by the superior and medial branches of the lateral, medial, and middle genicular arteries. In addition, a peripheral, vascularized, synovial fringe expands over the femoral and tibial surfaces of the menisci. However, it does not confer any vascularity to the meniscal tissue itself (Fig. 1.1). It is important to also note that the posterolateral aspect of the lateral meniscus at the popliteal hiatus is deficient of peripheral vessels as well as the synovial fringe. In contrast, the anterior and posterior horns of the menisci are covered with vascular synovial tissue and appear to be well vascularized.[1] At birth, the meniscus is completely vascularized throughout its entirety, even to its rim. However, by 9 months, the inner one-third becomes avascular and, by 10 years of age, the child's meniscus resembles that of an adult,[2,3] with the lateral meniscus having 10-25% of its outer rim vascularized, and the medial meniscus, 10-30%. The so-called "red-red" zone of an adult meniscus is estimated to be 3 mm from the peripheral attachment and, conversely, the "white-white" avascular zone was >5 mm. In between, from 3 to 5 mm, was a variable zone in which the amount of vessel infiltration changed from specimen to specimen. This discovery was vital to the understanding of which meniscal tears may have the potential to heal and is a key ingredient in determining whether a meniscal repair is indicated or not.

Not only were the anatomic studies showing us that meniscal repairs were viable, but biomechanical studies also demonstrated the importance of menisci function within the knee. Its role as a load-sharing structure that distributes forces and centers the condylar surfaces were elucidated in various studies.[2,4,5] It was also shown that the menisci reduced the joint contact forces within the knee, thereby reducing the rate of wear and degenerative arthritis.[6] Mechanoreceptors were also found to exist in the periphery of the meniscus, leading to the theory that they had a role in propioception of the knee as well.[2,7] Studies in post-total menisectomy knees have shown sequelae of early degenerative joint disease,[6,8] all stressing the importance of reestablishing the anatomy of damaged meniscus, whenever possible.

Studies on the ultrastructure of the meniscus have helped educate us on how to treat meniscal tears once the determination is made to perform a repair. Collagen fibers are arranged in various patterns, with the majority lining up circumferentially throughout the meniscus (Fig. 1.2).[9] These longitudinal fibers are oriented such that they resist the significant hoop stresses that the meniscus encounters during natural movement. Radial collagen fibers essentially "tie" the circumferential fibers together into bundles, which add stability and strength to the overall structure.[10] As result, repairing longitudinal tears, such as bucket-handle meniscal

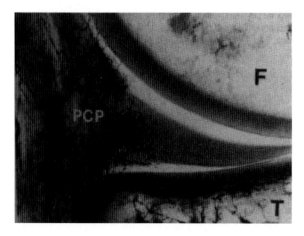

Fig. 1.1. Human Meniscus prepared by tissue clearing (Spalteholz) technique. A perimeniscal capillary plexus begins in the capsular and synovial tissues and supplies the outer 10-25% of the menisci

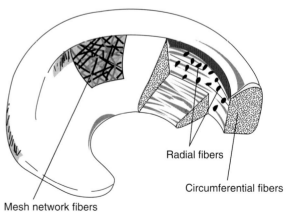

Fig. 1.2. Arrangement of collagen fibers within the human meniscus

tears, require reapproximating these circumferential collagen fibers. This is the proposed theory as to why the vertical mattress suture has been shown to have the highest load-to-failure strength.[11]

Indications for Repair

Patient Selection

Preventing complications begins as soon as one suspects a meniscal tear in a patient. This entails a detailed interview to rule out other causes of knee pain and entities that can mimic meniscal tears. The majority of meniscus tears can be diagnosed with a thorough history and physical examination. Once the diagnosis is made, standard radiographs are helpful in assessing knee alignment, and whether or not osteoarthritis is present. MRI is often helpful with characterizing the location and type of tear preoperatively, as well as identifying associated injuries, such as anterior cruciate ligament (ACL) injuries or subchondral bone injury and edema. Indications for repair include vertically oriented traumatic tears located in the peripheral 3 mm at the red-red zone (Fig. 1.3). Additionally, minimal degenerative changes in both the meniscus and surrounding cartilage are requirements for repair in order to maximize the chance of success. As with any surgery, proper indications reduce one's risk of failures and/or complications. Concomitant injuries, particularly, with ACL reconstructions, introduce healing cytokines and growth factors that have been shown to increase the rates of healing.[12]

Once the decision is made that a repair of a meniscal tear is possible, a thorough discussion is done with the patient regarding the risks and benefits of the surgery, as well as the rehabilitation requirements and expected outcomes. Informing patients of additional incisions is also recommended to prevent this from being a surprise in the recovery room. Following this, the surgeon needs to decide on his preferred method of repair. We recommend being facile at a number of different methods of repair and ensuring that the operating room at the hospital or surgery center has the appropriate tools and devices.

Intraoperative Details: Preventing Complications and Avoiding Pitfalls

Setting up

For the majority of our knee arthroscopic surgeries, we prefer general anesthesia over regional or local anesthesia, mainly due to the ability to have patients completely relaxed, free from muscular contractions, which permits the surgeon to open the medial compartment with valgus stress against a proximal, lateral thigh post, or in a figure-4 position for the lateral compartment. We try to avoid inflating the tourniquet during the procedure, as this helps assess whether the tear-site is vascularized. Nevertheless, a tourniquet is routinely placed on the upper thigh and the patient is positioned supine with the knee resting in extension. Prophylactic preoperative antibiotics (1 g of a first generation cephalosporin, if not allergic) are given intravenously

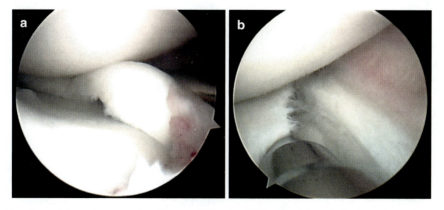

Fig. 1.3 Bucket-handle medial meniscus tear in a 15-year-old female. (**a**) Tear extends to the body of the meniscus and is easily displaced by a blunt trocar. (**b**) Displaced tear located at the periphery of the meniscus, within 3 mm of the meniscosynovial junction

approximately 30 min prior to incision. Finally, a "time-out" is performed with the cooperation of the nursing and anesthesia staff to identify the patient and the correct operative limb.

Diagnostic Arthroscopy

An important aspect of our standard arthroscopy protocol is the sole use of a gravity pressure head for inflow instead of a high-pressure pump. This gentle lavage of Lactated Ringers solution placed on an intravenous pole reduces the amount of imbibed fluid within the surrounding tissue while reducing postoperative pain and swelling. A standard diagnostic arthroscopy is performed through the anterolateral viewing portal. The anteromedial working portal is localized with a spinal needle to ensure optimal access to the pathology. A third outflow portal is not routinely used. In tight knees, the lateral meniscus can be seen relatively easily in the figure-4 position. However, the medial meniscal peripheral edges can be more difficult to visualize. Options to help visualization of this area include entering the medial side with the arthroscope through the intercondylar notch or using a 70° arthroscope. Alternatively, a posteromedial or posterolateral portal can be used. Most of the time, maximum valgus pressure with the thigh post and the knee near full extension suffices to allow visualization.

Preparation of Meniscal Repair Site

Regardless of the technique chosen for repair, it is crucial to prepare the meniscal repair site to maximize its chance for healing. In this regard, we liken the repair of a meniscus tear to fixation of a nonunion of a bony fracture. Without proper preparation of the nonunion site, operative treatment may fail. For successful healing to occur in both situations, a good blood supply is critical as well as the formation of a stable repair construct. First, removal of fibrous tissue creates a surface milieu more conducive to healing. We recommend rasping the edges of the meniscus tear to remove nonviable tissue and to create a bleeding bed (Fig. 1.4). Often, using a small motorized arthroscopic shaver with minimal or no suction (to avoid overly aggressive debridement) can assist in freshening the ends of the tears. Rasping of the paramensical synovium may also induce more

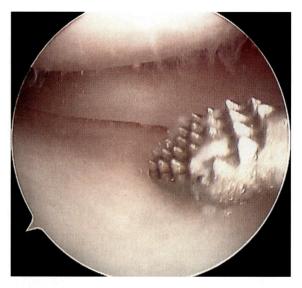

Fig. 1.4 Preparation of meniscal tear using an arthroscopic rasp to debride and stimulate the repair site

blood vessel formation. Finally, trephination is an effective alternative to establishing a healthy blood supply.[13,14] We routinely pass a needle through the peripheral fragment (either outside-in or inside-out) to help bring bleeding into the repair site (Fig. 1.5).

In particularly tight, varus knees, it can be difficult to gain enough exposure in the medial compartment during the meniscal repair to avoid damaging the articular surface. In such cases, we have found it helpful to perform a modified "pie-crust" of the MCL to help

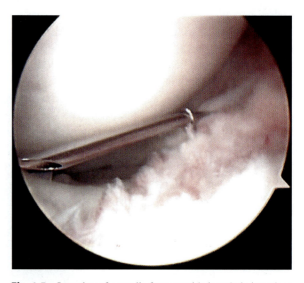

Fig. 1.5 Insertion of a needle from outside in to help introduce blood to the repair site as well as provide temporary fixation during the repair

open the joint space while providing a solid, valgus stress. To perform this, a 14-gauge angiocath needle, instead of a scalpel, is inserted into the MCL from outside through the skin. Without removing the angiocath needle from the skin, we pass the needle through the MCL multiple times in different places and at different levels. After placing a valgus force on the knee, the MCL should lengthen but remain in continuity. If a complete or partial MCL tear is iatrogenically incurred, then we immobilize the knee for 6 weeks in a hinged knee brace, but do not significantly alter the postoperative rehabilitation protocol. We believe this to be the "lesser of two evils," because we feel long-term results can be improved if damage to the articular cartilage can be prevented at the expense of a temporary MCL attenuation, which can heal uneventfully.

Techniques to stabilize a fracture site can also come into play when performing a meniscal repair. As with fractures, we strive for compression of the repair site. This helps minimize motion at the tear and promotes a stable healing environment. Placing the sutures or repair devices perpendicular to the tear also simulates fixation of a bony fracture. For this, we usually insert the fixator device or suture needle from the contralateral portal, while observing through the ipsilateral portal, in order to obtain sufficient compression, similar to an interfragmentary screw. It is imperative to create a meniscus repair stable enough to withstand the forces imparted during flexion and extension of the knee and postoperative weight bearing. At the end of a repair, the instruments are removed and the knee is taken through a few cycles of range of motion. The arthroscope is then reinserted to verify and document that the repair remains intact.

Enhancement Agents

In addition to proper preparation of the meniscal repair site, healing of the tear can be enhanced by the addition of either a fibrin clot or a platelet-rich plasma (PRP), both derived from a small sample of the patient's own blood. The fibrin clot has been widely used for many years and has been shown to be effective in supplementing meniscal repairs.[15-17] In a similar fashion, the Platelet-Rich Fibrin Matrix™ (PRFM) system (Cascade, Devon, United Kingdom) can potentially improve healing rates of meniscal repairs.

The PRFM system has the theoretic advantage of placing a more highly concentrated set of autologous

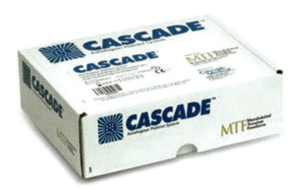

Fig. 1.6 Cascade™ with sample of patient's blood after centrifugation

growths factors (i.e., PDGF, VEGF, EGF, FGF) directly to the repair site, which has been shown to play important roles in musculoskeletal development and repair[18-20] and may provide a regenerative effect in meniscal cells.[21] In addition, because of the density of the precipitate, the PRFM is easier to suture and deliver into the knee than a fibrin clot.

In this technique, approximately 5–10 cc of the patient's blood is collected and taken from its sterile vial container to be centrifuged for 6 min. The supernatant is removed and the concentrated precipitate is prepared on a sterile back table (Fig. 1.6). A small, 3-0 absorbable suture is placed through the PRFM using a whipstitch or Bunnell stitch. For delivery of the PRFM through the portal, a metal skid or cannula along with an arthroscopic grasper is utilized to facilitate its passage. Alternatively, a knot pusher can be used to gently advance the PRFM to the repair site. Once the PRFM is placed within the meniscus tear, the repair is completed using either the suture-based repair techniques or one of the various available fixation devices described below, thereby, securing the enhancement agent into the meniscal repair (Figs. 1.7 and 1.8). Early studies have shown promise in human clinical trials[22] and future outcome studies will determine the effectiveness of these enhancement products.

Fixation Devices

There were several first generation fixation devices developed that were potentially useful for meniscal repairs (e.g., Arrow™, Hornet™, Dart™, Clearfix Screw™). These rigid devices utilized barbs or threads

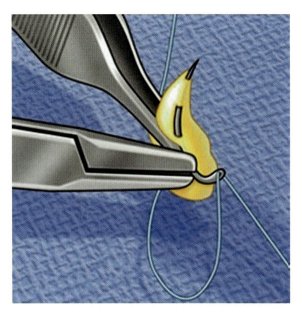

Fig. 1.7 A small, 3-0 absorbable suture is placed through the PRFM using a whipstitch or Bunnell stitch

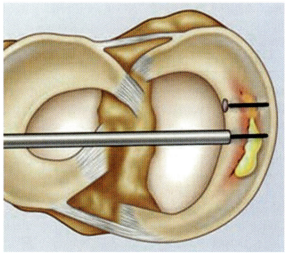

Fig. 1.8 Illustration of PRFM placed within meniscal tear, secured by a standard suture-based second generation fixation device

that crossed the tear site to bring the edges together. At first, these devices appeared to have many advantages compared to traditional suture repairs, such as a low rate of complications and failure rates varying from 5 to 12% at about 2 years.[23–27] Other advantages included not having to create an accessory incision and less postoperative pain. The procedure was simple and done quickly, and did not require the use of an assistant. Unfortunately, the senior author's results[28] at 4.5 years using the first generation fixators revealed unacceptable failure rates (28%) as well as other significant complications. The most common complication consisted of chondral scoring, fixator breakage, insertion problems, and significant postoperative joint line irritation from the fixator. Our results were also supported by Dudich et al. who demonstrated a similar 29% failure rate[29] and they have also abandoned the use of first generation meniscal fixators.

Subsequently, a second wave of meniscal fixators was developed. These suture-based, second-generation devices incorporate a dual anchor, absorbable implant system, connected together by a suture with a pretied, sliding locking knot. One or both anchors are placed through the tear and the capsule; then the pretied knot is tensioned, allowing for compression of the tear. Peripheral, vertically oriented meniscal tears in the posterior two-thirds are ideal for use of these fixators.

Currently, the most popular suture-based fixator is the FasT-fix™ (Smith & Nephew, Andover, MA) which is composed of two absorbable poly-l-lactic acid anchors with an attached 0 nonabsorbable suture (Fig. 1.9a, b). The FasT-fix is available on delivery needles with three curves (+22°, 0°, and −22°), allowing the surgeon to select the device with the angle needed to best approach the repair. We have found that the +22° needle is the most commonly used needle and, rarely, is the 0° needle required. The only time we have felt the need to use the −22° curved needle is in addressing incomplete, undersurface tears. The angle is ideal for passing sutures through the bottom half of the meniscus without the need to penetrate the superior surface, with the knot being tied, also, on the undersurface. The curved needles also enable the surgeon to simultaneously manipulate the needle to engage the meniscus and reduce the tear before passing the suture. Occasionally, the smoothness of the meniscal surface can cause the insertion needle to skive and, potentially, damage the articular surface. With a twisting motion, similar to the "pinch-tuck" technique for arthroscopic capsular plication, both edges of the tear can be successfully interlocked during the repair.

Preparation of the surfaces is performed in a fashion similar to preparation of a bony nonunion of a fracture, as previously mentioned. With large and particularly unstable tears, we recommend reducing the tear first by inserting a spinal needle from outside via a separate incision and passing a suture through the

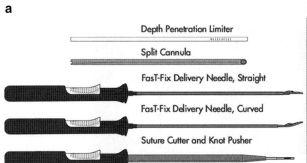
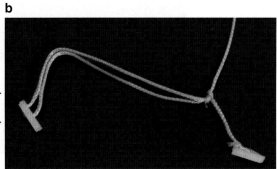
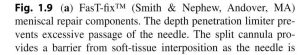

Fig. 1.9 (**a**) FasT-fix™ (Smith & Nephew, Andover, MA) meniscal repair components. The depth penetration limiter prevents excessive passage of the needle. The split cannula provides a barrier from soft-tissue interposition as the needle is introduced through arthroscopic portals. The delivery needle comes in angles of 0, −22, and +22°. (**b**) The FasT-fix anchor is composed of two 5-mm PLLA anchors connected by a pretied, sliding nonabsorbable No. 0 polyester suture

meniscal tear. The suture is then retrieved via an anterior working portals and a mulberry knot is tied and pulled back to provisionally hold the tear reduced.[30] Choosing the portal and angle of entry that is most perpendicular to the tear direction helps ensure a stable repair. This is usually accomplished through the contralateral portal. In addition, the contralateral portal entry reduces the risk of inadvertent damage to the popliteal neurovascular bundle, as the needle points away from the back of the knee (Figs. 1.10a, b). Once the portal is chosen, a snap or mosquito clamp is used to spread apart the soft tissue to prevent fat pad entrapment. The device also comes with a blue plastic cannula that allows a smooth passage of the implant and needle by the fat pad and into the joint.

The first suture implant is deployed after the initial pass of the suture needle through the capsule (Fig. 1.10c). To ensure that the anchor is completely through to the outer rim, we recommend gently pulling on the suture before inserting the second anchor. The surgeon should see the peripheral tear edge pull back, compressing the edges of the tear together. The FasT-fix device comes with a depth gauge that limits the penetration of the needle. This is useful in the beginning when one is first learning how to use the device but, once the surgeon is able to "feel" capsular penetration of the needle, the blue depth gauge is no longer needed. Once the needle and implant is past the capsule, the needle is brought back into the intra-articular space and the second implant is advanced into the ready position. The surgeon must make sure that the second implant is fully deployed by pushing the trigger with the surgeon's thumb until a "click" is heard (Fig. 1.10d, e).

Incomplete deployment of the second anchor can lead to dislodgement of the implant during insertion and is quite common, especially in the learning phase of the device. The second pass through the capsule layer can be configured in either a vertical, horizontal, or oblique orientation. When creating vertical sutures, the first pass is superior, often over the meniscus, directly into the capsule (Fig. 1.10g, h). Placement of the second implant inferiorly facilitates tensioning and cutting of the knot. The needle is then removed and the free suture end is pulled to slide the knot into the repair site. Compression of the repair site is enhanced by securing the sliding knot with an arthroscopic knot pusher and can be adjusted at this point before cutting the suture (Fig. 1.10i, j).

Another suture-based meniscal fixator available is the Rapid-Loc ™ system (DePuy Mitek, Inc., Raynham, MA), which comes with an absorbable or nonabsorbable anchor (Fig. 1.11a). The technique is very similar to other all-inside repair systems with the same ease of insertion and the ability to compress the meniscal tear surface. One advantage of the Rapid-Loc system is that only one pass of the needle is required through the capsule for fixation, thereby, reducing the risk of damage of vital neurovascular structures. The insertion needle comes in angles of 0, 12, and 27°. In addition, a metal skid provided in the set helps avoid scuffing of the articular surface and dragging the fat pad into the needle (Fig. 1.11b). An absorbable "top hat" gives a surface area of compression to the repair site; it is also available in nonabsorbable PLLA, and, in this version, is slightly lower in profile, which is what we prefer.

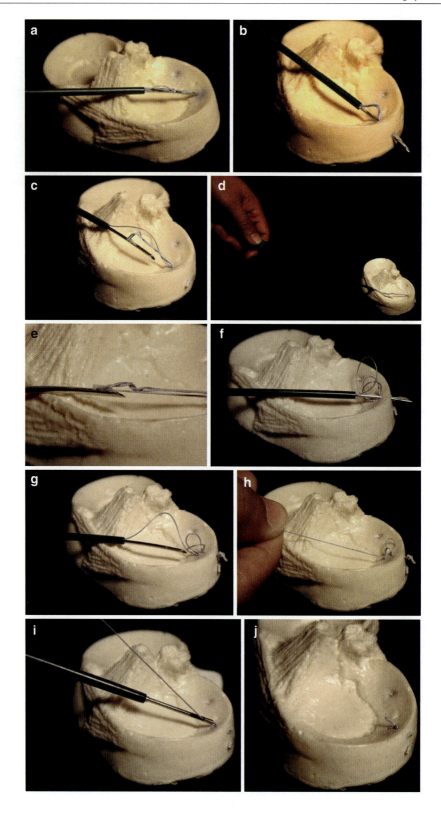

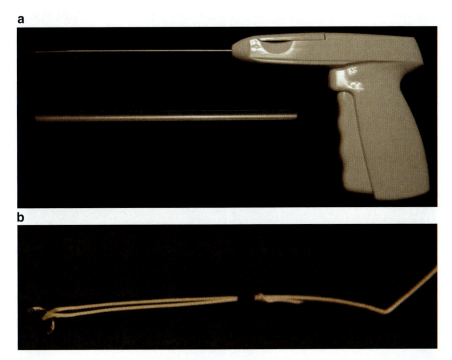

Fig. 1.11 (a) Rapid-Loc™ (Depuy Mitek) system includes the Meniscal Applier and a metal skid. (b) The Rapid-Loc is comprised of a soft tissue "backstop" (*left*) and a "tophat" (*right*) made of absorbable PLLA or PDS and a connecting suture made of either a nonabsorabable No. 2 Ethibond (Ethicon, Somerville, NJ) or an absorbable 2/0 Panacryl suture (Ethicon)

During insertion of the curved Rapid-Loc needle and its metal skid into the knee, the trailing suture is kept under slight tension, preventing the "top hat" anchor from sliding off the tip of the deployment needle (Fig. 1.12a-d). After insertion of the needle across the tear and capsule, the trigger is pulled to deploy the backstop anchor. The depth of penetration is limited by a built-in stop. The trailing suture is loaded onto the tensioning–cutting instrument and the top hat is brought down to the repair site with a gentle push–pull maneuver to allow slight compression of the repair site. At this point slight puckering of the repair site is often desired, as the top-hat sinks slightly into the body of the meniscus.

Inevitably, the orthopedic surgeon will encounter tears of a more complex configuration. With multidirectional tears, the use of multiple meniscal fixators usually suffices to create a stable repair. The key is to arrange the sutures perpendicular to the direction of the tear in order to capture and coapt the collagen fibers (Fig. 1.13). Horizontal cleavage tears, in our opinion, are considered stable because they do not displace with normal motion of the knee, but rather, reduce on top of themselves during weight-bearing compression. Therefore, we do not routinely repair stable horizontal cleavage tears. Unstable horizontal, degenerative cleavage tears are excised and debrided similar to routine partial menisectomies and are not normally repaired. Radial tears usually require multidirectional repairs and, in some cases, a formal open repair to stabilize all the components of the tear.

Fig. 1.10 (a) A longitudinal tear on a meniscal model is best approached from the contralateral portal to provide perpendicular fixation and avoid vital posterior neurovascular structures. (b) Insertion of the device through the capsule far enough to allow the anchor to flip. A depth limiter can be used (not shown) to prevent overpenetration of the needle. (c) The anchor flips after the needle is withdrawn during the first pass of the implant. A gentle tug is done to ensure that the anchor has properly engaged the capsule. (d) Deployment of the second implant is performed by sliding the *yellow* tab with the thumb until an audible "click" is heard. (e) Position of a properly deployed second anchor. (f) Second pass of needle superior to the tear to create a vertical mattress repair. (g) Withdrawal of the needle allows the second implant to engage the capsule and releases the pretied, sliding suture. (h) Gentle pulling of the free end slides the knot down and compresses the repair site. (i) Further compression can be performed using an arthroscopic knot pusher prior to being cut. (j) Final configuration of FasT-fix implant

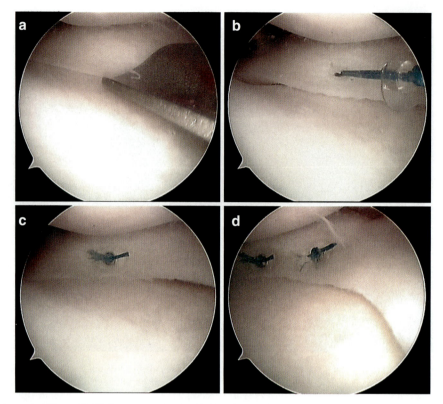

Fig. 1.12 (a) A metal skid provided helps protect the chondral surfaces during insertion of the meniscus applier and implant. (b) Once the backstop anchor is deployed and the capsule is captured, a gentle "push–pull" maneuver is performed to bring the "tophat" down to the repair site. (c) Final position of the "tophat" after compression with a slight puckering at the repair site. (d) A second implant is placed approximately 5 mm apart for optimal fixation

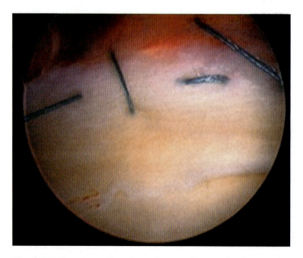

Fig. 1.13 Intraoperative view of a complex meniscal tear using FasT-fix sutures in multiple directions

Inside-Out Repair Techniques

Formal suture repairs are still considered by many the gold standard treatment option. Although no Level I evidence exists recommending their use, many level 4 studies show them to be an effective alternative.[13,31,32] Our experience with open repairs mainly exists with large, severely displaced, sometimes deformed, bucket handle tears and in revision cases after failed repairs with various all-inside devices. The ability to place multiple vertical mattress sutures makes the repair construct extremely stable. Obviously, the main concern is for neurovascular damage and pain and stiffness from the incision site postoperatively.

Anatomy At-Risk

The typical inside-out repair is usually performed for the posterior or middle third tears of the medial or lateral meniscus. With the patient in the supine position, a standard diagnostic arthroscopy is completed at which point the decision to repair the meniscal tear is done. To help identify the best incision site, we use the arthroscope to transilluminate the surface anatomy. The most common neurovascular injury on the medial side involves the saphenous nerve, its infrapatellar

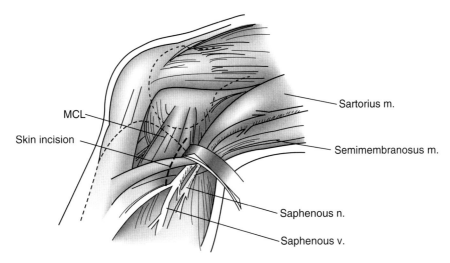

Fig. 1.14 Medial approach for inside-out meniscal repair. With the knee in flexion[33]

branch, and, less commonly, the sartorial branch. The common peroneal nerve is the most commonly damaged structure on the lateral side. In order to reduce the risk of capturing these nerves during the repair, one must clearly visualize the capsule and tie sutures directly onto to the capsule.

For posterior third meniscal repairs, the knee is flexed to 90° to bring the saphenous nerve posteriorly with the pes anserius on the medial side and, laterally, to bring the common peroneal nerve posteriorly. A 4–5 cm skin incision is made after transillumination of the skin with the arthroscope (Fig. 1.14).[33] The approach is carried anterior to both the direct head of semimembranosis and the medial gastrocnemius muscles. Retracting the semitendinosis and satorius posteriorly also helps prevent injury to the nerves. A retractor or pediatric vaginal speculum is inserted into the incision. Once the structures posterior to the capsule have been retracted, the zone-specific cannulae are inserted through the contralateral portal. Then, a long meniscal repair needle, loaded with a nonabsorbable 2-0 suture, is inserted through the cannula and out through the capsule. The needle is brought out posteriorly until it is deflected by the retractor or pediatric speculum. An assistant is required to pull the needle out through the capsule. Unfortunately, needle sticks can occur during this phase of the procedure, especially if the needle misses the speculum. The use of a Mosquito clamp or small clamp to extract the needle when the tip is visualized outside the capsule helps to decrease this risk.

A vertical mattress suture pattern is performed to capture the circumferential fibers, thereby, providing the strongest repairs.[34] One needle is placed on the superior surface of the meniscus and the other, through the inferior surface. Alternatively one limb is placed through the tear and the other just superior to the meniscus. This provides the best compression with largest amount of contact surface area. Introducing the needles from the contralateral portal minimizes the chance of injury to the posterior neurovascular structures (by directing the needles away from the back of the knee) while creating a repair construct that is most perpendicular to the tear. We routinely space multiple sutures approximately 5 mm apart for optimal fixation. The sutures are then tied under direct visualization onto the capsular tissue along with direct arthroscopic visualization of the repair inside the joint. An important point to remember is that even if an ACL reconstruction is done concomitantly, the sutures should be tied immediately after the repair, and before the ACL reconstruction is completed. If the repair is not stable enough to survive the motions of the ligament reconstruction, then it would likely fail postoperatively.

Lateral meniscus suture repairs are performed in a similar fashion as medial-sided repairs. The incision for the posterolateral retractor approach is conducted with the knee in flexion to move the common peroneal nerve posteriorly (Fig. 1.15a). The dissection continues anterior to the biceps femoris muscle and posterior to the iliotibial band and lateral collateral ligament. Retracting the biceps femoris posteriorly protects the common peroneal nerve. In addition, the surgeon must retract the lateral gastrocnemius posteriorly to visualize the needle coming out through

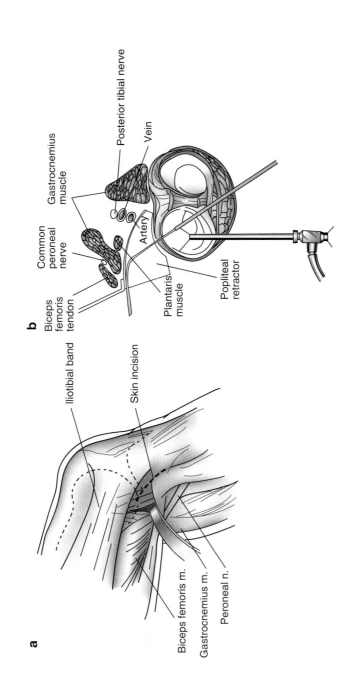

Fig. 1.15 (a) Lateral approach for inside-out meniscal repair.[33] (b) Popliteal retractor deflecting needle during posterolateral meniscal repair. The retractor is placed anterior to the common peroneal nerve, biceps femoris, and lateral gastrocnemius muscle[35]

the capsule, avoiding any neurovascular structures (Fig. 1.15b).[35]

Outside-in Repair Technique

Outside-in techniques are also a quick, simple, and effective alternative for meniscal repairs. They are best used for anterior and/or body meniscal tears, which are more difficult to access with a standard posterior inside-out repair. In addition, there are no major neurovascular structures in harms way when addressing anterior meniscal tears. We avoid this technique in posterior horn tears because it is not possible to introduce a repair construct that is somewhat perpendicularly oriented. To begin this method of repair, the surgeon inserts the arthroscope through the contralateral portal to identify the area of meniscus to be repaired. Our preferred method of an outside-in repair is performed using the Mensicus Mender II™ (Smith & Nephew, Andover, MA). Included in the set are two spinal needles (one curved and one straight) and a small wire loop attached to the tip of a stylet (Fig. 1.16a). The two needles are inserted from outside across the meniscus tear under direct visualization. The wire loop is then introduced through one needle and is hooked around the other needle, through which a 2-0 PDS suture is delivered (Fig. 1.16b, c). As the two needles are subsequently pulled out, a loop is created and can easily be tied over the capsule using a small incision.

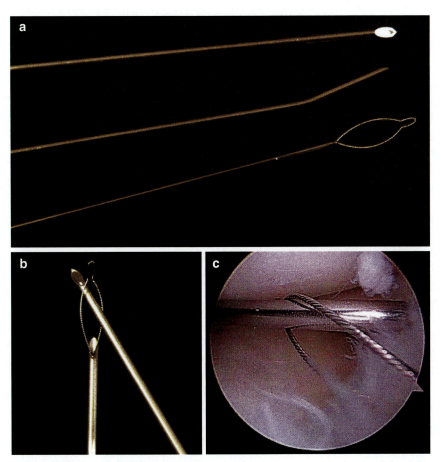

Fig. 1.16 (a) Meniscus Mender II™ (Smith & Nephew) set for outside-in repairs includes a straight and curved needle and a small wired loop. (b) Depiction of the Meniscal Mender needle passing through the wire loop. (c) Outside-in repair with wire looped around needle. A suture is passed through the needle and is hooked by the wire. After the wire and needle are removed, a loop is formed across the meniscus tear

Postoperative Pain Control Protocol

Pain control is often overlooked as an important factor in the immediate postoperative period. Each surgeon has their own preferences and each institution has their own protocol. All standard arthroscopies including those with isolated meniscal repairs undergo general anesthesia. If an ACL reconstruction is performed with the repair, then a femoral nerve block is administered preoperatively. We also inject the knee and portal sites with a mixture of 0.5% bupivicaine with epinephrine and Duramorph for pain control. We have also abandoned the use of various pain pumps because of reports of chondrolysis. If the surgeon chooses to use the pain pumps, then we recommend placing the pump extra-articularly and at a low dose to prevent this devastating complication.

Postoperative Rehabilitation

Our rehabilitation regimen begins with a period of immobilization with a knee immobilizer and toe-touch weight-bearing with crutches to avoid potential early failure for the first 2 weeks. To prevent arthrofibrosis, we recommend, beginning at week 3, initiating range of motion exercises only when seated or in the supine position. Progressive weight-bearing is allowed in weeks 3 and 4. Full weight-bearing with unrestricted low-impact walking and/or stationary bicycle is allowed at 4 weeks. Squatting is delayed until 4 months to reduce the forces across the repair. Finally, as with ACL reconstructions, cutting and pivoting sports are allowed at 6 months. When done concurrently with an ACL reconstruction, we make concessions with the ACL rehabilitation and follow our meniscal repair protocol, for the first month, after which the rehab is gradually progressed under standard ACL protocols.

Complications

Early complications in meniscal repairs mainly stem from complications from knee arthroscopy in general. To prevent infection, we routinely give preoperative, prophylactic antibiotics (1 g of cefazolin intravenously approximately 30 min prior to incision; if penicillin allergic, 1 g of vancomycin or 900 mg of clindamycin intravenously can substitute). Diligence with hemostasis can help reduce the incidence of postoperative hemarthroses and stiffness. A higher rate of arthrofibrosis can be seen when meniscal repairs are done concomitantly with ACL reconstruction[36] and with inside-out sutures that capture a significant amount of capsular tissue, which is not seen with fixators or outside-in repairs. Other less common complications such as, deep vein thrombosis (DVT) and avascular necrosis, are treated in a standard manner. Our protocol is to place every patient undergoing a meniscal repair on 81 mg of aspirin for 6 weeks for DVT prophylaxis.

Damage to the saphenous nerve or either of its branches is more controversial. We recommend observation in the majority of cases with the anticipation that the sensory nerve will either regenerate itself or become permanent. However, if there is suspicion that the suture placed during an inside-out repair was tied over the nerve, some recommend immediate exploration and decompression of the nerve. Similarly, if any nerve damage is encountered with the peroneal nerve in lateral open repairs, immediate revision surgery and open exploration are recommended as soon as the problem is recognized. Vascular injuries to major vessels require an immediate intraoperative vascular consult with either direct repair or arterial bypass surgery.

Short-term failures are generally due to loss of fixation of the repair site. This can occur for a variety of reasons, either from inadequate fixation, poor vascularity, overly aggressive physical therapy, unanticipated trauma, or noncompliance with the outlined rehabilitation program. Postoperative restrictions (i.e., avoidance of squatting for 4 months) must be repeatedly emphasized to the patients, especially when patients are pain free. We believe that by performing the steps discussed above from patient selection to likening the repair to fixation of a bony nonunion, one can minimize complications to a significant degree. In cases where a repair has failed, the options include either an attempt at a revision meniscal repair if the tissue is not degenerated where an open technique is usually required, or performing a partial or subtotal meniscectomy, as necessary (Fig. 1.17a-c).

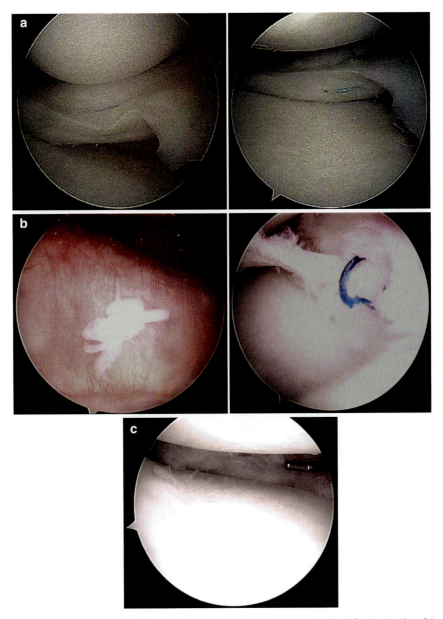

Fig. 1.17 (a) Medial meniscus repair performed with an all-inside technique using the FasT-fix implant in a 24-year-old female. (b) Failed meniscal repair with loose body remnant of a FasT-fix implant 19 months after her initial surgery. (c) Intraoperative image after removal of loose body and partial medial menisectomy

Conclusion

Although it is not known how long a repair needs to heal or how much strength a repair needs to have, meniscal repairs, when done properly and for the correct indications, have a very high success rate. Historically, open repairs were the mainstay of treatment and, still, are effective procedures with excellent outcomes. However, less invasive, all-inside implants are emerging as a viable alternative because of their ease of insertion and lower overall complication rate. With the older generation fixators, chondral injury, implant breakage, and prominent hardware are common complications. However, manufacturers have focused on improving these fixators by producing implants with lower profile heads and faster resorption rates. In addition to advances in implant technology, development of meniscal repair enhancement products, such as PRP, may also increase healing rates and improve clinical outcomes of meniscal repairs. In conclusion, we believe that if the proper steps are taken before, during, and after performing meniscal repairs, regardless of the technique chosen, then a very satisfying outcome with a low rate of complications can be expected.

References

1. Arnoczky S, Warren R (1982) Microvasculature of the human meniscus. Am J Sports Med 10:90-5
2. Greis P, Bardana D, Holstrom M et al (2002) Meniscal injuries. Basic science and evaluation and management. J Am Acad Orthop Surg 10:168-87
3. Clark C, Ogden J (1983) Development of the human knee joint. J Bone Joint Surg 65A:538
4. Ahmed A, Burke D (1983) In vitro measurement of static pressure distribution in synovial joints. Part I: Tibial surface of the knee. J Biomech Eng 105:216-25
5. Radin E, de Lamotte F, Maquet P (1984) Role of the menisci in the distribution of stress in the knee. Clin Orthop Relat Res May(185):290-4
6. Wilson W, van Rietbergen B, van Donkelaar C et al (2003) Pathways of load-induced cartilage damage causing cartilage degeneration in the knee after menisectomy. J Biomech 36:845-51
7. Dye S, Vaupel G, Dye C (1998) Conscious neurosensory mapping of internal structures of the human knee without intra-articular anesthesia. Am J Sports Med 26:773-7
8. Fairbank T (1948) Knee joint changes after meniscectomy. J Bone Joint Surg 30:664
9. Bullough P, Munuera L, Murphy J et al (1970) The strength of the menisci of the knee as it relates to their fine structure. J Bone Joint Surg Br 52:564-7
10. McDevitt C, Webber R (1990) The ultrastructure and biochemistry of the mensical cartilage. Clin Orthop Relat Res Mar(252):8-18
11. Post W, Akers S, Kish V (1997) Load to failure of common meniscal repair techniques: Effects of suture technique and suture material. Arthroscopy 13:731-6
12. Cannon W Jr (1996) Arthroscopic meniscal repair. In: McGinty JB, Caspari RB, Jackson RW et al (eds) Operative Arthroscopy, 2nd edn. Lippincott-Raven, Philadelphia, PA, pp 299-315
13. De Haven K, Arnoczky S (1994) Meniscal repairs: instructional course lecture, American Academy of Orthopaedic Surgeons. J Bone and Joint Surgery 43
14. Fox J, Rintz K, Ferkel R (1993) Trephination of incomplete meniscal tears. Arthroscopy 9(4):451-5
15. Henning C, Lynch M, Yearout K et al (1990) Arthrscopic meniscal repairs using exogenous fibrin clot. Clin Orthop Relat Res Mar(252):64-72
16. Arnoczky S, Warren R (1988) Meniscal repair using an exogenous fibrin clot. An experimental study in dogs. J Bone Joint Surg 70:1209-17
17. Wolf B, Rodeo S (2004) Arthroscopic meniscus repair with suture: inside-out with fibrin clot. Sports Med Arthrosc Rev 12:15-24
18. Newman A (1998) Current concepts: Articular cartilage repair. Am J Sports Med 26:309-24
19. Winterbottom N, Kuo J, Reich C et al (2002) Antigenic response to bovine thrombin exposure during surgery; a prospective study of 309 patients. J Appl Res 2:2-14
20. Li X, Tjwa M, Moons L et al (2005) Revascularization of ischemic tissue by PDGF-CC via effects on endothelial cell and their progenitors. J Clin Invest 115:118-27
21. Ishida K, 5 et al (2007) Regenerative effects of platelet-rich plasma on meniscal cells in vitro and its in vivo application with biodegradable gelatin hydrogel. Tissue Eng 13:1103-12
22. DeBerardino T, 3 (2007) Biologic enhancement for meniscal repair (platelet-rich plasma). Tech Knee Surg 6(3):168-71
23. Gill S, Diduch D (2002) Outcomes after meniscal repair using the meniscus arrow in knees undergoing concurrent anterior cruciate ligament reconstruction. Arthroscopy 18:569-77
24. Petsche T, Selesnick H, Rochman A (2002) Arthroscopic meniscus repair with bioabsorbable arrows. Arthroscopy 18:246-53
25. Hurel C, Mertens F, Verdonk R (2000) Biofix resorbable meniscus arrow for meniscal ruptures: results of a 1-year follow-up. Knee Surg, Sports Traumatol, Arthrosc 8:46
26. DeHaven K (1999) Meniscal repair. Am J Sports Med 27(2):242-50
27. Henning C, Clark J, Lynch M (1988) Arthroscopic meniscal repair with posterior incision. Instr Course Lect 37:209-31
28. Kurzweil P, Tifford C, Ignacio E (2005) Unsatisfactory clinical results of meniscal repair using the meniscus arrow. Arthroscopy 21(8):905-7
29. Lee G, Diduch D (2005) Deteriorating outcomes after meniscal repair using the meniscus arrow in knees undergoing concurrent anterior cruciate ligament reconstruction: Increased failure rate with long-term follow-up. Am J Sports Med 33:1138-41
30. Kurzweil P (2008) Meniscus Repair with Meniscal Fixators. Master Techniques in Knee Surgery, 3rd edn. Lippincott Williams & Wilkins, Philadelphia, PA, pp 89-97
31. Rockborn P, Gillquist J (2000) Results of open meniscus repair. Long-term follow-up study with a matched uninjured control group. J Bone Joint Surg Br 82(4):494-8
32. DeHaven K, Lohrer W, Lovelock J (1995) Long-term results of open meniscal repair. Am J Sports Med 23(5):524-30
33. Jackson D (ed) (2003) Master Techniques in Orthopaedic Surgery: Reconstructive Knee Surgery, 2nd edn. Lippincott Williams & Wilkins, Philadelphia, PA, pp 57-71
34. Shelbourne K, Johnson G (1993) Locked bucket handle meniscal tears in knees with chronic anterior cruciate deficiency. Am J Sports Med 21:779-82
35. Medvecky M, Noyes F (2005) Surgical approaches to the posteromedial and posterolateral aspects of the knee. J Am Acad Orthop Surg 13:121-8
36. Reish M, Kurzweil P (2007) FasT-Fix meniscus repair. Tech Knee Surg 6(3):161-7

Editors' Comments (Meniscus Repair)

Unstable Bucket Handle Tears

For complete, unstable bucket handle tears, we continue to recommend use of a mini open approach for repair, to achieve optimal secure fixation. Although current arthroscopic "all-inside" fixation devices have come a long way, they can still be difficult to use on the undersurface of the meniscus, and may not always be able to achieve a vertical suture orientation, which has been shown to provide a mechanically superior repair. When possible, we recommend staggering vertical sutures above and below the meniscus. In addition, anterior horn suturing is difficult if not impossible with the all-inside devices. With a mini open approach using an inside-out repair technique, all of these issues can be addressed. In addition, the inside-out technique is still the only method of repair that does not leave a knot or implant on the articular surface of the meniscus.

Fast Fix Device

Several important tricks can assist in use of this device. To ensure that the second part of the implant is fully deployed, we recommend using a clamp to push the trigger until a click is heard and/or the trigger is maximally deployed. There is significant resistance on the trigger, and thumb pressure alone may be inadequate. If one is going to only stock one size of this implant, we recommend the 20° curve, which is most versatile.

Finally, a percutaneously placed spinal needle is very useful in order to lift the meniscus to assist with undersurface fixation of tears with this device, and can also be used to reduce the meniscus into proper position while inserting the fixation device.

Postoperative Rehab

Our approach to rehab is somewhat more aggressive than the authors. With inside-out repair, or all-inside meniscal repair devices that have suture crossing the repair, we feel comfortable with immediate weight-bearing as tolerated with a locked knee brace. Direct axial loading exerts a compression force across the repair, and would not be expected to affect healing. The brace is kept locked for 4 weeks for weight-bearing and at night. Patients may otherwise open the brace for range of motion exercises. We have not had problems utilizing this protocol for 17 years

Fibrin Clot

The use of a fibrin clot remains controversial. No statistically significant benefit has ever been demonstrated with its use. In addition, when we used to utilize blood clots to enhance repair, we were unimpressed with the security of the clot fixation. On the other hand, healing of meniscal tears repaired at the time of ACL reconstruction have universally been shown to have better healing rates than isolated meniscal repairs. Our interpretation of this data is that perhaps the stem cells released at the time of notchplasty and reconstruction are responsible for these improved healing rates. For this reason, we abrade or microfracture the notch at the time of isolated meniscal repairs to stimulate bleeding as well as to release bone marrow stem cells.

Zone-Specific Meniscal Repairs

Cannulae

Because of the differing anatomy of the medial and lateral compartments, the opposite knee cannulae needs to be used when repairing the posterior horn of the lateral meniscus. Thus, a left posterior cannula works better on the right knee posterior lateral horn, and vice versa. For medial meniscus tears, the right posterior cannulae is used for the right knee medial meniscus, as designed.

Fluid Management During Inside-Out Repairs

We have found that complex bucket handle repairs can best be performed with the fluid turned off, and the suction on the inflow cannula. This eliminates frustrating extravasation and difficult fluid management.

Additional Tips

Because of the curve of the cannulae, always make your incision slightly distal to the joint, and carefully dissect out the soft tissue to ensure clean passage of the needles.

Always make sure to identify the infrapatellar branch of the saphenous nerve during suture tying and closure to avoid a neuroma.

If the posterior horn/root sutures are very difficult to pass or retrieve, consider an all-inside repair device for this area.

For lateral repairs, try to avoid capturing the popliteus with your sutures.

For repairs performed with acute ACL/MCL injuries, be careful with your dissection and valgus stress. If the MCL is tenuous, consider repairing the menscus with absorbable 2-0 PDS sutures tied over the sartorious facia, rather than dissect all the way to the disrupted MCL.

It is helpful to have designated meniscal rasps available to abrade the meniscus edge to help promote repair. We prefer the Bowen rasps, which are small, ball tipped rasps and come in various angles.

Complex Repairs

In patients under 40, we have been aggressive in performing complex repairs. This includes radial repairs that extend to the vascular zone, nondegenerative horizontal tears, and multidirectional tears which extend to the vascular zone. We also will perform repairs up to 5 mm from the capsular attachment for acute tears if the meniscal tissue demonstrates good integrity, stimulating healing by "trephining" the meniscus with an 18 gauge spinal needle to create multiple vascular access channels. Radial tears and horizontal tears are repaired with horizontal sutures, after stimulating bleeding in an outside technique. In addition, posterior root avulsions can be potentially addressed with a 4.5-mm bony tunnel drilled into the posterior root insertion with an ACL guide from the proximal tibia and passage of suture through the root. Postoperative rehab for these cases is much slower, with nonweight-bearing for 6 weeks since the axial loading forces created a potential distracting or shearing force on the repair in these situations.

Chapter 2
Avoiding and Managing Complications in Meniscus Transplantation

Benjamin Shaffer and J.R. Rudzki

Top 10 Pearls

- Preoperative planning to identify associated mechanical axis malalignment as well as ligamentous or chondral pathology will facilitate optimal outcomes.
- Appropriate sizing is critical and best performed with an AP and Lateral radiograph with a calibrating size marker to correct for magnification error as well as axial MRI to confirm the size estimate. The optimal meniscal allograft should be within 5-10% of the patient's native meniscus.
- Exposure with extensile parapatellar incisions to adequately visualize and accomplish graft passage is essential. In complex or revision cases, sub-periosteal incision and reflection of the adjacent peripheral portion (5%) of the patellar tendon insertion with resection of a small portion of the retropatellar fatpad may greatly facilitate adequate exposure.
- Intra-articular arthroscopic preparation for the procedure requires meticulous preparation of the retinacular portals, adjacent synovium, ligamentum mucusum, and retropatellar fatpad with an arthroscopic cautery device to ablate tissue that impedes visualization. During meniscectomy in preparation for allograft transplantation, it is helpful to leave a thin rim of meniscal tissue at the mensico-capsular junction to aid in appropriate identification of allograft placement and more closely reproduce native anatomy.
- Performing a notchplasty of the inferior 5-10% of the central portion of the ipsilateral femoral condyle may facilitate graft passage and minimize chondral trauma in a tight medial compartment, which would otherwise impede graft passage. Visualization of the posterior-central aspect of the associated tibiofemoral compartment for correct posterior plug or trough placement in the sagittal and coronal planes is imperative, and may be confirmed with intraoperative fluoroscopy.
- Marking the meniscal allograft at the anterior and posterior horns on the superior and inferior surfaces will greatly facilitate orientation during delivery and reduction of the meniscal allograft.
- Delivery sutures placed at the junction of the posterior horn and mid-body will assist in reduction and delivery of the meniscus to the appropriate position and decrease the risk of graft flippage or malorientation during reduction.
- Capsular abrasion with a meniscal repair device or whisker shaver may be helpful to obtain a bleeding surface at the menisco-capsular junction.
- Fixation for bone plug allografts is accomplished by shuttling sutures at the bone-meniscal root out of the reamed tunnels and tying over a bone-bridge. Alternatively, allograft dovetail or slot grafts with poor fixation may have their press-fit improved with the use of an interference anterior-to-posterior screw placed over a guide-wire.
- Meniscal transplant fixation is best achieved with an inside-out technique using a cannulated needle delivery system. This technique can be supplemented with all-inside meniscal repair devices. Despite the ease of use with these devices, optimal

B. Shaffer (✉)
WOSM, 2021 K Street, NW, Washington, DC, 20006, USA
e-mail: dr.shaffer@dcsportsmedicine.com

J.R. Rudzki
Department of Orthopedic Surgery, The George Washington University School of Medicine, Washington, Washington, DC, USA

stability is obtained with alternating sutures placed on the superior and inferior aspects of the meniscal allograft.

Introduction and Background

The importance of the meniscus to normal knee function, including load transmission, shock absorption, lubrication, and joint stabilization, is well established.[1] So too are the consequences of its removal, either by injury, meniscectomy, or repair failure.[2-4] Despite emphasis on its preservation, however, pain, impairment, and eventual arthritis following meniscectomy remain a significant clinical problem for many patients.[5] Fortunately, since 1984, meniscus transplantation has provided an effective treatment option in properly selected meniscus-deficient patients.[6-11] Although the long term chondroprotective benefit remains unproven, the ability of meniscus transplantation to relieve pain, restore function, and at the very least serve as a "bridge" procedure for symptomatic patients without other recourse is well established.

However, meniscus transplantation is not without risks or complications. Optimal results demand careful patient selection as well as surgical precision. Risks of transplantation include persistent or worsening of pain, swelling, stiffness, infection, nerve injury, mechanical failure, risk of disease transmission, and an approximately 30% rate of return to the operating room for subsequent (partial or total) meniscectomy.[8,9,12-14] In addition, meniscus transplantation is usually accompanied by some additional concomitant procedure(s), such as articular cartilage restoration, realignment, or stabilization, which may potentially increase the surgical risks. The purpose of this chapter is to delineate the pitfalls and problems associated with meniscus transplantation, and emphasize considerations and techniques by which they can be minimized and/or avoided.

Functional Anatomy at Risk

- The meniscus is an important structure in normal knee function, providing stress protection across joint surfaces.
- Since symptomatic relief of transplantation theoretically requires replicating the normal meniscus, understanding its normal attachment sites is critical.

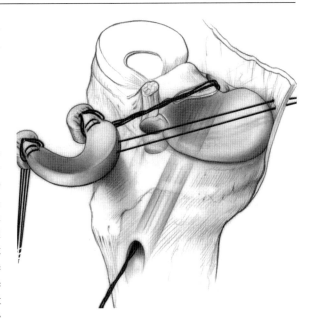

Fig. 2.1 Two tunnel technique for medial meniscal allograft transplantation. Additional tunnels for concomitant ACL or PCL reconstruction make precise tunnel placement critical to prevent tunnel blow-out or convergence. (Reproduced with permission from Klimkiewicz JJ, et al. Meniscal Surgery 2002 Update: Indications and techniques for resection, repair, regeneration, and replacement. Arthroscopy 2002;18:14-25)

An extensive knowledge of the relevant regional anatomy is imperative for an allograft meniscal transplantation to most closely approximate restoration of native anatomy. Intraoperatively, visualization may occasionally be sub-optimal and concomitant procedures may require multiple tunnel placements (Fig. 2.1). Therefore, a detailed understanding of the native anatomy will help the surgeon best accomplish the procedure when these and other variables might impede performance of a routine procedure. The medial meniscus covers approximately 30% of the tibial plateau, has an estimated mean width of 9–10 mm, which increases from anterior to posterior, and thickness of 3–5 mm. The lateral meniscus covers approximately 50% of the tibial plateau, has a mean width of 10–11 mm, and thickness of 3–5 mm. The medial meniscal horn insertion sites are more anterior and posterior than the lateral meniscus whose insertion sites are separated by only 6–10 mm (Fig. 2.2). Pollard et al. studied the anatomical considerations regarding meniscal width and length relevant to transplantation. The authors reported that the net meniscal width roughly equals the coronal distance

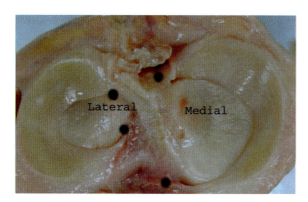

Fig. 2.2 Anatomy of the meniscal horn insertion sites

from the tibial eminence peak to the periphery of the metaphysis on a standard anteroposterior view. Meniscal AP length, however, was reported as approximately 80% of the sagittal length of the plateau medially and 70% of the plateau laterally on a standard lateral radiograph.[15] In a morphologic study of 48 cadaveric knees, Berlet et al. identified four types of insertions for the anterior horn of the medial meniscus.[16] In this study, 59% of the anterior horn tibial insertions were located in the flat intercondylar region of the tibial plateau and 24% were located on the downward slope from the medial tibial plateau to the intercondylar region. The authors concluded that these findings may explain a predisposition for meniscal allograft subluxation or extrusion, which may manifest as anterior knee pain. While this suggestion requires further study, a thorough knowledge of the variability of anterior horn insertion anatomy can facilitate meniscal allograft harvest and transplantation. We recommend consideration of a suture anchor to augment anterior horn fixation in situations where the anterior horn location or fixation may place the graft at risk for extrusion.

The medial meniscus is attached to the capsule via the meniscotibial and coronary ligaments as well as to the deep fibers of the medial collateral ligament. The lateral meniscal attachments are different and include connections to the meniscofemoral ligaments and popliteo-meniscal fasciculi, which are not reproduced with meniscal allograft transplantation.[17,18] With regard to load transmission, the medial meniscus transmits approximately 50% of the tibiofemoral joint load and the lateral meniscus transmits approximately 70%.[19] The medial meniscus transmits approximately 50% of the compressive load in extension but 85% at 90° of flexion, which may influence surgeon-specific rehabilitation protocols.[20] The medial meniscus plays a role in joint stability, with an increase in anterior tibial translation noted after medial meniscectomy in the ACL-deficient knee.[21] In addition, increased varus and valgus stress and angulation may be observed after medial and lateral meniscectomy. After partial meniscal excision, the increase in local contact stress has been estimated at 65% in comparison to 235% after complete excision.[22] Although several studies have demonstrated the ability of meniscal allograft transplantation to improve the tibial contact mechanics over that of the meniscectomized knee, the true extent of the chondroprotective effects are as yet unknown.

Complications

With few exceptions,[23] complications associated with meniscus transplantation are usually culled from retrospective Level IV-evidence case series.[11,12,24-27] Assessment of their true incidence is, therefore, somewhat difficult. But in review of the literature, the most common postoperative complication is a compromised outcome because of residual, recurrent, or worse pain and/or impairment. In our personal experience, such compromised postoperative outcomes are often due to ill-considered indications, failure to recognize established contraindications, or failure to anticipate, recognize, or definitively address intraoperative technical problems.

Complications with meniscus transplantation can occur at any stage of the procedure, including the preoperative, intraoperative, or postoperative period. Attention in each stage is important to avoid unnecessary problems. Although these discrete time frames permit better understanding of the specific steps along the way where problems are encountered, it must be recognized that, in fact, suboptimal clinical outcome or untoward experience may be multifactorial, such as a combination of preoperative errors in patient selection and intraoperative technique.

Preoperative Considerations

Several preoperative factors influence the propriety of considering a patient a candidate for meniscus transplantation. Some are intuitive, but others require experience specific to this procedure. Generally, they include factors unique to the patient, graft, and operative preparation. Each requires attention.

Patient-Specific Factors

The ideal indication for meniscus transplantation is a physiologically young (under 50) patient with symptoms attributable to their meniscus insufficiency, unresponsive to nonoperative treatment, and with healthy articular surfaces, neutral alignment, and normal stability. Several authors have expressed concern for advanced chondral wear or arthrosis, which may predispose patients to graft extrusion or higher rates of failure.[8,12,28] Recently, Stone et al. presented their results of 47 meniscal allograft transplants in patients with moderate to severe arthrosis and reported success based on graft retention, pain relief, and functional improvement in 89.4% with a mean failure time of 4.4 years as assessed by Kaplan-Meier survival analysis.[29] Despite this report, the general consensus in the literature supports a conclusion that healthy articular surfaces, neutral alignment, and normal ligamentous stability play a significant role in achieving optimal outcomes.

Potential Pitfalls

A number of pitfalls are avoidable by careful preoperative evaluation:

1. *Do not perform a meniscus transplant in patients whose symptoms are **not** due to meniscus insufficiency*. Indications for meniscus transplantation are very specific. Patient symptoms must be related to meniscus insufficiency. Although this may seem self evident, proper selection requires a careful history and physical. Even in cases in which a subtotal meniscectomy has been performed, meniscus-deficient symptoms may not be present for 5–10 years postoperatively. So beware the early meniscectomized patient whose symptoms are not necessarily (or likely) due to the meniscectomy. Symptoms may be due to patellofemoral or articular pathology, and treatment must be directed accordingly. In cases where the degree to which the meniscus insufficiency contribution to the patient's complaint is unclear, trial placement in an unloader brace (only good for the medial side) may provide prognostic insight. Distinguishing medial compartment overload from meniscus insufficiency is not easily delineated, however, by this unloading trial. Finally, a bone scan showing increased uptake in the affected compartment may be helpful in assessing overload due to meniscus deficiency.

2. *Do not perform meniscus transplantation in knees with "significant" articular cartilage pathology*. The key here is the definition of "significant." Although implantation in the face of arthritis may provide short-term relief, the most commonly cited cause of clinical failure is graft transplant in a knee that is either arthritic or in which there is Outerbridge III or greater chondral damage.[8,12,28] Osteophytes and exposed subchondral bone make for a hostile environment for the meniscus, which is subjected to inevitable damage and eventual meniscectomy. Avoid transplantation in patients with diffuse Grade IV changes, flattening of the femoral condyles, and significant osteophyte formation. Although transplants are ideally not performed in patients with significant chondral wear, in reality, few patients with symptomatic meniscus insufficiency have healthy articular surfaces. The advent of chondral resurfacing techniques, such as osteochondral reconstruction with autograft or allograft transplants, and cell-based therapy such as Autologous Chondrocyte Implantation, have permitted some relative relaxation of the stringent criteria for meniscus transplantation in the face of chondral pathology.[30] Cartilage restorative procedures are appropriate for select contained focal chondral lesions, performed either concomitantly or as a staged procedure with meniscus transplantation. Larger lesions with poor shoulders, or knees with bipolar disease, however, remain relative contraindications to transplantation. If there is any question about articular cartilage integrity, consider diagnostic evaluation before ordering the graft. Preoperative

assessment of cartilage integrity requires AP and PA flexion weight bearing films, as well as evaluation of previous operative reports and when available, arthroscopic photos or video clips.

3. *Do not perform a meniscus transplant in a malaligned knee.* Any malalignment must be addressed to avoid overload and graft failure.[31] For example, placement of a medial meniscus in a varus knee predisposes to failure through increased medial compartment stresses. In the medial compartment, consideration must be given to a concomitant or staged approach in which a proximal tibial (opening medial or closing lateral wedge) osteotomy[32] is followed by meniscus transplantation. Conversely, lateral meniscus insufficiency with valgus alignment must be addressed through a distal femoral opening wedge osteotomy, again either concomitantly or as a staged procedure. The degree of correction is less than with traditional osteotomy strategies for unicompartmental arthritis, attempting to provide sufficient realignment to unload the compartment. Many patients with malalignment already have some element of arthritis and may not be appropriate candidates for transplantation. Furthermore, osteotomy may relieve symptoms sufficiently such that meniscus transplantation (either concomitantly or staged) is unnecessary. If staged or performed concomitantly, realignment must precede transplantation. Alignment is anticipated preoperatively through evaluation of gait, stance, and preoperative full-length standing films (Fig. 2.3).

4. *Avoid transplantation in the face of instability.* Meniscus insufficiency is often accompanied by ligamentous pathology, particularly involving the anterior cruciate ligament (ACL). Bucket-handle meniscal tears are commonly associated with ACL tears. Resection of these bucket tears, either primarily or following failure of meniscus repair, may lead to a combined pattern of meniscus and ACL insufficiency. Failure to recognize instability will likely lead to meniscus allograft failure, as has been observed in meniscus repair in ACL-deficient knees, whose failure rate has been reported at up to 35%.[8,21,24,31,33–35] Conversely, patients with chronic ACL and meniscus insufficiency may benefit from a combined procedure to include meniscus transplantation with the ACL reconstruction. This is because restoration of stability through ACL reconstruction

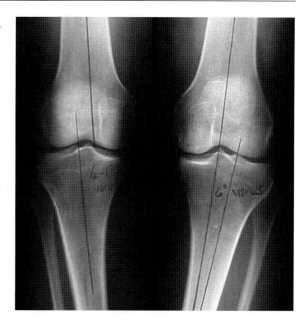

Fig. 2.3 Weight-bearing knee radiographs (long-cassette cropped for clarity) to evaluate mechanical axis

alone is often not achievable in the medial meniscal-deficient knee. Such biomechanical interdependence has been demonstrated in the lab as well as with clinical outcome data.[21,33–37] This is one circumstance in which meniscus transplantation may be considered in the absence of typical meniscus deficient symptoms, and is seen predominantly on the medial side. If staged, meniscus transplantation is best performed after a stabilization procedure.

5. *Do not perform meniscus transplants in knee "abusers".* Attempting to improve symptoms and decrease impairment are not necessarily the same as returning patients to their "preinjury" level of activity. Many patients are capable of resuming an active lifestyle, which can include impact activities such as running, tennis, soccer, and basketball. However, the risks and complications of this procedure are less clearly justified in patients whose goal is to return to aggressive and/or highly competitive impact load sports. In addition, this procedure requires patient strict compliance with postoperative therapy, postop activity restrictions, and finally, realistic expectations.

6. *Do not perform meniscal transplants prophylactically.* Given the known consequences of meniscectomy, particularly in the young patient, there is temptation to consider prophylactic implantation in this "at risk" population. However, any preventative

benefit of meniscus transplantation is unproven. Given that long term chondroprotective advantage is not yet established, and the potential for complications is well established, prophylactic implantation cannot be recommended or justified. Recently, T2 mapping Magnetic resonance imaging has emerged as a potential tool to facilitate the identification of patients with chondral overload after meniscectomy who may be good candidates for consideration of meniscal allograft transplantation.

7. *Consider other patient factors in decision making.* Patient age, weight, activity demands, expectations, and compliance are all factors that should be considered when weighing the merit of any procedure, but especially complex reconstructions such as meniscus transplantation.

Graft-Specific Considerations

Risk of disease transmission has focused attention on methods of graft procurement and processing. Current tissue banking methods require compliance with CDC-established standards for harvesting, testing, and storing meniscal tissue.[38] Although these have lowered, they have not eliminated the risk. Storage alternatives have included fresh, fresh frozen, cyropreserved, and lyophilized. Fresh tissue has not proven superior clinically to fresh frozen, and is limited in supply. Lyophylized (freeze-dried) tissue is somewhat brittle and upon immersion in saline expands to a somewhat unpredictable size. Furthermore, this method has been associated with graft "shrinkage" following implantation.[7,32] For these reasons, fresh and lyophilized tissues are no longer used in meniscus transplantation. At this time, there does not appear to be any clinical outcome difference between the use of fresh frozen or cryopreserved tissue. Newly developed proprietary techniques by which disease transmission risk can be further decreased have been recently introduced but as of yet have no clinical track record. Currently, in the absence of tissue banking uniformity, the surgeon needs to be familiar with the alternative banks, their procurement, and processing methods. If combining meniscus transplantation with allograft osteoarticular or ligament reconstruction, consideration can be given to trying to obtain "same donor" graft source, though this is not commonly possible.

Graft sizing is essential to ensure a good fit and approximate the optimal load transmission characteristics of the native meniscus[39–42] (Fig. 2.4). Unfortunately, no uniform standard currently exists by which preoperative measurement can assure ideal fit. Furthermore, the threshold for tolerance of size mismatch in which the donor tissue does not "fit" is unknown, though it is estimated to be within 5% of the length and width of the meniscal dimensions[12,43–46] (Fig. 2.3). Reliance on plain X-ray and even MRI have shown to have a high rate of inaccuracy.[44] Our current preoperative protocol

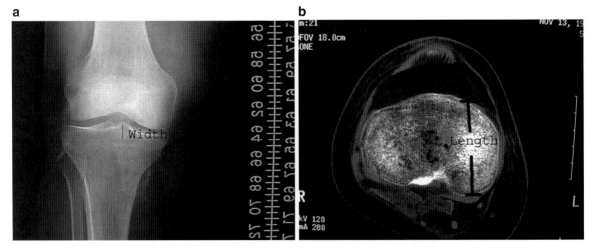

Fig. 2.4 (**a**) Appropriate meniscal sizing is critical. Weight-bearing antero-posterior radiograph is used to measure medial-lateral meniscal width. (**b**) An axial CT or MR image may be used to facilitate measurement of meniscal AP length

estimates medial lateral "width" by measuring from the eminence to the peripheral margin of the affected compartment on a true AP radiograph with magnification marker. Measurement of meniscal "length" relies on use of CT scan, obtained preoperatively. The protocol is to obtain 2 mm continuous axial cuts, beginning at the intercondylar eminences and extending to the tibial tubercle. Anterior–posterior bone dimension is measured from the mid-anterior to the mid-posterior cortical rim, using the most proximal "slice" from the articular surface that shows the dense cortical outline of the relevant compartment.

Regardless of the care with which the surgeon estimates appropriate meniscal dimensions, accuracy also depends upon the method by which the tissue bank has measured their meniscus specimen. Good communication between the surgeon and tissue bank are necessary to ensure they are using the same measurement parameters. However, ultimately we do not know the importance of other meniscal dimensions on knee biomechanics, including height, radial width, and shape. Therefore, although attempt at anatomic replacement is preeminent, truly replicating the normal meniscus is not achievable at this time. A recent study by Stone et al. suggests their may be a role for correlating values predicated on gender, height, and weight in sizing meniscal allograft for transplantation.[47]

Operative Instrumentation

In addition to standard knee arthroscopic instruments, transplantation requires knee retractors and meniscal repair instrumentation. Medial transplants most commonly are performed using bone plugs (Fig. 2.1), necessitating use of an ACL guide, guide pin, and cannulated reamers for tunnel placement. Availability of 6 and 7 mm diameter reamers is especially helpful in tight medial compartments for passage of a smaller posterior bone plug. Laterally, a slot or dovetail technique require specific instrumentation for an optimal graft press-fit (Fig. 2.5). Finally, surgeon preparation and training are prerequisite for success with this technically demanding procedure. Training in a learning center environment, surgical facility, and observation of an experienced clinician can all facilitate performance of this technique.

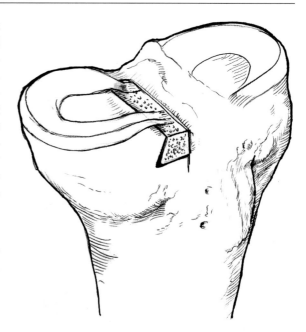

Fig. 2.5 Lateral meniscal allograft in prepared trough for wedge press-fit (courtesy of Arthrex, Naples, Fl)

Intraoperative Considerations

Pitfalls can occur during any step of the procedure, including remnant meniscectomy and rim preparation, graft preparation, tunnel establishment, graft passage, and graft fixation. Anticipating problems at each step improves the opportunity for a smooth and effective procedure.

Diagnostic Arthroscopy, Remnant Meniscectomy, and Rim Preparation

1. *Perform an arthroscopy* to confirm absence of the meniscus and determine what other procedures if any may require treatment and adjustment of your plan. Ideally, arthroscopic assessment confirms rather than reveals additional structural abnormalities.
2. *Preserve some of the menisco-capsular tissue when removing remnant meniscus.* Some remnant meniscus, perhaps 2-3 mm, should remain as a site for identifying and occuring transplant attachment (Fig. 2.6). This is particularly true laterally, where enthusiastic resection may lead to inadvertent graft extrusion

when the graft is attached peripherally to the deficient capsule. Do not remove the meniscal horn attachments, which serve as a good reference when establishing tunnels. Finally, remove the remnant anterior body of the meniscus via the anterior arthrotomy (used in meniscus transplant passage) rather than an unnecessary and protracted arthroscopic resection.
3. *Ensure thorough rim preparation.* Failure to prepare the rim risks nonhealing and eventual graft failure. As performed for a meniscus repair, a shaver or rasp is used to maximize peripheral healing by thorough meniscocapsular abrasion to generate a healing response.

Graft Preparation

1. *Take care in preparing graft.* Medially, bone plugs are most commonly used for bone fixation. Care in plug preparation at this step will facilitate subsequent graft seating and proper orientation (Fig. 2.7). The posterior bone plug should be prepared such that their orientation will be anatomic when introduced into an approximately 45–60° bone tunnel. It should be no more than 6 or 7 mm in diameter, no more than 7 or 8 mm in length, and bullet-shaped for easy tunnel entry. Greater diameter or longer plugs risk graft passage, especially in a tight medial compartment, inadequate graft seating and graft fracture. Ensure strong sutures are placed both in the meniscal soft tissue and the bone plugs themselves. Ideally, the sutures should emerge from the apex of the bone plugs so that when tensioned, they will pull down easily into its tunnel. The anterior bone plug can be fashioned larger because it is inserted into the anterior tunnel under direct visualization. In situations where graft passage through the knee is difficult, the surgeon may elect to introduce the graft from a posteromedial approach. In such a situation, the anterior bone block will require paring down to facilitate its passage under the condyle to the front of the knee.

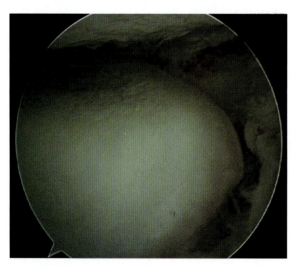

Fig. 2.6 Meniscal rim preservation to localize proper placement of meniscal transplant

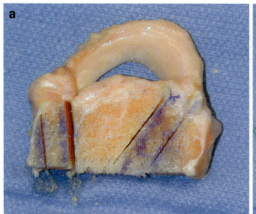
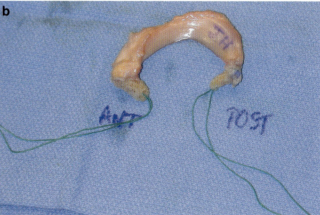

Fig. 2.7 (**a**) Preparation of medial meniscal allograft bone plugs. (**b**) Prepared bone plugs and identification of the anterior and posterior horns as well as the superior surface with initials

Because of the anterior and posterior horn proximity, lateral meniscus transplants are usually performed using a continuous block of bone seated into a slot or trough (Figs. 2.2 and 2.5). Special instrumentation has been developed to ensure templating of the dowel or dove-tail shaped bone block so that it mates the trough. Poor graft preparation will lead to inadequate seating of the bone block. Difficulty in medial meniscus graft passage using the bone plug technique has led to the development of a slot or dovetail technique similar to that used laterally. Careful templating of the bone block is necessary during this step to ensure subsequent passage and seating. The primary disadvantage of using a bone bridge or slot technique medially is that it requires placement through some of the ACL footprint (Fig. 2.8). When performing a concomitant ACL reconstruction, this strategy has merit. But in isolated medial transplanatation, undermining the medial ACL footprint for graft placement seems unwise.

Tunnel Establishment

Medially, the bone plug technique is most commonly employed, and requires making two tunnels. The posterior tunnel is the most challenging because it requires anatomic positioning for ideal graft placement. Most medial compartments are relatively tight and thus variably accessible for identification and guide placement.

Tricks to Establish Posterior Plug Tunnel in MM Transplant

1. *Preserve the normal posterior horn attachment* during rim preparation, making this anatomic landmark available for identification of the normal insertion site. Anatomic references show that the insertion is just medial and anterior to the most anterior fibers of the PCL.
2. *Introduce the ACL guide through the anteromedial portal.* Ensure that you are familiar with the guide design so that the pin will emerge at the intended site. Establish an angle in the sagittal plane that approximates the prepared plug, but modify the angle as necessary to avoid convergence with a concomitantly performed proximal ACL tunnel.
3. Visualize the posterior horn attachment site. Consider establishment of a posteromedial portal through which the scope can be introduced, permitting direct visualization of the horn. While viewing from the back, the guide is placed anteriorly.

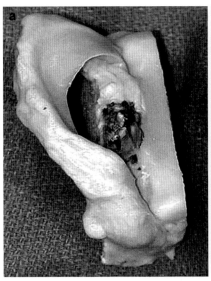 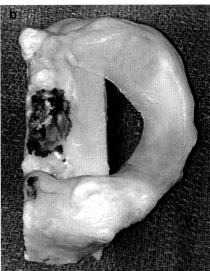

Fig. 2.8 Medial meniscal horn anatomy in reference to ACL tibial insertion (Reproduced with permission from Sekiya JK. Meniscal allograft transplantation. J Am Acad Ortho Surg 2006;14:170)

Tricks to Establish Anterior Plug Tunnel in MM Transplant

1. *Do not establish the tunnel until the graft has been passed and anatomically seated.* The tunnel is then made based on where the horn and bone plug are positioned, rather than forcing them to insert at the normally anatomic site.
2. *Drill and ream the anterior tunnel through the anterior arthrotomy incision.* Direct the cannulated reamer at a 45° angle posteriorly. The preshaped anterior bone plug can usually be tamped into place with an interference fit and not require fixation. If the graft is insecure, a small bioabsorbable (or metal) interference screw can be used. Another alternative is to pass the sutures in the bottom of the bone plug through a small drill hole in the anteromedial proximal tibia. These sutures can then be secured by use of a button or tied to sutures from the posterior bone plug tunnel.

Tricks When Using a Dovetail/Slot Technique in MM Transplant

1. *Use this technique with caution*, it undermines the ACL footprint
2. If you must use this technique, *do it in association with ACL reconstruction*, in which the graft and ACL can share the graft origin.
3. Ensure that trough position, length and shape is sufficient to properly match the contoured graft.

Lateral transplants are nearly always performed with slot/trough/dovetail technique. Each requires some variation on the recipient site for the graft bone block, and try to capitalize on the concept of interference bony fixation. Initial slot technique required laborious templating on the back table and intraoperative free-handed preparation. Fixation required sutures tied over the proximal anteromedial tibia. Subsequent refinements in lateral transplant technique included a "keyhole approach" to contain the bone block through interference fit of mated parts (Fig. 2.9). However, it required considerable skill to ensure anatomic position. The fiddle factor intraoperatively led to the simple designs most com-

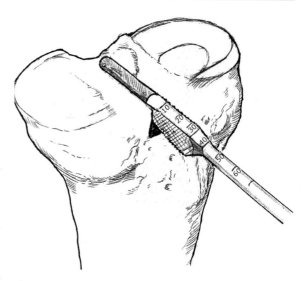

Fig. 2.9 Preparation of the trough for lateral meniscal transplant for Arthrex Dovetail technique (courtesy of Arthrex, Naples, Fl)

monly used today, including the dovetail, or slot technique, the simplest and easiest approach to lateral transplantation.

Tricks When Using a Dovetail/Slot Technique in LM Transplant

1. *Make sure the slot is truly co-linear* with the anterior and posterior horns. Anatomic placement demands that the horn origins replicate normal anatomy. Unfortunately, such co-linear placement is often unachievable through a conventional anterolateral arthrotomy because of impingement by the patellar tendon's lateral margin. Variability in the patellar tendon's tibial tubercle attachment and tendon width make the exact line of placement different for each patient.
2. *Use a spinal needle percutaneously to confirm co-linear placement* of the intended slot. The anterolateral incision/artrotomy should be made directly over this site, which is often over the lateral to midthird of the patella tendon. Begin the slot with the use of a shaver or burr to clarify the trajectory for replicating the meniscal horn insertion sites (Fig. 2.10).

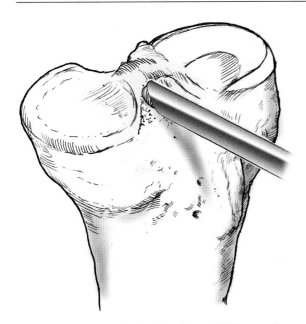

Fig. 2.10 Trough creation begins with establishing a co-linear plane along the meniscal horn insertion sites with a motorized burr or shaver

3. *Make the slot through a split in the patellar tendon if necessary.* After determining the ideal angle to ensure both anterior and posterior horns are co-linear and replicate normal anatomy, incise the patella tendon and make the bone slot through this window.
4. *It should not be too short or too long.* The prepared bone block should be made such that the posterior bone block has been pared down so that there is no excess protruding beyond the posterior horn itself. Thus, the slot must be prepared to a depth that upon graft placement replicates the proper position of the graft. If the slot is not sufficiently deep for example, the posterior horn will not sit properly under the posterior medial articular cartilage. If the slot is too long, the graft can break out the back of the posterior tibial wall, compromising fixation and risking graft extrusion from poor positioning. The most important part of graft and tunnel preparation in the slot technique is to ensure that the graft is co-linear with the anatomic attachment sites, and that it is placed to a depth that also replicates these attachments. Failure to do so requires refashioning of the graft and/or slot until it is properly seated.
5. *When performing plug technique for a medial transplant, make the anterior tunnel after graft passage.* Despite preoperative sizing, the graft is sometimes short, with the anterior horn (and bone plug) attachment site shy of the patients' normal anatomic insertion. When encountering such a situation, the priority is to ensure the graft is properly seated and lying within the joint as would a normal meniscus, and then making an anterior bone plug tunnel that accommodates the graft. Sometimes, in cases of significant graft/knee mismatch, the anterior tibial tunnel must be established 1–2 cm proximal to its normal insertion to accommodate the graft.

Graft Passage and Seating

This step offers the greatest opportunity for surgical frustration and intraoperative "delay-of-game". Medial grafts using bone plugs are the most challenging surgical step, particularly in tight medial compartments. Several tricks are useful to facilitate graft passage and positioning, and avoid the otherwise predictable struggle with the uncooperative graft.

Tips for Graft Passage and Seating Using Medial Bone Plug Technique

1. *Ensure proper graft and tunnel preparation in the first place.* Avoid a "toggling" effect in which the bone plug is pulled like a molly bolt against the top of the posterior tunnel, instead ensuring the bone plug goes into its tunnel in a co-linear manner. This is facilitated by ensuring that the sutures emerge from the tip of the posterior plug rather than the side. A beath needle drilled down the center of the plug from the meniscal side to the tip of the bone allows such suture "centering". Make sure the tip of the graft is "bullet" shaped and that the plug is downsized by a millimeter or so relative to the tunnel diameter.
2. *Improve medial compartment access by addressing the MCL.* Several strategies have been described, including trephinating of the deep capsule with controlled stretching of the MCL, as well as detachment and reattachment of the MCL. Controlled MCL lengthening can be easily performed using a #11 blade percutaneously or with a 14 gauge angiocatheter. Under direct visualization, several

transverse slits are made in the capsule. The application of valgus stress usually yields improved visualization and access. Detachment of the femoral MCL attachment with its bone plug was described early in the evolution of medial reconstructions, permitting improved access but requiring refixation.[9] We suspect this technique is of greater theoretic benefit than practically useful. It may be a worthwhile consideration if other measures preclude sufficient access for graft passage. Another option to help open the medial compartment is with an external fixator.[48] Although we have limited experience using this technique, we consider it as another bail-out strategy if other techniques are unsuccessful at providing adequate access for passage. When used, unicortical threaded pins must be well fixed on the femoral and tibial sides, bridged by a fixator, which is gradually lengthened to open up the joint. Make sure the pins are placed sufficiently proximal and distal to the joint so they do not obstruct access posteromedially at the site of either meniscus repair or subsequent graft passage from a posteromedial approach (see later).

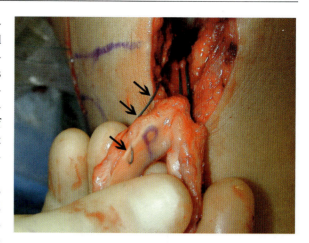

Fig. 2.11 Prepared medial meniscal allograft with guide suture to maintain orientation (arrows)

3. *Perform a "notchplasty."* With the use of a small burr (4.5 or 5.5 mm), a small amount of bone is removed from the medial femoral condyle, along an anterior-posterior line that is directly superior to the posterior horn of the medial meniscus. Removal of 4–5 mm of bone will demonstrate the posterior horn much more easily, as well as provide access for the posterior bone plug passage. This maneuver is routinely performed.

4. *Use a "guide" suture to maintain graft orientation.* When passing the graft, a suture placed at the posteromedial corner permits another means by which the graft remains oriented. Without this suture, the graft can flip in the notch, preventing visualization and seating (Fig. 2.11).

5. *Introduce the graft from a posteromedial approach.* This method has been advocated by Harner and others.[23,49] Its advantage is that it permits entrance and seating of the bone block directly into the posterior tunnel. However, there are limitations with this technique, including the need for an adequate capsulotomy and posteromedial exposure, in addition to the potential for difficulty with graft passage of the anterior plug from posterior to anterior. If the graft is passed from back to front, the plugs ought to be fashioned such that the anterior bone plug is pared down or chamfered with a rongeur to facilitate passage.

If difficulty is encountered in attempting anterior bone plug passage, consider using a disposable cannula or extending the anterior incision. The cannula, whose internal diameter must exceed the diameter of the bone block, is positioned into the anteromedial arthrotomy and directed along the medial gutter. The graft is loaded into the cannula and pulled anteriorly, delivering the plug for insertion.

6. *Ensure easy entrance of plug into posterior tunnel* by removing any soft tissue from the tunnel's rim and using a small rasp through the tunnel to chamfer and smooth the intraarticular aperture. A narrow diameter Gore-Smoother (Gore and Associates, Flagstaff, AZ) may be helpful.

7. *Do not discard bone plugs.* Historically, some authors have advocated removal of bone plugs and fixing the horn attachment sites with sutures only.[31,50] Certainly this "trick" simplifies meniscus transplantation. However, strong biomechanical evidence demonstrates the importance of preservation of bone blocks to minimize the risk of meniscal extrusion.[51] Paletta et al. reported increased mean contact pressures of 220–360% without horn fixation, and noted these levels were similar to complete meniscectomy.[51] In this study, the authors reported a 55–65% decrease in peak local contact pressure with bone plug fixation. Alhalki and Howell et al. studied three methods of fixation for medial meniscal transplant in a cadaveric biomechanical study, examining the effects on tibial contact mechanics.[52] The authors reported that bone plug fixation restored

the contact mechanics most closely to normal, and similar to the conclusions of Paletta et al., recommended anatomic bone plug fixation for optimal restoration of tibial contact mechanics.

Tips for Graft Passage and Seating Using Medial or Lateral Bone Block Technique

1. *Be cautious while using bone block technique on the medial side.* This procedure, unless accompanied by ACL reconstruction, encroaches on the ACL footprint. Violation of a normal anatomic structure (ACL) to facilitate meniscal transplant healing is not indicated. Theoretic benefit of using the bone block technique is preservation of the normal shape of the meniscus and avoidance of the complications of bone plug passage. But the risks of using a bone block, in addition to compromising the ACL footprint, include inaccurate positioning of the bone graft, from which there is no "bail out," and sizing error, in which the graft fails to sit properly. Accommodation of the graft to the knee, as is achievable when using plugs and the anterior body/horn is slightly nonanatomic, is not an option.
2. *Ensure accurate slot or dovetail.* When using either medial or lateral bone block technique, there is little room for size or position inaccuracy. Care must be taken to ensure the bone block is prepared and placed such that the horn attachment sites directly replicate the attachments of the meniscus. The bone block must be prepared with attention to ensure that it has the same width, height, and length as the corresponding trough.
3. *If the block does not pass easily, ensure that there is no soft tissue interposition and down-size graft for an easier fit.* Regardless of which compartment is being replaced, soft tissue must be removed from the bone tunnels or trough, particularly at the aperture, to facilitate graft passage.

Graft Fixation

Most transplants rely on a combination of bone and soft tissue fixation. Traditional medial implantation relies on use of bone plugs anteriorly and posteriorly to secure bony fixation, augmented by peripheral capsular fixation. Opportunities for intraoperative pitfalls abound during graft fixation.

1. *Meniscus repair is best performed using an "inside-out" technique.* Although there are many described procedures to repair meniscal tears, none have better strength or durability than the standard vertical-mattress suture repair. The ability to balance the repair using sutures on both the superior and inferior meniscal surface further ensures maintainance of orientation (Fig. 2.12). Because the graft is typically introduced through an anteromedial or anterolateral arthrotomy, suture of the anterior and mid-body can be easily accomplished using #2-0 nonabsorbable braided suture on a small curved-cutting needle. Alternatively, some authors have advocated using a percutaneous "outside-in" technique for the mid and anterior body. Although "all inside" meniscal fixators have been successfully used with meniscus repairs, their use in meniscus transplantation requires discretion. Hybrid techniques using both fixators and inside-out sutures may be an acceptable compromise.
2. *Bone fixation is critical to graft stability and prevent extrusion.* Although several authors have advocated removal of the bone plugs for the sake of expediency, it is our distinct impression that firm bony fixation is important for maintaining graft orientation, providing stability during heal-

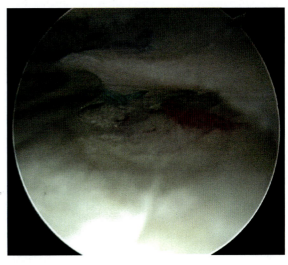

Fig. 2.12 Balancing suture on undersurface of meniscal transplant placed with zone-specific inside-out cannula

ing, and most importantly, to minimize the risk of meniscus extrusion.[51] Without secure horn attachments, peripheral graft translation or extrusion may occur.
3. *If the block is loose or fractures, consider augmenting fixation.* Alternative strategies include use of suture, suture anchors, or interference screw fixation. Sutures can be placed through the bone blocks, passed through drill holes in the anteromedial tibia and tied over a bone bridge or a button. Suture anchors may be similarly used. Interference fixation has also been described to securely fix the bone block within the trough/slot, though we have not found this routinely necessary.[52]

Concomitant or Staged Procedure Considerations

Performing procedures concomitantly has advantages. For example, the arthrotomy necessary for meniscus passage can serve to simultaneously provide access for osteoarticular transplantation. Performance of both procedures permits a combined canvalescence and subjects the patient to only one procedure and one anesthetic. Disadvantages of concomitant procedures, however, include increased surgery and tourniquet duration, complexity of the procedure, convergence of tunnels with ACL reconstruction or at the site of osteotomy, and a more difficult and prolonged recovery. Concomitant surgery also requires experience with each procedure. If staged, meniscus transplantation should be deferred as the second procedure.

Postoperative Considerations

Most postoperative protocols rely on a period of protected weight-bearing for two weeks, followed by gradual weight-bearing.[53] Noncompliance with premature weight bearing may risk bone graft stability, peripheral soft tissue fixation, and lead to failure. Premature return to athletic activities, particularly those including impact and torsional loading, further jeopardize the transplant. Appropriate patient selection and education are crucial to avoid compromising outcome.

Revision Surgery

Little data is available regarding revision meniscal transplantation.[54] However, critical components to consider in such a setting include identifying any comorbid conditions that require attention and may have been responsible for graft failure. For example, a failed graft in an arthritic knee need not be revised with yet another transplant, and ligamentous instability or malalignment should be addressed prior to revision transplantation in an appropriate candidate. Identification of the cause of failure is critical.

Technically, the steps for revision are the same as those in primary reconstruction, with the overt exception of possible bone stock compromise. A critical point to recognize is the need for adequate exposure if performing a lateral meniscal allograft in a trough. After a previous procedure, scar tissue and adhesions in the region of the retropatellar fat pad and anterior retinaculum may significantly impair visualization and access. Arthroscopic evaluation and debridement of previous meniscal remnant, assessment of articular cartilage and ligament status, are important components that deserve pre-revision assessment. Any bone defects can be addressed at this time with auto or allograft bone. A second stage approach for revision is probably best delayed approximately four months to permit bone incorporation.

Clinical Results

In 1989, Milachowski et al. reported superior results in patients who underwent deep frozen meniscal allograft transplantation in comparison to lyophilized grafts in a study of 22 grafts with average 14 month follow-up.[7] The authors performed second-look arthroscopy in 15 patients and reported shrinkage in one of five deep-frozen grafts, compared with nine of ten lyophilized grafts. In addition, the authors reported 90% good and excellent clinical results in their group of deep-frozen grafts compared with <40% good and excellent results in the lyophilized group. Garrett reported the results of 6 isolated meniscal transplantations and 37 transplantations in combination with either an ACL reconstruction or an osteotomy. At minimum two-year follow-up (range: 2–7 yrs), the authors reported a well-healed meniscal rim and no significant graft shrinkage in 20 of the 28 patients evaluated with repeat arthroscopy.[12] Van Arkel and DeBoer presented their results of 23 meniscal allograft transplants in 25 patients with second-look arthroscopy in 12 patients and found seven cases with complete healing and the remaining five with partial healing.[14] They noted seven patients with degenerative changes, three frank failures, and concluded that better clinical outcomes were associated with stable knees and normal alignment. These authors subsequently presented average five-year follow-up data on 63 transplants in 57 cases and reported cumulative survival rates of 76%, 50%, 67% for lateral, medial, and combined, respectively, and suggested that medial survival may improve when combined with ACL reconstruction in ACL-deficient patients.[24] Noyes et al. evaluated 96 fresh-frozen irradiated grafts in 82 patients.[55] Twenty-nine menisci failed within 24 months after implantation, and second-look arthroscopy and/or MRI data from all 96 allografts showed that 22% of the grafts healed, 34% healed partially, and 44% failed.

Carter examined 38 of 46 meniscal transplants with second-look arthroscopy at 24–73 months and reported four cases of failure and four cases of shrinkage.[25] Verdonk et al. reported on the results of 54 meniscal allografts in 51 patients at mean 4.6 year follow-up.[9] On the basis of Hospital for Special Surgery Knee Scores, patients less than three years from surgery had pain relief and improved function – however, these results deteriorated at three years. Magnetic resonance imaging of 39 grafts revealed normal shape and position; however, there was poor correlation between MRI and clinical outcome. Goble et al. reported the results of 47 cryopreserved meniscal allograft transplants in 45 patients.[13] The authors reported a well-healed and functional meniscus in 10 of the 13 patients who underwent second-look arthroscopy and graft biopsies from eight cases demonstrated an average of 80% viable meniscal tissue. Ryu et al. retrospectively studied the results of 26 meniscal allografts (16 lateral and 10 medial) in 25 patients at 12–72 months follow-up and reported improved function and reduced pain.[27] Recently, Farr et al. presented a case series of 29 patients who underwent meniscal allograft transplantation and autologous chondrocyte implantation (ACI).[30] Four patients failed before the 2-year follow-up (14%) and required revision surgery and three patients were lost to follow-up. Sixteen patients underwent concomitant procedures including tibial tubercle osteotomy, anterior cruciate ligament reconstruction, and high tibial osteotomy. The authors reported statistically significant improvement in the standardized outcome surveys, visual analog pain, satisfaction, and Lysholm scores. No significant differences were noted in any subgroup (medial vs. lateral, isolated vs. concomitant, or unipolar vs. bipolar). They concluded that allograft meniscal transplantation in combination with ACI demonstrates improvement in both symptoms and knee function at minimum two-year follow-up. However, it is important to note these outcomes are less favorable than the literature-reported outcomes of either procedure in isolation.

Cole et al. presented their results of 44 meniscal allograft transplants in 39 patients evaluated at minimum 2-year follow-up using the Lysholm, Tegner, International Knee Documentation Committee, Knee Injury and Osteoarthritis Outcome Score, Noyes symptom rating and sports activity, and SF-12 scoring systems.[10] Four transplants failed early (9%), leaving 40 transplants in 36 patients for review. Twenty-one menisci were transplanted as isolated procedures (52.5%) and 19 were combined with other procedures (47.5%) to address concomitant chondral pathology. The authors reported statistically significant improvements in standardized outcome surveys as well as visual analog pain and satisfaction scales. Overall, 77.5% were completely or mostly satisfied and 90% were classified as normal or nearly normal using the International Knee Documentation Committee knee examination score at final follow-up. No significant differences were reported between the medial and lateral subgroups or the isolated and combined subgroups. The authors concluded that meniscal allograft transplantation alone or in combination with other procedures results in reliably improved in knee function and pain at minimum 2-year follow-up.[10] Noyes et al. reported their results from 40 cryopreserved meniscal allograft transplants in 38 patients evaluated at mean 40-month follow-up.[8] Twenty-five of the 40 underwent a concomitant ligament reconstruction of osteochondral autograft procedure. Meniscal allograft characteristics were assessed subjectively, clinically, and with magnetic resonance imaging. Thirty-four (89%) patients rated their knee as improved. Pain with daily activities reduced from 79% prior to surgery (30 patients) to 11% (four patients) at time of latest follow-up and 76% (29 patients) resumed light low-impact sports. The authors reported that concomitant procedures improved knee function without increasing the rate of complications. In their MRI assessment of meniscal allograft characteristics, the authors reported the allograft menisci were normal in 17 knees (43%), altered in 12 (30%), and failed in 11 (28%).

Conclusion

Meniscus transplantation provides an effective option for treating symptomatic meniscal-deficient patients. The current evidence-based literature demonstrates the ability of meniscal transplantation to reduce pain and increase function. Despite these encouraging findings, the long-term function of meniscal transplants and any chondroprotective effects remain unknown. Careful patient selection and technical precision are essential in performing these procedures. Anticipating intraoperative pitfalls will facilitate successful surgical technique, and help minimize complication risks.

References

1. Fithian X, Kelly M, Mow V (1990) Material properties and structure-function relationships in the menisci. Clin Orthop 252:19-31
2. Fairbank TJ (1948) Knee joint changes after meniscectomy. J Bone Joint Surg Br 30:664-70
3. McGinty J, Geuss L, Marvin R (1977) Partial or total meniscectomy. A comparative analyisis. J Bone Joint Surg Am 59:763-6
4. Gillquist J, Oretorp N (1982) Arthroscopic partial meniscectomy. Technique and long-term results. Clin Orthop. 167:29-33
5. Bolano L, Grana W (1993) Isolated arthroscopic partial meniscectomy. Functional radiographic evaluation at five years. Am J Sports Med 21:432-7
6. Milachowski K, Weismeier K, Erhardt W et al (1987) Transplantation of the meniscus: An experimental study in sheep. Sportverletzung Sportschaden 1:20-4
7. Milachowski K, Weismeier K, Wirth C (1989) Homologous meniscal transplantation: Experimental and clinical results. Int Orthop 13:1-11
8. Noyes F, Barber-Westin S, Rankin M (2004) Meniscus transplantation in symptomatic patients less than fifty years old. J Bone Joint Surg Am 86:1392-404
9. Verdonk P, Demurie A, Almqvist K et al (2005) Transplantation of viable meniscal allograft. Survivorship analysis and clinical outcome of one hundred cases. J Bone Joint Surg Am 87:715-24
10. Cole B, Dennis M, Lee S et al (2006) Prospective evaluation of allograft meniscus transplantation: A minimum 2-year follow-up. Am. J Sports Med 34:919-27
11. Hommen J, Applegate G, Del Pizzo W (2007) Meniscus allograft transplantation: Ten-year results of cryopreserved allografts. Arthroscopy 23:388-93
12. Garrett J (1993) Meniscal transplantation: A review of 43 cases with two to seven year follow-up. Sports Med Arthrosc Rev 1:164-7
13. Goble E, Kane S, Wilcox T et al (1996) Meniscal allografts. In: McGinty JB, Caspari RB, Jackson RW, Poehling GG (eds) Operative arthroscopy, 2nd edn. Lippincott-Raven, Philadelphia, PA, pp 317-31
14. van Arkel E, de Boer H (1995) Human meniscal transplantation. Preliminary results at 2 to 5-year follow-up. J Bone Joint Surg Br 77:589-95
15. Pollard M, Kang Q, Berg E (1995) Radiographic sizing for meniscal transplantation. Arthroscopy 11:684-7
16. Berlet G, Fowler P (1998) The anterior horn of the medial meniscus. An anatomic study of its insertion. Am J Sports Med 26:540-3
17. Johnson D, Swenson T, Livesay G et al (1995) Insertion-site anatomy of the human menisci: Gross, arthroscopic, and topographical anatomy as a basis for meniscal transplantation. Arthroscopy 11:386-94
18. Simonian P, Sussmann P, van Trommel M et al (1997) Popliteomeniscal fasciculi and lateral meniscal stability. Am J Sports Med 25:849-53
19. Seedholm B, Hargreaves D (1979) Transmission of load in the knee joint with special reference to the role of the menisci: Part II. Experimental results, discussions, and conclusions. Eng Med Biol 8:220-8
20. Ahmed A (1992) The load-bearing role of the knee menisci. In: Mow V, Anoczky S, Jackson D (eds) Knee meniscus: Basic and clinical foundations. Raven Press, New York, NY, pp 59-73
21. Levy I, Torzilli P, Warren R (1982) The effect of medial meniscectomy on anterior-posterior motion of the knee. J Bone Joint Surg Am 64:883-8
22. Baratz M, Fu F, Mengato R (1986) Meniscal tears: The effect of meniscectomy and repair on intraarticular contact areas and stress in the human knee-A preliminary report. Am J Sports Med 14:270-5
23. Brand J, Johnson D (2001) Complications and pitfalls in meniscal transplantation. In: Malek M (ed) Knee Surgery-Complications, pitfalls, & salvage. Springer-Verlag, New York, NY, pp 60-73
24. Van Arkel E, De Boer H (2002) Survival analysis of human meniscal transplantations. J Bone Joint Surg Br 84:227-31
25. Carter T (1999) Meniscal allograft transplantation. Sports Med Arthrosc Rev 7:51-62
26. Rath E, Richmond J, Yassir W et al (2001) Meniscal allograft transplantation. Two- to eight-year results. Am J Sports Med 29:410-4
27. Ryu R, Dunbar V, Morse G (2002) Meniscal allograft replacement: A 1-year to 6-year experience. Arthroscopy 18:989-94
28. Cole B, Carter T, Rodeo S (2002) Allograft meniscal transplantation. Background, techniques, and results. J Bone Joint Surg Am 84:1236-50

29. Stone K, Walgenbach A, Turek T et al (2006) Meniscus allograft survival in patients with moderate to severe unicompartmental arthritis: A 2- to 7-year follow-up. Arthroscopy 22(5):469-78
30. Farr J, Rawal A, Marberry K (2007) Concomitant meniscal allograft transplantation and autologous chondrocyte implantation: Minimum 2-year follow-up. Am J Sports Med 35:1459-66
31. Van Arkel E, De Boer H (1995) Human meniscal transplantation: Preliminary results at 2 to 5-year follow-up. J Bone Joint Surg Br 77:589-95
32. Cameron J, Saha S (1997) Meniscal allograft transplantation for unicompartmental arthritis of the knee. Clin Orthop 337:164-71
33. Rubman M, Noyes F, Barber-Westin S (1998) Arthroscopic repair of meniscal tears that extend into the avascular zone: A review of 198 single and complex tears. Am J Sports Med 26:87-95
34. Eggli S, Wegmuller H, Kosina J et al (1995) Long-term results of arthroscopic meniscal repair: An analysis of isolated tears. Am J Sports Med 23:715-20
35. Cannon W Jr, Vittori J (1992) The incidence of healing in arthroscopic meniscal repairs in anterior cruciate ligament-reconstructed knees versus stable knees. Am J Sports Med 20:176-81
36. Graf K Jr, Sekiya J, Wojtys E (2004) Long-term results after combined medial meniscal allograft transplantation and anterior cruciate ligament reconstruction: Minimum 8.5-year follow-up study. Arthroscopy 20(2):129-40
37. Papageorgiou C, Gil J, Kanamori A et al (Mar 2001) The biomechanical interdependence between the anterior cruciate ligament replacement graft and the medial meniscus. Am J Sports Med 29:226-31
38. McAllister D, Joyce M, Mann B et al (2007) Allograft update: The current status of tissue regulation, procurement, processing and sterilization. Am J Sports Med 35:2148-58
39. Alhalki M, Hull M, Howell S (May 2000) Contact mechanics of the medial tibial plateau after implantation of a medial meniscal allograft: A human cadaveric study. Am J Sports Med 28:370-6
40. Rankin M, Noyes F, Barber-Westin S (2006) Human meniscus allografts' in vivo size and motion characteristics: Magnetic resonance imaging assessment under weightbearing conditions. Am J Sports Med 34:98-107
41. Dienst M, Greis P, Ellis B et al (2007) Effect of lateral meniscal allograft sizing on contact mechanics of the lateral tibial plateau: An experimental study in human cadaveric knee joints. Am J Sports Med 35:34-42
42. Huang A, Hull M, Howell S (2003) The level of compressive load affects conclusions from statistical analyses to determine whether a lateral meniscal autograft restores tibial contact pressure to normal: A study in human cadaveric knees. J Orthop Res 21(3):459-64
43. Pollard M, Kang Q, Berg E (1995) Radiographic sizing for meniscal transplantation. Arthroscopy 11:684-7
44. Shaffer B, Kennedy S, Klimkiewicz J, Yao L (2000) Preoperative sizing of meniscal allografts in meniscal transplantation. Am J Sports Med 28:524-33
45. Carpenter J, Wojtys E, Huston L et al (1993) Preoperative sizing of meniscal allografts. Arthroscopy 9:344
46. McDermott I, Sharifi F, Bull A et al (2004) An anatomical study of meniscal allograftsizing. Knee Surg Sports Traumatol Arthrosc 12:130-5
47. Stone K, Freyer A, Turek T et al (2007) Meniscal sizing based on gender, height, and weight. Arthroscopy 23:503-8
48. Kurtz C, Bonner K, Sekiya J (2006) Meniscus transplantation using the femoral distractor. Arthroscopy 22:568e1-3
49. Johnson D, Swenson T, Harner C (1994) Meniscal reconstruction using allograft tissue: An arthroscopic technique. Oper Tech Sports Med 2:223-31
50. Garrett J, Stevensen R (1991) Meniscal transplantation in the human knee. A preliminary report. Arthroscopy 7:57-62
51. Paletta G, Manning T, Snell E et al (1997) The effect of allograft meniscal replacement on intra-articular contact area and pressures in the human knee. A biomechanical study. Am J Sports Med 25:692-8
52. Alhalki M, Howell S, Hull M (1999) How three methods for fixing a medial meniscal allograft affect tibial contact mechanics. Am J Sports Med 27:320-8
53. Farr J, Meneghini R, Cole B (2004) Allograft interference screw fixation in meniscus transplantation. Arthroscopy 20:322-7
54. Fritz J, Irrgang J, Harner C (1996) Rehabilitation following allograft meniscal transplantation: A review of the literature and case study. J Orthop Sports Phys Ther 24:98-106
55. Rath E, Richmond J, Yassir W et al (2001) Meniscal allograft transplantation: Two- to eight-year results. Am J Sports Med 29:410-4
56. Noyes F, Barber-Westin S, Butler D et al (1998) The role of allografts in repair and reconstruction of knee joint ligaments and menisci. Instr Course Lect 47:379-96

Editors' Comments (Meniscal Allograft)

We have found that the best way to pass sutures accurately through the small bone plugs for medial meniscus transplants is to drill with a Keith needle. A suture is passed through the meniscus tissue, and then threaded through the bone plug using the Keith needle after drilling.

Another trick to assist in passage of the meniscus allograft is to burr down part of the tibial emminence. This can be performed in combination with "notchplasty" of the lateral aspect of the medial femoral condyle or alone.

Preoperatively, an unloader brace can be helpful in differentiating "malalignment pain" from the pain of meniscal insufficiency. If considerable relief occurs in a varus knee following brace use, serious consideration should be paid toward performing a staged procedure with the osteotomy as the first intervention.

When passing the meniscal graft with the control suture at the junction of the posterior horn and the body, a slotted cannula is best used (with a nitinol needle) as the passage device. The slotted cannula allows for removal of the passage device without having to sever the passing suture.

To help maintain the normal hoop stresses of the meniscus, we measure the native A–P distance from the anterior to posterior horn as it exists on the donor tibial block, prior to preparing the medial meniscus bone plugs. This way, we can have some measurement to use as to where to place the anterior horn once the posterior horn has been passed.

With the bone block, or slot technique, it is best to err as mesial (close to midline) as possible so as to avoid graft extrusion.

We have found that with a 7-mm wide bone block that the footprint of the ACL can usually be avoided on the medial side, making the slot technique a viable option for medial meniscus transplantation as well as for lateral meniscus transplantation. With a previously placed ACL graft, the use of a slot technique becomes much more difficult due to the medially angled tibial tunnel, which is usually placed directly through where the slot needs to be created. This is the one situation where a plug technique is absolutely required.

If a block breaks during passage, there are several bail out options. First, one can simply pass the broken block, and if there is a good press fit, the block should heal even if cracked. If the fit is compromised, pass a suture through each half of the block and retrieve the sutures through drill holes in the anteromedial tibia, and tie over the cortex utilizing a button. Another option is to use two interference screws passed from anterior to posterior. One is passed posteriorly enough to fix the posterior fragment, and the second one passed more anteriorly to fix the anterior fragment.

Because the bone blocks are quite small, we have found that standard interference screws are too large. We have successfully used small bioabsorbable suture anchors as interference screws, which also provides sutures that can be used to further secure the horns.

Patients that have pain after meniscus transplantation may have partial detachment or small areas of failed healing to the capsule. If patients have pain more than 6 months postoperatively, we obtain an MR intraarticular arthrogram to evaluate healing, and have successfully gone back and reinforced several grafts in areas of inadequate healing. Be careful while evaluating a postoperative MRI on a meniscus transplant, since revascularization can be misinterpreted as re-tearing. Some patients following transplantation will develop symptomatic but minor rim tears that can also be treated quite simply with partial meniscectomy.

Chapter 3
Avoiding and Managing Complications in Cartilage Restoration Surgery

Bert R. Mandelbaum, Joshua A. Johnston, and Jason M. Scoop

Top 10 Pearls

- Know the "personality" of the particular articular cartilage defect.
- Small (<2 cm²), well-contained or shouldered lesions have the best potential prognosis regardless of the restorative method used.
- Malalignments, ligament instabilities, and meniscal injury or deficiency must be identified and addressed to ensure an effective and durable repair.
- Symptomatic improvement can take up to 6 months following cartilage restoration surgery and progressive improvement can be expected for at least 2 years.
- Chronic pain following microfracture or autologous implantation surgery may not represent failure of the cartilage restoration, but rather stress reaction secondary to subcortical insufficiency.
- Atraumatic graft insertion in osteochondral auto- and allograft transplantation is essential to avoid lack of peripheral integration.
- Transplant the minimal amount of bone necessary to fill the defect in osteochondral allograft transplantation.
- Obtain hemostasis of the defect bed prior to implanting autologous chondrocytes.
- Meticulous preparation of the periosteal patch with complete debridement of adherent fat and connective tissue may minimize graft hypertrophy.
- Use the "sandwich technique" in deep lesions treated with autologous chondrocyte implantation.

Introduction and Background

"From Hippocrates to the present age, it is universally allowed that ulcerated cartilage is a troublesome thing and that, once destroyed, is not repaired." The Scottish physician William Hunter said this in a paper presented to the Royal Society in 1743. Over 260 years later, articular cartilage lesions of the knee remain a "troublesome thing." Articular cartilage defects (ACDs) of the knee are frequently observed. Curl and coworkers described 53,569 hyaline cartilage lesions in 19,827 patients undergoing knee arthroscopy.[1] Similarly, a prospective survey of 993 consecutive knee arthroscopies demonstrated evidence of articular cartilage pathology in 66%.[2] Articular cartilage lesions are frequently associated with acute ligament or meniscal injuries, traumatic patellar dislocations, and osteochondral injuries or may develop from chronic ligamentous instability or malalignment.[3-6] Articular cartilage has little intrinsic reparative and regenerative capabilities. If not successfully treated or left untreated, symptomatic articular cartilage lesions may further breakdown and result in premature osteoarthritis of the joint. Pain, swelling, and mechanical symptoms that are associated with such lesions, especially larger and chronic lesions, can cause significant disability that may limit employment, sport participation, and activities of daily living. Treatment options for the treatment

B.R. Mandelbaum (✉)
Santa Monica Orthopaedic and Sports Medicine Foundation, 1301, 20th Street, Suite 150, Santa Monica, CA, 90404, USA
e-mail: bmandelbau@aol.com

J.A. Johnston
Orthopedic Surgery, Santa Monica Orthopedic and Sports Medicine Group, Santa Monica, CA, USA

J.M. Scopp, MD
Peninsula Orthopedic Associates, Salisbury, MDaryland, USA

of articular cartilage lesions include debridement, marrow stimulation techniques (abrasion chondroplasty, microfracture, drilling), osteochondral allograft, osteochondral autograft (OATs), and autologous chondrocyte implantation (ACI).

The best way to avoid complications in the treatment of ACDs is a rational and systematic approach to their care. This chapter will review our evaluation, classification, rationale, and algorithm for treatment of ACDs. We will discuss our approach to the common complications encountered when treating ACDs as well as technique-specific complications. Finally, we will look ahead to novel treatment strategies that have the potential to minimize some of the most commonly encountered treatment complications.

Complications

Preoperative Assessment of the Patient with an Articular Cartilage Defect

The most important issue in the management of articular cartilage disorders is an accurate and uniform characterization of the local, regional, systemic, and familial factors that contribute to the disease process. Subjective and objective tools can be used to assess both the lesion and the disease process. The first step in avoiding complications in the treatment of ACDs involves using the preoperative assessment to provide insight to the appropriate and specific treatment profile for each patient.

Avoiding complications in the treatment of ACDs begins with an accurate and thorough patient history. Important details include the patient's age, age at which the injury occurred, the defect etiology, mechanism of injury, and prior surgical interventions. Patients will often complain of nonspecific symptoms including activity-related pain, swelling, and loss of motion. If the defect involves a detached or loose body, mechanical catching and/or locking may be described. A high index of suspicion is important in patients with acute hemarthrosis, acute or chronic ligamentous instability, patellar dislocation or maltracking, or lower extremity malalignment. Medical and family history of inflammatory arthritides such as lupus, rheumatoid arthritis, and human leukocyte antigen (HLA)-B27 associations are important factors to consider in treatment planning. Endocrine disorders including thyroid, diabetes, obesity, estrogen-deficiency, and collagen disorders such as Ehlers-Danlos and Marfan syndromes are known chondral modifiers and are important details in the patient's history.

Subjective clinical survey outcome tools are used to create a reliable, reproducible score that is used to stratify each patient along the continuum of articular cartilage disorders. Subjective outcome measurements can provide insight into the specific and appropriate treatment profile. The consistent use of the same instruments allows meaningful assessment at baseline and follow-up. Various instruments have been used to stratify the subjective assessment of ACDs and osteoarthritis. To date, there has been no effort to organize the subjective assessment tools to reflect the continuum that exists when describing articular cartilage disorders and there is no consensus regarding an ideal scoring system. Patient population, age, and activity level are different; these differences are reflected in the scores. In the senior author's (BRM) clinical practice, all patients who are evaluated for knee pain complete several standardized subjective clinical outcome tools including the Cincinnati, IKDC Subjective Knee Form, International Cartilage Repair Society (ICRS) rating scale, and the Knee Injury and Osteoarthritis Outcome Score (KOOS). In addition, a quality of life survey, the Rand Short Form (SF)-36 is helpful to optimally define the impact of the problem and interventions on the patient's psychological and emotional lifestyle.

Objective assessment of ACDs begins with a thorough physical examination. Physical examination of the knee provides a functional assessment of articular cartilage status and provides insight on the knee macroenvironment. Important elements include range of motion, effusion, and joint line tenderness. Lower extremity malalignment, ligamentous laxity, and meniscal integrity are crucial factors to be considered and must be addressed to minimize complications and maximize outcomes in the treatment of ACDs.

Diagnostic techniques for the measurement of the structural integrity of cartilage of the knee include plain radiography and magnetic resonance imaging (MRI). Because cartilage is not visible on plain radiographs, the joint space width seen on weight-bearing X-rays has been employed as a proxy for cartilage lesions. Standard radiologic projections include weight-bearing anteroposterior (AP), flexed 45° posteroanterior (PA), patellofemoral, and lateral views. Calculation of mechanical axis and patellofemoral alignment is essential in the pre- and postoperative assessment. The accuracy, reliability, and sensitivity to change in plain radiographs in patients with articular cartilage disorders can be optimized by correcting for magnification errors, adhering to published protocols for radiographic technique, and using microfocal magnification and computerized interpretation of digitized radiographs. Despite these protocols and techniques, radiographs remain unable to detect subtle changes in cartilage defects, chondropenia, and early OA. In spite of these limitations, plain radiographs remain the primary outcome measurements of choice for all studies of cartilage disorders of the knee.

MRI of articular cartilage continues to evolve. Cartilage sensitive MRI presents a sensitive, specific, and accurate tool for noninvasive assessment of articular cartilage injury. Images should be obtained in three planes; using fast spin echo imaging with a repetition time of 3,500–5,000 ms and moderate echo time provides high contrast resolution among articular cartilage, subchondral bone, and joint fluid. Besides preoperative diagnosis, cartilage sensitive MRI can be very helpful for postoperative evaluation of cartilage repair. Even with cartilage specific sequencing, MRI may not detect a considerable number of chondral lesions especially partial thickness lesions. MRI techniques continue to rapidly improve and the latest techniques will not only predictably define subtle cartilage lesions, but also detect changes in the matrix, such as glycosaminoglycan content (Fig. 3.1).

The preoperative assessment of the patient with an articular cartilage disorder gives the surgeon an accurate and uniform subjective and objective characterization of the local, regional, systemic, and familial factors that contribute to the disease process. It is essential to comprehensively and systematically assess the lesion and disease process for strategic therapeutic and prognostic purposes.

Arthroscopic Assessment

Arthroscopy remains the gold standard for the assessment of articular cartilage lesions. Arthroscopy provides direct visualization of articular cartilage and the knee macroenvironment. This data can be combined with subjective and objective findings obtained during the history and physical examination to fully define and classify the local, regional, and systemic factors that may influence lesion progression, joint degeneration, or defect regeneration. The International Cartilage Repair Society (ICRS) has developed a comprehensive method of documentation and classification (Figs. 3.2 and 3.3).

Chondropenia

While the natural history of chondral injury of the knee is not well defined, it is apparent that a loss of articular

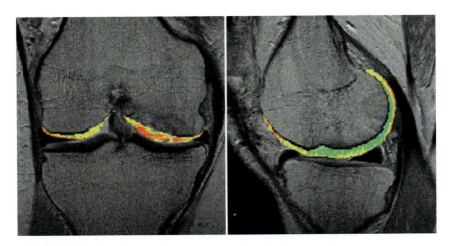

Fig. 3.1 Matrix-specific MRI

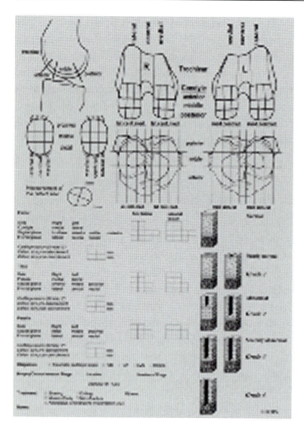

Fig. 3.2 ICRS comprehensive classification of articular cartilage defects

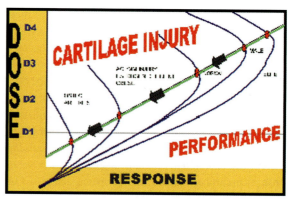

Fig. 3.4 Dose–response curve of articular cartilage

Modified International Cartilage Repair Society (ICRS) Grading System	
Injury Grade	Modified ICRS
0	Normal cartilage
1a	Soft indentation
1b	Superficial fissures and cracks
2	Lesions extending down to <50% of cartilage depth
3a	Defects extending down >50% of cartilage layer
3b	Defects down to calcified layer
3c	Defects down to but not through the subchondral bone layer
3d	Delamination
4	Severely abnormal; with penetration through subchondral plate

Fig. 3.3 Modified ICRS grading system

integrity through injury, pathologic loading, and aging can cause degenerative changes over time. Intact articular cartilage possesses optimal load bearing characteristics and adjusts to the level of activity. In the healthy patient, a positive linear dose-response relationship exists for repetitive loading activities and articular cartilage function (Fig. 3.4). However, studies indicate that this dose-response curve reaches a threshold and that activity beyond this threshold can result in maladaptation and injury of articular cartilage.[7] High-impact loading above this threshold has been shown to decrease cartilage proteoglycan content, increase levels of degradative enzymes, and cause chondrocyte apoptosis.[8–11] If the integrity of the functional weight-bearing unit is lost, either through acute injury or chronic microtrauma, a chondropenic response is initiated that can include loss of articular cartilage volume and stiffness, elevation of contact pressures, and development or progression of ACDs. Concomitant pathologic factors such as ligamentous instability, malalignment, meniscal injury of deficiency, and medical history of inflammatory arthritis, endocrine disease, or collagen disorders can further support the progression of the chondropenic cascade. Without intervention, chondropenia leads to progressive deterioration of articular cartilage function and may ultimately progress to osteoarthritis. The senior author (BRM) has proposed a new cartilage score, the Chondropenia Severity Score (CSS), which takes into account the chondropenic curve (Fig. 3.5). The CSS involves the objective assessment of meniscal injury as well as the size and the number of cartilage lesions in each anatomic location of the knee. The senior author (BRM) has been using the CSS in all arthroscopies over the last 2 years and studies are ongoing to determine the relationship of the CSS to patient outcomes and prognosis.

CHONDROPENIA SEVERITY SCORE (CSS)

Patello-Femoral Cartilage:		Medial Compartment Cartilage:		Lateral Compartment Cartilage:	
Patella:		MFC:		LFC:	
Normal	10	Normal	10	Normal	10
Grade Ia	8	Grade Ia	8	Grade Ia	8
Grade Ib	6	Grade Ib	6	Grade Ib	6
Grade IIa	5	Grade IIa	5	Grade IIa	5
Grade IIb	3	Grade IIb	3	Grade IIb	3
Grade IIIa	2	Grade IIIa	2	Grade IIIa	2
Grade IIIb	1	Grade IIIb	1	Grade IIIb	1
Grade IV	0	Grade IV	0	Grade IV	0
Trochlea:		MTP:		LTP:	
Normal	10	Normal	10	Normal	10
Grade Ia	8	Grade Ia	8	Grade Ia	8
Grade Ib	6	Grade Ib	6	Grade Ib	6
Grade IIa	5	Grade IIa	5	Grade IIa	5
Grade IIb	3	Grade IIb	3	Grade IIb	3
Grade IIIa	2	Grade IIIa	2	Grade IIIa	2
Grade IIIb	1	Grade IIIb	1	Grade IIIb	1
Grade IV	0	Grade IV	0	Grade IV	0
Meniscus:	n/a	Meniscus:		Meniscus:	
		100% remaining	20	100% remaining	20
		>2/3 remaining	15	>2/3 remaining	15
		1/3 – 2/3 remaining	10	1/3 – 2/3 remaining	10
		<1/3 remaining	5	<1/3 remaining	5
		0% remaining	0	0% remaining	0
					TOTAL CSS
SUMS:					

Fig. 3.5 Chondropenia severity score

Intraoperative Complications

Treatment Algorithm: The Chondropenic Pathway

The most common complication in cartilage restoration surgery is clinical failure with patient dissatisfaction due to continued pain, swelling, and mechanical symptoms. Clinical failure has generally been reported in the 5–35% range depending on the particular patient profile, lesion characteristics, and treatment modality. This complication can be minimized by the careful selection of the appropriate and comprehensive treatment profile for the specific articular cartilage lesion and the disease process. A comprehensive analysis of the local, regional, and systemic factors related to the ACD is used to develop a treatment plan. The orthopedic surgeon must understand the complexities of articular cartilage biochemistry, biomechanics, physiology, and the natural course of the lesion

We have created flow charts summarizing the primary and secondary treatment options in femoral and patellofemoral defects (Tables 3.1 and 3.2). A chondropenic pathway has been developed for the management of ACDs which takes into account the local, regional, and systemic factors that contribute to the disease process.

While a full review of the treatment algorithm is beyond the scope of this chapter, several important general principles are essential. The limited ability of articular cartilage for spontaneous repair has been well documented.[12,13] Following the acute injury and the resultant tissue necrosis, the lack of vascularization of articular cartilage prevents the physiologic inflammatory response to tissue injury. The absent potential for replication and repair by the intrinsic mature chondrocytes and lack of recruitment of extrinsic undifferentiated repair cells results in a qualitatively and quantitatively insufficient repair cartilage. Repetitive loading of the injured articular cartilage results in further cellular degeneration with accumulation of degradative enzymes and cytokines, disruption

Table 3.1 Femoral defects

Treatment options			
Microfracture	++	++	+
O.C.G.	++	++	−
Allograft	−	−	++
A.C.I.	−	−	++
Treatment options			
Microfracture	++	+	−
O.C.G.	++	++	−
A.C.I.	−	++	++
Allograft	−	−	++

−Treatment no recommended, + acceptable treatment, ++ optimal treatment
[a]Appropriate treatment is staged to avoid compromise of postoperative rehabilitation

Table 3.2 Trochlear and/or patellar defects

Treatment options		
Rehabilitation	++	++
Microfracture	++	++
Lateral release	+	+
Treatment options		
A.C.I.	+	++
Fresh allograft	−	++
Lateral release	+	+
P.F. realignment	+	++

−Treatment no recommended, + acceptable treatment, ++ optimal treatment of collagen ultrastructure, increased hydration, and fissuring of the articular surface. These biochemical and metabolic changes mimic the early changes seen in osteoarthritis.

Partial thickness lesions do not heal; they remain static as there are no biological mechanisms to create a reparative cascade. Full thickness lesions heal with fibrous Type I fibrocartilage that lacks organization and composition to maintain wear characteristics and integrity for the long term. Defects <2 cm^2 that are well contained or shouldered may be asymptomatic and nondegenerative for a long unspecified amount of time thus having the best potential prognosis. Defects >2 cm^2 that are poorly contained or shouldered have a lower probability of regenerative success which translates into pain, swelling, and lower levels of function.

Treatment options can broadly be classified as reparative (marrow stimulation techniques including abrasion chondroplasty, drilling, and microfracture), restorative (OATs, mosaicplasty, and osteochondral allograft transplantation), or regenerative (ACI). Reparative techniques, while relatively simple with minimal associated morbidity, are limited in that the repair tissue is "hyaline-like" fibrocartilage and clinical results likely deteriorate over time. Restorative and regenerative techniques have the potential to "reset" the patient's baseline on the chondropenia curve (Fig. 3.4) and halt the progression of the chondropenia cascade. Restorative techniques provide a hyaline cartilage repair but are limited in size due to donor site morbidity in the case of OATs procedures or carry the inherent risks and concerns of fresh-frozen allograft tissue in the case of osteochondral allograft transplantation. While regenerative techniques have had encouraging clinical and histologic results and avoid donor site morbidity, ACI can be limited by lesion depth, are technically difficult, require a staged procedure, and have cost/reimbursement issues. Regardless of the articular cartilage procedure of choice, malalignments, ligament instabilities, and meniscal injury or deficiency must be identified and addressed to ensure an effective and durable articular cartilage repair. Performing simultaneous adjuvant procedures avoids prolonged rehabilitation and should be considered whenever appropriate.

Some general intraoperative complications are extremely rare and readily avoidable with maintenance of general compliance and safety standards. Wrong-site surgery has been addressed by the American Academy of Orthopaedic Surgeons in an advisory statement recommending preoperative marking of the operative site and complying with institutional protocols such as "time-outs." Neurovascular injuries are extremely rare in cartilage restoration surgery; the most common being a neuropraxia injury to the infrapatellar branch of the saphenous nerve. Patients undergoing open procedures should be counseled appropriately regarding the rare possibility of nerve injury.

Technique-specific complications will be addressed in a separate section.

Postoperative Complications

Rehabilitation

The rational and systematic care of ACDs continues in the postoperative period. Appropriate postoperative rehabilitation promotes the ideal physiologic environment for the differentiation and incorporation of the reparative or the restorative tissue. The postoperative course represents a balance between protection of the cartilage repair and initiation of appropriate and specific rehabilitation. Rehabilitation should be started in a safe and timely manner to decrease the risks associated with prolonged immobilization and deconditioning including stiffness, weakness, venous thrombosis, and loss of function. Standard postoperative protocols have been developed with these trade-offs in mind.

Every patient has a specific and unique rehabilitation protocol depending on lesion location, size, and concomitant procedures; what follows are our general guidelines. All cartilage restoration patients are initially made touch down weight-bearing with two-crutch assistance for 6 weeks followed by progression to full weight-bearing as symptoms allow. During the first 6 weeks postoperatively, patients are started on a self-directed home rehabilitation program consisting of simple exercises to maintain motion and strength. At 2 weeks postoperatively, closed kinetic chain exercises such as stationary biking are allowed; limited arc strengthening exercises are also initiated in the range of motion that avoids loading of the repaired lesion. Patients are referred to a formal professionally monitored physical therapy program after 6 weeks for a standardized program to regain motion, strength, proprioception, and sport-specific functional training.

In general, low-impact activities are started at 3 months, running at 4 months, and cutting and pivoting activities at 9–12 months; functional restoration with return to high-impact athletic or professional activities is expected by 12–14 months. Patients treated for patellar or trochlear lesions are kept in a knee immobilizer for the first 2 weeks postoperatively and allowed to weight bear as tolerated in the brace immediately, but otherwise follow the standard protocol. Patients who undergo an ACI procedure of the distal femur or proximal tibia use a continuous passive motion machine (CPM) 8 h a day for the first 2 weeks. Continuous passive motion provides cartilage nutrition and avoids the development of adhesions. Cold therapy is used during the first 2 weeks to decrease pain and swelling, then used as needed if symptoms dictate.

It is also essential that both the surgeon and the patient maintain patience during the postoperative period as significant clinical improvement can occur slowly. We emphasize to our patients that symptomatic improvement can take up to 6 months following cartilage restoration surgery and that progressive improvement can be expected for at least 2 years.

Infection

Deep infection is an uncommon but potentially devastating complication of cartilage restoration surgery. The intraarticular proteolytic enzymes associated with septic arthritis of the knee will readily degrade both native articular cartilage and repair tissue. Although most would agree that antibiotic prophylaxis is indicated for open, complex procedures such as ACI and osteochondral allograft implantation and for "high-risk" patients such as those with diabetes, immune disorders, history of infection, and skin disorders, routine antibiotic prophylaxis for arthroscopic surgery of the knee and shoulder has recently become a somewhat controversial issue.[14,15] Complications can be associated with routine use of prophylactic antibiotic administration including allergic reactions, antibiotic-induced diarrhea (including *Clostridium difficile* infection), and the potential induction of antibiotic-resistant organisms.

The ultimate goal on any surgical intervention is to minimize morbidity and maximize the probability of successful outcome. The risk of infection following arthroscopic surgery is multifactorial and antibiotic prophylaxis is only one facet. To complicate matters further, postoperative infection has the potential for litigious behavior and antibiotic prophylaxis has been proposed in pay-for-performance measures affecting orthopedic surgeons. We feel the benefits of antibiotic prophylaxis outweigh the potential side effects. In the senior author's (BRM) practice, routine antibiotic prophylaxis is used with a first generation cephalosporin (Ancef) or an aminoglycoside (Vancomycin) in the case of documented penicillin allergy; two additional days of oral antibiotic prophylaxis are used in cases utilizing open surgery.

The surgeon must have a high index of suspicion for deep infection as successful treatment requires early and aggressive treatment. If septic arthritis is suspected, an aspiration should be performed under sterile conditions and the fluid sent for appropriate studies including Gram stain, culture (including aerobic, anaerobic, AFB, and fungal cultures), cell count with differential, and crystal analysis. Any indication of acute infection warrants urgent irrigation and debridement. Broad spectrum intravenous antibiotics should initially be administered, followed by organism-specific treatment as the cultures dictate. Often, an infectious disease consultation is warranted to direct and monitor the appropriate course of treatment. In cases in which allograft or autograft tissue transfer has been used, an initial effort should be made to preserve the restorative tissue. However, in cases of resistant or recurrent infection, the restorative tissue often must be sacrificed to cure the infection. In the case of infections associated with allograft tissue implantation, public health and regulatory agencies should be notified to facilitate an investigation if deemed appropriate.

Deep Venous Thrombosis and Pulmonary Embolism

Another uncommon but potentially devastating complication of articular cartilage restoration surgery is pulmonary embolism. Anticoagulative prophylaxis for deep venous thrombosis (DVT) is also extremely controversial. While a full review of DVT prophylaxis is beyond the scope of this chapter, a discussion of the potential complications associated with cartilage restoration surgery would be incomplete without a brief summary. We provide DVT prophylaxis to patients with a documented history of DVT or in cases of known hypercoagulative states or disorders. All patients wear thigh-high TED hose for the first week postoperatively and immediate mobilization is encouraged.

Patients with inappropriate calf pain and swelling following cartilage restoration surgery should be evaluated with duplex ultrasound, magnetic resonance angiography, or venography. A positive study for proximal DVT or PE should be treated with anticoagulative therapy under the supervision of a medical doctor, hematologist, or vascular surgeon.

Technique-Specific Complications

General

Regardless of the specific treatment modality used, adherence to meticulous surgical technique is essential to ensure optimal results and avoid preventable complications. Full descriptions of the various cartilage restoration techniques are available. We will discuss our techniques for avoiding complications in cartilage restoration surgery and dealing with intraoperative complications if they occur.

Marrow Stimulation Techniques

The key to all marrow stimulation techniques (microfracture, drilling, and abrasion chondroplasty) is the establishment a stable marrow clot in the optimal environment to promote mesenchymal stem cell differentiation. Microfracture as described by Steadman presents an improvement of earlier marrow stimulation techniques.[16] This technique includes debridement of the cartilage lesion to stable cartilage margins, careful removal of the calcified cartilage layer, and micropenetration of the subchondral bone using commercially available instrumentation. Four-millimeter wide subchondral bone bridges are maintained for preservation of the subchondral bone plate integrity and function. Release of blood and marrow fat droplets from the microfracture holes results in the formation of a clot in the cartilage defect that contains pluripotent marrow-derived mesenchymal stem cells. The mesenchymal stem cells produce a mixed fibrocartilage repair tissue that contains varying amounts of type II collagen. Critical components of the procedure include debridement of all pathologic articular cartilage to form a stable perpendicular edge of healthy viable cartilage, thorough and complete removal of the calcified cartilage layer, and visualization of adequate marrow elements flowing into the lesion after microfracture has been performed.

Compared with other cartilage restoration techniques, microfracture is technically simple, has limited invasiveness, low associated morbidity, and short postoperative rehabilitation. Microfracture is most successful in small, acute lesions. The major complication of microfracture surgery is deterioration of knee function. Decreasing pain scores, Tegner scores, and IKDC scores after 2 years has been described by several investigators in 47–80% of athletes.[17–20] The reason for this functional decline has not yet been identified. Clinical evidence suggests that repair cartilage volume plays a critical role for durability of functional improvement after microfracture as deterioration of knee function occurs primarily in patients with poor repair cartilage fill at second look arthroscopy or on postoperative MRI. MRI evaluation after microfracture has shown that the majority of the lesions demonstrate depressed repair cartilage morphology. Incomplete peripheral integration with persistent gaps between the native and repair cartilage is observed in 53–96%. Lack of peripheral integration increases vertical shear stresses between repair and native cartilage and promotes repair cartilage degeneration. In addition, subchondral bony overgrowth can occur in 25–40% resulting in a relative thinning of the overlying repair cartilage with biomechanical implications for the repair cartilage function and durability[17,21] (Fig. 3.6). We have observed a number of clinical failures due to intralesional osteophytes.

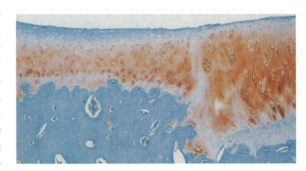

Fig. 3.6 Histology of osseous overgrowth following microfracture with relative thinning of reparative tissue

In these lesions, an "island" of exophytic bone is surrounded by otherwise healthy appearing fibrocartilage reparative tissue. The intralesional osteophyte is usually small and treated simply with abrasionplasty of the lesion and revision microfracture as previously described.

Chronic lesions with subchondral sclerosis can be more difficult to treat. In chronic lesions with subchondral sclerosis, we make a relatively deeper penetration with the awl in the center of the lesion then proceed with microfracture as previously described. Aggressive debridement of the subchondral bone can compromise its integrity leading to the potential complication of stress reactions and chronic pain. Symptoms duration of >12 months is a negative predictor of successful outcome in microfracture surgery.[20]

Current research is directed at identifying and improving the factors that lead to insufficient repair cartilage volume after microfracture.

Osteochondral Autograft Transplantation and Mosaicplasty

Autograft transplantation provides a hyaline cartilage repair by harvesting cylindrical osteochondral grafts from areas of limited weight-bearing, such as the peripheral trochlea, and transfer into small to midsize (1–4 cm^2) defects of the weight-bearing cartilage using a press-fit technique.[22,23]

Restoration of concave or convex articular cartilage surfaces can be technically demanding and short-term fixation strength and load-bearing capacity may deteriorate early.[24] Incongruity and graft height mismatch can result in significant elevation of contact pressures.[25] Graft harvest and implantation must be perpendicular to the articular surface to avoid obliquity and step off at the surface. If a graft is inserted too deep, a second recipient hole can be drilled adjacent to the initial graft and an arthroscopic probe is used to elevate the graft. Peripheral chondrocyte death from mechanical trauma at the graft and recipient edges can lead to lack of peripheral integration with persistent gap formation.[26,27] Recipient holes should be dilated, especially in stiff bone to allow easy atraumatic graft insertion. Donor side morbidity has been described; however, long-term morbidity appears to be low.[28-30] Donor site morbidity may be minimized by using smaller plugs from the medial trochlea or lateral trochlea distal to the sulcus terminalis.[31] OAT transfer is limited to defects <4 cm^2 due to limitations in available donor tissue. It is also limited to lesion depths of no greater than 1 cm due to limitations in the available donor sites and problems with fixation. Autograft transplantation techniques are effective and durable techniques for hyaline articular cartilage resurfacing of small to moderate size chondral and osteochondral defects of the weight-bearing articular cartilage in patients with short preoperative intervals and without established degenerative changes.

Osteochondral Allograft Transplantation

Osteochondral allografts have been successfully used for the treatment of large and deep chondral and osteochondral lesions from acute trauma, osteochondritis dissecans, avascular necrosis, and joint degeneration. Fresh osteochondral allografting transplants mature hyaline cartilage, with viable chondrocytes that survive hypothermic storage and subsequent transplantation while maintaining their metabolic activity and sustaining the surrounding collagen matrix.

By debridement and removal of host bone from the area of the chondral or osteochondral lesion, a recipient site is initially prepared. A size- and depth-matched osteochondral allograft is then harvested and placed into the recipient bed by either screw fixation or press-fit technique.[32,33] This technique provides a hyaline cartilage repair. Since chondrocyte viability, matrix composition, and mechanical properties of hypothermically stored cartilage grafts has been shown to deteriorate rapidly, implantation should be performed as a fresh graft within 28 days of graft harvest.[34] Several studies have shown that the transplanted bone is readily incorporated by the host with good articular cartilage function. However, recent survival analysis revealed deterioration over time with 95% survival at 5 years, 80% at 10 years, and 65% at 15 years.[35] Better outcomes are seen with unipolar lesions, without malalignment, rigid fixation, and age <60 years.[36]

Critical components of the surgical procedure include restoration of the mechanical environment with concomitant procedures when indicated, transplanting the minimal amount of bone necessary, simplifying the procedure with the use of dowels, avoidance of impaction at implant insertion, and use of rigid internal fixation when needed.

Complications unique to osteochondral allograft transplantation include the potential for disease transmission, immune reactions, and limitations of available donor tissue. Immune responses may be a component in the rare complication of osseous failure of the graft. To minimize the risk of immune reactions, the minimal amount of bone necessary to fill the defect should be transplanted and high pressure saline washing of the allograft is recommended to remove marrow elements from the osseous portion of the graft. The allogenic chondrocytes seem to be immunoprivileged and long-term in vivo viability has been demonstrated. Allograft safety has significantly improved over the last 15 years. Basic criteria for donor screening and procurement of tissue is set by the Food and Drug Administration (FDA) and the American Association of Tissue Banks (AATB). Routine cultures of the graft at the time of transplantation are not recommended as they are not sufficiently sensitive and specific for allograft contamination and only add a layer of confusion in the case of infection. It is essential that the surgeon has a good working relationship with a known and trusted tissue bank. Osteochondral allograft transplantation can be logistically challenging. While every effort is made to size match the donor tissue, sizing mismatches can occur complicating successful anatomic recreation of the articular surface.

The allograft should be cut to the proper depth as calibrated from the lesion at 12, 4, and 8 o'clock. If the graft is malpositioned, it can be removed with a terminally threaded retrieval pin and repositioned. The tolerance of the grafts can be quite small and a graft site dilator should be used in stiff bone to facilitate atraumatic insertion. It is better to have an atraumatically placed "looser" graft that requires adjuvant fixation than a "tight" press-fit graft that requires significant impact to place. Large lesions can be treated with two allograft dowels overlapped in a "snowman" fashion (Fig. 3.7).

In the event of massive allograft contamination (i.e., dropping the graft on the floor) and insufficient tissue remains to harvest a second graft, the contaminated graft can be immersed in sterilization solution and implanted. Treatment of massive graft contamination has been described in the ACL reconstruction literature but not specifically in the case of osteochondral allografting.[37,38] Studies have shown that a 4% chlorhexidine gluconate soak may be more effective in sterilizing grafts than bacitracin/polymyxin or 10% povidone-iodine solutions soaks. There are several reports of chondrolysis following the use of chlorhexidine in the knee,[39,40] however, recent literature has shown that brief (1 min) exposure of human articular cartilage to 0.05% chlorhexidine solution does not impair cartilage metabolism.[41] Every attempt should be made to avoid massive graft contamination. The surgeon who prepared the osteochondral graft should remain in possession of the graft and personally transfer the graft from the graft preparation area to the surgical field. While studies have shown that massively contaminated ACL grafts can be secondarily sterilized with antibiotic soaks, we cannot recommend secondary sterilization and implantation of a massively contaminated graft. The safest course of action in this case may be a second staged procedure when another osteochondral allograft becomes available.

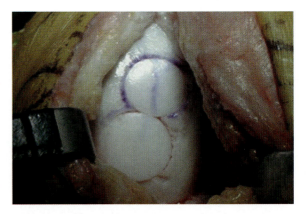

Fig. 3.7 Large articular cartilage defect treated with "snowman" technique (courtesy of W. Bugbee)

Autologous Chondrocyte Implantation

ACI is a two-stage procedure. The first stage involves a thorough diagnostic arthroscopy and chondrocyte graft harvest. Implantation of the cultured chondrocytes is performed in a second stage after 2–6 weeks. Autologous chondrocyte transplantation has been described as a successful technique for hyaline-like restoration of full-thickness articular cartilage lesions in the knee by several investigators with long-term durability of improved knee function up to 11 years postoperatively.[42-44]

Key components of the procedure include identification of concomitant joint pathology, proper chondrocyte graft harvest, preparation of the cartilage defect, periosteal patch preparation, and chondrocyte delivery.

Adjuvant procedures such as ligament reconstruction, osteotomies, and meniscal allograft implantation should be performed at the second stage to avoid repetitive surgical trauma and prolonged rehabilitation and promote the patient's return to preoperative activity.

In the first stage, harvesting of 200–300 mg of normal articular cartilage is obtained from a lesser weight-bearing area of the injured knee, generally the medial or lateral superior ridge of the femoral condyle or intercondylar notch. The intercondylar notch is preferred for patellofemoral lesions. Using cartilage that has been debrided from the cartilage defect as graft is not recommended since chondrocyte quality from this area has been shown to be inferior. Graft procurement is done best with an angled or ring curette. The grafted cartilage tissue is sent for standardized commercial isolation and culturing of chondrocytes. A sufficient number of cells should be obtained for the size of the defect (range 4–12 million cells). Chondrocyte viability is routinely tested and should be >95% before implantation.

At the second stage, the cartilage defect is debrided back to a healthy cartilage margin. Debridement of the calcified cartilage should be carefully performed without violation of the subchondral bone plate. Violation of the subchondral bone may affect the biomechanical integrity of the bone plate and may introduce bleeding and development of fibrous repair tissue in the treated defect. If bleeding is encountered, hemostasis of the defect bed can be achieved by application of epinephrine, thrombin, or fibrin glue.

An appropriately sized periosteal flap is then harvested, generally from the proximal medial subcutaneous border of the tibia. The periosteal flap is then sutured flush to the surrounding rim of articular cartilage using interrupted 6-0 Vicryl (Ethicon, Inc., New Brunswick, NJ) with the cambium layer facing into the defect. We generally oversize the periosteal patch by 1–2 mm circumferentially compared with our ACD template to ensure adequate coverage. In areas where the cartilage rim is thick such as the patella or the distal femur, the periosteal flap should not be "sewn down" to the subchondral bone as this creates a step-off at the articular surface. If the cartilage lesion is uncontained, minisuture anchors can be used to create a lesion contained by the periosteal patch. Meticulous preparation of the periosteal patch with complete debridement of adherent fat and connective tissue is recommended to minimize the risk of graft hypertrophy.

Chondrocyte delivery is performed after the periosteal rim is sealed with fibrin glue. A water tight test is performed with saline prior to injecting the cultured chondrocytes. Following cell injection, the remaining corner of the periosteal flap is secured with sutures and sealed with fibrin glue. Very large defects can be treated with segmental delivery of chondrocytes into separate periosteal compartments to promote an even distribution of chondrocytes in the ACD.

Deep lesions (>1 cm) are treated with the "sandwich technique"[42] (Fig. 3.8). The osseous defect is filled with cancellous bone graft from iliac crest or proximal tibia to the level of the subchondral plate. One periosteal flap sized for the defect is then anchored with the cambium layer facing toward the joint using fibrin glue applied between the periosteal flap and the bone graft. A second-sized periosteal flap is then placed facing into the defect and secured to the surrounding cartilage with interrupted 6-0 Vicryl (Ethicon, Inc., New Brunswick, NJ). The rim is again sealed with fibrin glue and the cultured chondrocytes then implanted between the two periosteal flaps.

Complications after autologous chondrocyte transplantation are rare. Complications generally associated with arthrotomy and protected weight-bearing such as stiffness, DVT, or infection may principally occur. Infection, venous thromboembolism, or nerve injury have not been observed in published series of ACI. Intraarticular adhesions have been described in 0–10 % and are frequently the result of intraarticular hematoma or harvesting femoral periosteum from the suprapatellar pouch region. If symptomatic, it can be treated successfully by manipulation under anesthesia or arthroscopic lysis of adhesions.

Hypertrophy of the implanted periosteum presents the most frequently observed complication after autologous

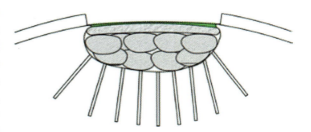

Fig. 3.8 ACI sandwich technique

chondrocyte transplantation. This complication usually presents itself 3–9 months postoperatively with localized pain, and complaints of knee catching by the patient. Hypertrophy of the graft is seen in up to 63% of postoperative magnetic resonance images but described as clinically symptomatic in only 13–15%.[42–47] hypertrophy can be minimized by meticulous preparation of the periosteal patch with complete debridement of adherent fat and connective tissue. Symptomatic hypertrophy can be effectively treated by arthroscopic chondroplasty.

Partial detachment of the graft may occur and becomes symptomatic. Management involves arthroscopic debridement and trimming of any protruding areas of the graft. Rarely, complete delamination may occur and is usually associated with premature weight-bearing. The incidence of traumatic delamination is higher in athletes which are subjecting the graft to high joint loading and shear forces. Careful monitoring for periosteal hypertrophy with restricted progression of joint loading or prophylactic arthroscopic debridement may reduce the risk for delamination in this high demand population.

Graft failure has been described in 6–7%. Grafts usually fail between 12 and 24 months after surgery and frequently show central degeneration. Treatment with revision chondrocyte implantation has been shown to be effective in many cases. All patients with graft failure should be carefully evaluated for the presence of subtle instability, axial malalignment, or patellar maltracking, which has been shown to lead to lower success rates after autologous chondrocyte transplantation.

Revision Surgery

Revision surgery generally follows the treatment algorithm as described above. It is especially important to fully understand the mechanism of failure of the index procedure. As previously described, exogenous causes of cartilage restoration surgery including malalignments, ligament instabilities, and meniscal injury or deficiency must be identified and addressed to ensure an effective and durable articular cartilage repair. Infection must always be ruled out as a cause of surgical failure in cases of persistent pain and effusion especially if associated with erythema, persistent or prolonged wound drainage, or systemic signs of infection.

A complication unique to revision surgery is dealing with previously placed skin incisions. In general, laterally based flaps at the knee should be avoided and the most lateral previous incision that facilitates the planned procedure should be used. When multiple incisions are present and there is concern for skin necrosis, the initial incision should be made without tourniquet inflation to facilitate inspection of the skin edges. If skin viability remains a concern after inspection of the skin edges, a delayed incision technique can be performed as described in the total joint arthroplasty literature. The skin incision is made and flaps are elevated in preparation for an arthrotomy. The wound is then closed and allowed to heal. If there is no skin necrosis, the planned procedure is performed through the same incision at 4–6 weeks. Advocates of this technique postulate that this not only tests the viability of the skin flaps but also promotes increased collateral circulation secondary to the healing process. We have a low threshold for a plastic surgery consultation when warranted. If skin necrosis occurs following cartilage restoration surgery, then it is important to keep the skin sealed for as long as possible to allow the capsulotomy to heal and prevent deep infection. Range-of-motion exercises are stopped and the knee is immobilized in a removable splint or brace to facilitate wound inspection. Persistent drainage warrants an immediate plastic surgery consultation. Surgical options include excision and primary closure of the defect, wound vac dressings followed by split thickness skin grafting, and gastrocnemius muscle flaps with split thickness skin grafting.

Future Directions

Second-generation techniques for cell-based, biologic articular cartilage repair are rapidly developing. These techniques use three-dimensional scaffolds from numerous biologic (collagen, hyaluronate, alginate), carbohydrate-based (polylactide, polyglycolide), or mineral-based (tri-calcium-phosphate, hydroxyapatite) polymers and materials. The scaffolds can be seeded with chondrocytes or chondroprogenitor cells in vitro and then implanted into the defect. The use of three-dimensional scaffolds has the potential to reduce complications associated with autograft and allograft transfer techniques and minimize surgical-related morbidity secondary by facilitating all-arthroscopic techniques and decreasing surgical times. The scaffolds may also be biologically manipulated to enhance chondrocyte proliferation and maturation. In the future, chondrocyte cell lines may be optimized to select for enhanced cartilage-forming capacity. Finally, studies investigating the chondrogenetic potential of mesenchymal stem cells suggest that cartilage formation is possible using stem cells from a variety of tissue sources. In addition to surgical developments, accelerated rehabilitation programs are currently being investigated to determine whether returning patients to activity faster can be done without compromising the patient's long-term functional improvement. Overall, the rapidly developing area of cell-based articular cartilage repair remains very promising and exciting. Close interdisciplinary collaboration between basic scientists, bioengineers, clinicians, and physiotherapists will ensure continued rapid improvement and development of biologic cartilage repair methods that can reliably generate hyaline cartilage, reduce surgical morbidity, and provide durable clinical improvement.

References

1. Curl W, Drome J, Gordon E et al (1997) Cartilage injuries: A review of 31516 knee arthroscopies. Arthroscopy 13:456-60
2. Aroen A, Loken S, Heir S et al (2004) Articular cartilage lesions in 993 consecutive knee arthroscopies. Am J Sports Med 32:211-5
3. Moti A, Micheli L (2003) Meniscal and articular cartilage injury in the skeletally immature knee. Instr Course Lect 52:683-90
4. Smith A, Tao S (1995) Knee injuries in young athletes. Clin Sports Med 14:629-50
5. Mandelbaum B, Browne J, Fu F et al (2000) Articular cartilage lesions of the knee. Am J Sports Med 26:853-61
6. Piasecki D, Spindler K, Warren T et al (2003) Intraarticular injuries associated with anterior cruciate ligament tear: findings at ligament reconstruction in high school and recreational athletes. Am J Sports Med 31:601-5
7. Kiviranta I, Tammi M, Jurvelin J et al (1992) Articular cartilage thickness and glycosaminoglycan distribution in the canine knee joint after strenuous running exercise. Clin Orthop Relat Res Oct(283):302-8
8. Jackson D, Lalor PA, Aberman H et al (2001) Spontaneous repair of full thickness defects of articular cartilage in a goat model. J Bone Joint Surg Am 83A:53-64
9. Lohmander L, Roos H, Dahlberg L et al (1994) Temporal patterns of stromelysin, tissue inhibitor and proteoglycan gragments in synovial fluid after injury to the knee cruciate ligament or meniscus. J Orthop Res 12:21-8
10. Arokoski J, Kiviranta I, Jurvelin J et al (1993) Long-distance running causes site-dependent of cartilage glycosaminoglycan content in the knee joint of beagle dogs. Arthritis Rheum 36:1451-9
11. Pearle A, Warren W, Rodeo S (2005) Basic science of articular cartilage and osteoarthritis. Clin Sports Med 24:1-12
12. Buckwalter J, Mankin H (1997) Articular cartilage. Part II: Degeneration and osteoarthrosis, repair, regeneration, and transplantation. J Bone Joint Surg Am 79:612-32
13. Vrahas M, Mithoefer K, Joseph D (2004) Long-term effects of articular impaction. Clin Orthop Relat Res Jun(423):40-3
14. Lubowitz J, Poehling G (2007) Arthrsocopy and antibiotics. Arthroscopy 23:1-3
15. Bert J, Giannini D, Nace L (2007) Antibiotic prophylaxis for arthroscopy of the knee: is it necessary? Arthrsocopy 23:4-6
16. Steadman J, Rodkey W, Singleton S et al (1997) Microfracture technique for full thickness chondral defects: Technique and clinical results. Oper Tech Orthop 7:300-4
17. Mithoefer K, Williams R, Warren R et al (2005) The microfracture technique for treatment of articular cartilage lesions in the knee: A prospective cohort evaluation. J Bone Joint Surg 87:1911-20
18. Gobbi A, Nunag P, Malinowski K (2005) Treatment of chondral lesions of the knee with microfracture in a group of athletes. Knee Surg Sports Traumatol Arthrosc 13:213-21
19. Blevins F, Steadman J, Rodrigo J et al (1998) Treatment of articular cartilage defects in athletes: an analysis of functional outcome and lesion appearance. Orthopedics 21:761-8
20. Mithoefer K, Williams R, Warren R, et al. (2005) High-Impact athletics after knee articular cartilage repair. A prospective evaluation of the microfracture technique. Presented at the 2005 Annual Meeting of the American Orthopedic Society for Sports Medicine (AOSSM), July 16, 2005, Keystone, Colorado
21. Mithoefer K, Willi3ams R, Warren R et al (2005) The microfracture technique for treatment of articular cartilage lesions in the knee: A prospective cohort evaluation. J Bone Joint Surg 87:1911-20
22. Bobic V (1996) Arthroscopic osteochondral graft in ACL reconstruction: A preliminary clinical study. Arthroscopy 3:262-4
23. Kish G, Modis L, Hangody L (1999) Osteochondral mosaicplasty for the treatment of focal chondral and osteochondral lesions of the knee and talus in the athlete. Rationale, indications, technique, and results. Clin Sports Med 18:45-66
24. Whiteside R, Bryant J, Jakob R et al (2003) Short-term load bearing capacity of osteochondral autografts implanted by the mosaicplasty technique: An in vitro porcine model. J Biomech 36:1203-8
25. Koh J, Wirsing K, Lautenschlager E et al (2004) The effect of graft height mismatch on contact pressures following osteochondral grafting. Am J Sports Med 32:317-20
26. Horas U, Pelinkovic D, Aigner T (2003) Autologous chondrocyte implantation and osteochondral cylinder transplantation in cartilage repair of the knee joint: A prospective comparative trial. J Bone Joint Surg Am 85:185-92
27. Huntley J, Bush P, McBurnie J (2005) Chondrocyte death associated with human femoral osteochondral harvest as performed for mosaicplasty. J Bone Joint Surg Am 87:351-60
28. LaPrade R, Botker J (2004) Donor-site morbidity after osteochondral autograft transfer procedures. Arthroscopy 20:e69-73

29. Hangody L, Fule P (2003) Autologois osteochondral mosaicplasty for the treatment of full thickness defects of weight bearing joints: Ten years of experimental and clinical experience. J Bone Joint Surg Am 85(Suppl 2):25-32
30. Gudas R, Kelesinskas R, Kimtys V et al (2005) A prospective randomized clinical study of mosaic osteochondral autologous transplantation versus microfracture for the treatment of osteochondral defects in the knee joint in young athletes. Arthroscopy 21:1066-75
31. Garretson R, Katolik L, Beck P et al (2004) Contact pressure at osteochondral donor sites in the patellofemoral joint. Am J Sports Med 32:967-74
32. Gross A (1997) Fresh osteochondral allograft for posttraumatic knee defects: Surgical technique. Oper Tech Orthop 7:334-9
33. Jamali A, Emmerson B, Chung C et al (2005) Fresh osteochondral allografts. Clin Orthop Relat Res Aug(437):176-85
34. Williams R, Dreese J, Chen C (2004) Chondrocyte survival and material properties of hypothermically stored cartilage: An evaluation of tissue used for osteochondral allograft transplantation. Am J Sports Med 32:132-9
35. Gross A, Shahsa N, Aubin P (2005) Long-term followup of the fresh osteochondral allografts for posttraumatic knee defects. Clin Orthop Relat Res Jun(435):79-87
36. Shasha N, Aubin P, Cheah H et al (2002) Long-term clinical experience with fresh osteochondral allografts for articular knee defects in high-demand patients. Cell Tissue Bank 3:175-82
37. Molica M, Nonweiller D, Evans J et al (2000) Contaminated anterior cruciate ligament grafts: The efficacy of 3 sterilization agents. Arthroscopy 16(4):373-8
38. Izquirdo R Jr, Edwin R, Bauer R et al (2005) A survey of sports medicine specialists investigating the preferred management of contaminated anterior cruciate ligament grafts. Arthroscopy 21(11):1348-53
39. Douw C, Bulstra S, Vandenbroucke J et al (1998) Clinical and pathological changes in the knee after accidental chlorhexidine irrigation during arthroscopy: Case reports and review of the literature. J Bone Joint Surg 80-B(3):437-40
40. Van Huyssteen A, Bracey D (1999) Chlorhexidine and chondrolysis in the knee. J Boint Joint Surg 81-B(6):995-6
41. Best A, Nixon M, Taylor G (2007) Brief exposure of 0.05% chlorhexidine does not impair non-osteoarthritic human cartilage metabolism. J Hosp Infect 67(1):67-71
42. Peterson L, Minas T, Brittberg M et al (2003) Treatment of osteochondritis dissecans of the knee with autologous chondrocyte transplantation. J Bone Joint Surg 85(Suppl 2):17-24
43. Knutsen G, Engebretsen L, Ludvigsen TC et al (2004) Autologous chondrocyte transplantation compared with microfracture in the knee. A randomized trial. J Bone Joint Surg Am 86:455-64
44. Peterson L, Brittberg M, Kiviranta I et al (2002) Autologous chondrocyte transplantation. Biomechanics and long-term durability. Am J Sports Med 30:2-12
45. Brittberg M, Lindahl A, Nilsson A et al (1994) Treatment of deep cartilage defects in the knee with autologous chondrocyte transplantation. N Engl J Med 331:889-95
46. Mithöfer K, Peterson L, Mandelbaum B et al (2005) Articular cartilage repair in soccer players with autologous chondrocyte transplantation: Functional outcome and return to competition. Am J Sports Med 33(11):1639-46
47. Mithöfer K, Minas T, Peterson L et al (2005) Functional outcome of knee articular cartilage repair in adolescent athletes. Am J Sports Med 33:1147-53

Editors' Comments (Articular Cartilage)

Microfracture

It is imperative to debride the lesion to stable vertical margins and to remove the layer of calcified cartilage in order to achieve optimal results with circumferential as well as bony integration. We have found that this requires certain specialized curettes to accomplish. We prefer to use small ENT (mastoid) curettes which are small, sharp, and available in curved angles. In addition, we occasionally use a reverse angled currette to clear the anterior margin of the lesion.

We also protect our microfractures with 4 weeks of nonweight-bearing and 3 months with an unloader brace. In our experience, premature return to activity is a common cause for failure. If the lesion is located in an area that will not make contact in full extension (trochlea, posterior femoral condyle, patella) we allow full weight-bearing immediately with a locked brace at zero°.

Microfracture of the patella is challenging due to the difficulty of access to a perpendicular angle and the mobility of the patella. We usually use the 90° awls on the patella, and manually drive the tip into the bone while stabilizing the patella. With hard bone this can be difficult. One should be prepared to consider an arthrotomy to flip the patella 90° to get a direct perpendicular shot if necessary.

Make sure to always verify that bleeding has been created by eliminating inflow pressure, draining the joint, or even placing suction on the scope cannula while observing the microfracture area.

OATS

How to help ensure a flush plug:

This is the most challenging part of any osteochondral plug procedure. Although there is no way to guarantee an exact fit, here are some pearls, which we have found useful:

1. It is easier to get a small plug to orient than a large one, since with a small plug any slight variation in angle of harvest is less pronounced. If you are having trouble getting a flush fit, you may consider use of several small plugs.
2. The radius of curvature of the edge of the condyle is more similar to the radius of curvature of the intercondylar notch. So for larger plugs (8–10 mm) we prefer to harvest from this location.
3. We harvest the donor plug. Then we raise the foot of the initially flexed OR table to the position that allows a direct perpendicular approach to the chondral lesion for removal of the recipient site plug. We keep the foot of the table at the exact same position for the graft insertion to help ensure a perpendicular fit.

If the plug is not exactly flush after insertion due to mismatch of radius or harvest angle, there are several options:

1. Impact the plug until no part of the plug is prominent, even if a portion of the plug is recessed. It has been demonstrated to be much better biomechanically for the knee to have a slightly recessed plug rather than a proud plug.
2. Remove the plug and reharvest a new plug with a better harvest angle.
3. If it is a larger plug, try to impact the high portion only with a small impactor. This may compress the bone or possibly crack the plug and will most likely have some negative effect on the chondrocytes, so do this with caution.

ACI

If you inadvertently tear the periosteum while harvesting or suturing, it is OK to simply repair the rent and salvage the periosteal graft. If you find that you do not have enough periosteum to cover the entire defect, it is OK to harvest a second patch of periosteum and to a patch quilt technique by sewing the two patches together.

If there is inadequate cartilage to sew on the edge of the defect, instead of using an anchor, one can attempt to sew through bone. Utilize a small cutting needle, manually create a passage through the bone, and then follow with the standard 6-0 Vicryl.

You may also consider using a synthetic patch that is becoming more readily available.

If you find an intralesional osteophyte following a previous microfracture, use a bone tamp to compress the ostephyte so that the bony base of the lesion is smooth. Removing the osteophyte in any other way causes significant bleeding in the lesion and risks fibrocartilage formation.

For lesions that extend very posterior, one may utilize mini suture anchors for the posterior sutures. Place bone wax in the drilled holes.

Place your final suture to close the remaining window in the periosteum for cell insertion, before actually inserting the cells. This way the suture is ready to tie immediately after cell insertion, to avoid excessive leakage of cells during final suturing.

When harvesting the periosteum, use a wet sponge to clean off fat and sweep away superficial fascia prior to harvesting the periosteum. It is much easier than trying to trim this away after harvesting.

If returning to the OR for periosteal hypertrophy, consider use of a whisker blade to avoid unintentionally aggressive debridement. We have also occasionally utilized a thermal wand to shrink the hypertrophied edges with low heat and no contact (plasma layer effect).

If there is partial delamination of the graft of less than a centimeter, consider microfracture for this small area.

Chapter 4
Avoiding and Managing Complications in ACL Reconstruction

Don Johnson and Olufemi Ayeni

Top 10 Pearls

- Educate patient of risks preoperatively, and if the complication occurs, involve the patient in the problem solving process until the complication is resolved.
- Accurate clinical exam is essential to ensure that all aspects of injury is recognized and treated, so that factors such as posterolateral corner injury are not missed.
- The surgeon should be familiar with several harvest, fixation, and surgical approaches to tackle intraoperative challenges.
- Before stripping the hamstring tendons while harvesting, pull on the tendons and watch for dimpling on the calf. If dimpling occurs, additional release of bands should be done.
- Avoid overruns when using the saw blade and harvesting the bone tendon bone graft. Bone graft the residual defect as much as possible.
- Use of the low anteromedial portal is an effective technique for obtaining accurate femoral tunnel placement when the transtibial technique is inadequate.
- Intraoperative fluoroscopy is very helpful for assessing tunnel, guide wire and fixation placement.
- At the completion of surgery, the graft should be tested clinically with pivot shift and lachman examinations, and a final arthroscopic evaluation of the graft throughout the arc of motion should be completed.
- In the revision setting, all previous reports and notes should be obtained. A CT scan is an invaluable tool when determining bone deficits.
- In a difficult primary reconstruction or revision ACL reconstruction, staging the procedure is a safe and effective technique to address all complexities.

Introduction and Background

Despite all the care and precision taken in diagnosing the injury and deciding the best approach, situations arise that cannot always be anticipated. The following sections describe an array of complications, their remedies, and certain precautions that will assist in preventing such occurrences.

Preoperative Factors

The timing of surgery has been a factor in determining range of motion postoperatively, and it has been shown that surgery within an acute time frame may increase the risk of arthrofibrosis.[1] Although specific times are arbitrary, consideration should be given to the "personality of the injury."

In cases of severe injuries, significant swelling, soft tissue damage, associated capsular or multiligamentous damage, it is better to delay surgery until the acute inflammatory phase resolves. Once the inflammation subsides, preoperative treatment should include physical therapy to obtain full range of motion (−3 to 125°) and quadriceps function. In isolated or less severe injury patterns, full range of motion should be achieved prior to surgery.

D. Johnson (✉)
Sports Medicine Clinic, Carleton University, Ottawa, ON, Canada, K1S5B6
e-mail: donnie@carletonsportsmed.com

O. Ayeni
Sports Medicine Clinic, Carleton University, Ottawa, Ontario, Canada

Before discussing surgery with the patient, it is important to determine the full extent of the injury, and despite a severe injury, a thorough knee examination should be completed, clinically and radiographically. *Associated injuries,* such as posterolateral corner disruption and/or meniscal injuries, make treatment more complicated. A complete diagnosis of all injured structures should be made and each considered individually depending on the extent of the damage. In the case of a capsular injury, one should be wary of an acute operation requiring arthroscopy because of the risk of compartment syndrome and associated fluid extravasation. In such cases, intermittent palpation of the extremity is important in assessing compartment pressure. When operating on the posterolateral corner, making the incision first allows the fluid to drain from the incision and prevents compartment syndrome.[2]

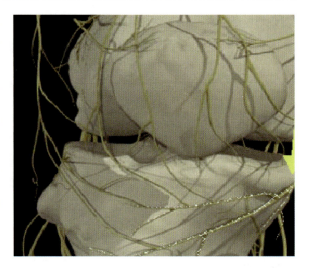

Fig. 4.1 Nerve plexus around the knee. *Arrow* indicates infrapatellar branch of saphenous nerve

Preexisting conditions, such as degenerative changes, should also be noted because they may affect prognosis and outcome.

Wrong site surgery has gained significant attention in the media of late, and of all the complications, this is the most avoidable. Institutional standards vary but include reviewing consent with patient, marking the operative limb preoperatively, taking a verifying "time out" before the procedure begins.[3,4]

Neurovascular injuries may occur at the time of injury and this should be diagnosed before the operation commences. Consultations with colleagues in adjunct services may be required in certain circumstances. However, care should also be taken in positioning the patient and all extremities should be padded appropriately. Hip hyperextension is a known risk for femoral nerve palsy because the nerve is stretched in this position.

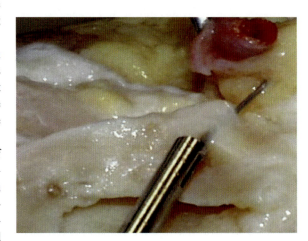

Fig. 4.2 Popliteal artery lies directly behind the posterior horn of the lateral meniscus

Functional Anatomy at Risk

- The saphenous nerve (Fig. 4.1) (infrapatellar branch) is responsible for anteromedial sensation of the knee in the majority of patients. It originates after the saphenous nerve emerges from the deep fascia of the thigh between the sartorius and gracilis. It then traverses the sartorius and joins the patellar plexus, curving distally and medially to the patella. There are numerous variations, and preservation of this nerve/plexus is difficult. It has been shown that harvesting the hamstrings through an oblique incision or using two horizontal incisions to harvest a bone tendon bone graft is less damaging to the nerve.

- The popliteal artery lies posteriorly to the posterior horn of the lateral meniscus (Fig. 4.2). A thin layer of fat separates this artery from the posterior capsule behind the posterior horn of the lateral meniscus. One should be careful when working at the back of the notch, or when repairing the posterior horn of the lateral meniscus, to avoid over penetration and damage to the artery.

Intraoperative Factors

Hamstrings autograft is commonly used and the complication associated with this particular graft harvest usage is *graft amputation* (Fig. 4.3).

Solution: When this problem occurs, there are three options: (1) proceed with a single tendon reconstruction; (2) use another graft source, or (3) use an allograft, if available. Trying to salvage the residual portion of the hamstring tendon is not recommended. The amputated graft can be used as an augment by stitching it to the other hamstring tendon that has been fully harvested. This converts the graft into a very useable three-strand graft. Trying to retrieve the residual portion of the amputated hamstring tendon is often frustrating, time consuming, and unsuccessful. This is due to the retraction of the tendon into the musculature in the posterior thigh. Also, further dissection can endanger the neurovascular structures present in the posterior aspect of the knee.

Prevention: Apart from knowledge of the harvest site anatomy, harvest technique is crucial. After exposing the hamstrings tendons sufficiently, care should be taken to apply an in-line pull on the hamstring tendons and make sure all fibrous bands attached to the medial head of the gastrocs are divided (Figs. 4.4 and 4.5). If the graft is free from fibrous bands, putting tension on the graft should cause no dimpling of the skin overlying the gastrocs muscle. Also, in the process of stripping the tendons, the tendon stripper should be aligned in the same direction as the tendon applying a constant force of pull on the hamstrings. If the graft has been amputated prematurely, conversion to an alternate graft, either autograft or allograft is indicated. This may include bone tendon bone grafts and/or allograft.

Patellar tendon autograft is the other gold standard and when harvesting the bone tendon bone graft, use a saw blade with a depth stop to minimize plunging. Then harvest in the order of patella bone block, tendon with a double bladed knife, and finally the tibial block to ensure the tendon fibres are in line with the bone blocks on both ends.

Problem: Complications may include fracturing of the bone plug, inadequate harvest of the bone plug, and fractures of the tibia or patella.

Solution: On the one hand, if the bone plug is inadequate, a "piggy back" grafting technique can be completed by bone grafting the deficient plug with bone from the coring reamer from the tibial tunnel. The newly added graft can be secured with heavy suture or fiber wire (Fig. 4.6). On the other hand, the graft may be reversed and the deficient site used like a soft tissue graft and secured to the tibia. The bone plug is inserted into the femur and the soft tissue side is secured, using a larger interference screw (Fig. 4.7). In addition, the soft tissue graft is sutured in krackow fashion and can be tied over a button or post on the tibia.[5]

Prevention: After making a longitudinal skin incision (medial to midline to avoid discomfort kneeling), an incision through the paratenon is completed. Alternately, two transverse incisions, one over the distal patella, and the other over the tibial tubercle can be made.

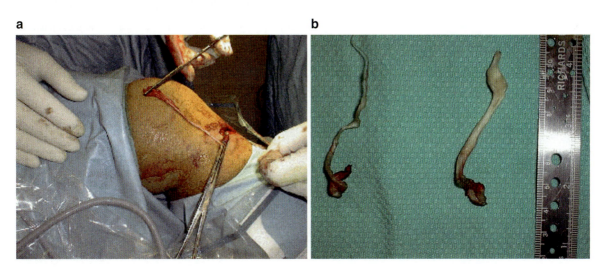

Fig. 4.3 Graft amputation

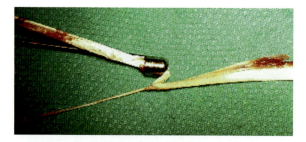

Fig. 4.4 The band to medial gastrocnemius that causes kinking of the tendon

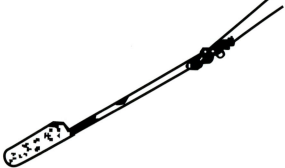

Fig. 4.7 Whip stitching of graft to use as soft tissue graft

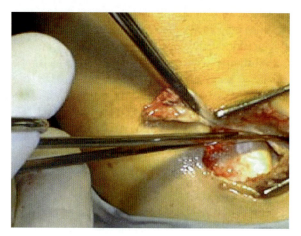

Fig. 4.5 Cutting the bands to the gastrocnemius fascia

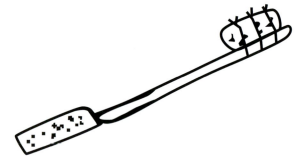

Fig. 4.6 Suturing a bone plug onto graft

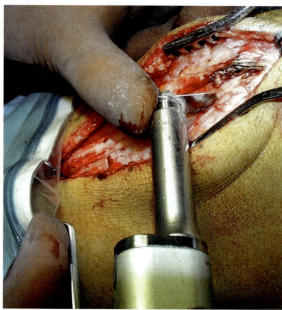

Fig. 4.8 Appropriate use of saw, minimizing overrunning of saw blade

These transverse incisions avoid damage to the infrapatellar branch of the saphenous nerve. The central third of the patellar tendon, with proximal tibial and patellar bone plugs, is harvested. The key technical step in successfully harvesting the graft includes safe use of the oscillating saw. This saw is used like a cast saw and it should have a 70° orientation to the coronal plane when harvesting the bone blocks (Fig. 4.8). Care should be taken to ensure that the same cut line is used, and multiple track marks are avoided. The aim is to have a trapezoidal-shaped graft and avoid the deep V-shaped graft that leaves a void, increasing the risk of stress fractures (Fig. 4.9). Likewise, overrunning with the saw and leaving transverse saw cuts on the patella increase the risk of stress fractures postoperatively (Fig. 4.10). Finally, the graft should be pried out carefully with a sharp, narrow osteotome. Damage to the articular cartilage beneath the graft can occur with overzealous use of the osteotome when removing the bone plugs.

Problem: *Dropping the graft* is another potential complication during the operation (Fig. 4.11).

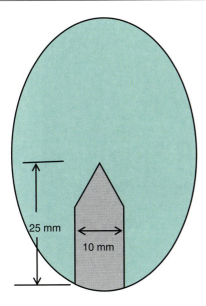

Fig. 4.9 Correct harvest technique with no overruns and trapezoidal graft shape

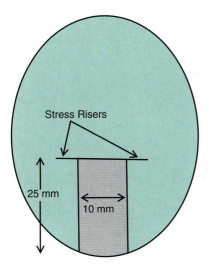

Fig. 4.10 Stress risers resulting from overrunning of saw

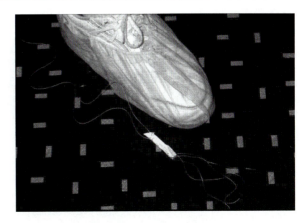

Fig. 4.11 Dropped graft

- Then, the graft is soaked in 4% chlorhexidine solution for 15 min and scrubbed with a new brush at the completion of soaking.
- Finally, the graft is placed in a triple antibiotic solution containing: 0.1% gentamycin, 0.1% clindamycin, and 0.05% polymyxcin for 15 min. At the completion of this protocol, the operation proceeds as planned.

Prevention: A "no touch" technique is the best way to avoid this risk (Fig. 4.12). The graft is handled in a sterile basin wrapped in moist, saline-soaked gauze, and a designated individual takes the graft to the back table for preparation. Finally, attaching the graft to a fixture on the back table provides extra assurance, in case someone lifts an instrument from the table with the graft sutures entwined in the instrument (Fig. 4.13). In several cases, the graft has been wrapped in a sponge on the back table, and the scrub nurse has thrown the sponge off the setup.

Problem: *Tunnel malposition* is a significant surgical error than will lead to early failure of surgical reconstruction (Fig. 4.14).

Solution: On the one hand, when a tibial tunnel is placed too anteriorly, it will impinge on the notch in extension and be tight in flexion. To deal with this, it is important to make the notch larger and chamfer the tunnel posteriorly to allow for translation of the graft. If the femoral tunnel is placed too anteriorly, the graft will be tight in flexion but loose in extension. To deal with this, a second tunnel can be drilled in the femur, provided that there is enough room to avoid confluence of the tunnels. If the femoral tunnel is only slightly anterior, then a trough can be created posterior to the original tunnel to allow for more accurate placement.

Solution: There are several ways of dealing with the dropped graft. Most involve cleansing the graft with a combination of antiseptic and antibiotic solutions.[6,7] Ultimately, the patient should be informed of the complication postoperatively, and monitored closely for possible infection. After retrieving the graft, our routine includes thorough irrigation and antibiotic treatment on a separate (contaminated) table.

- Specifically, the graft is cleansed in normal saline and a scrub brush used to remove debris on the graft.

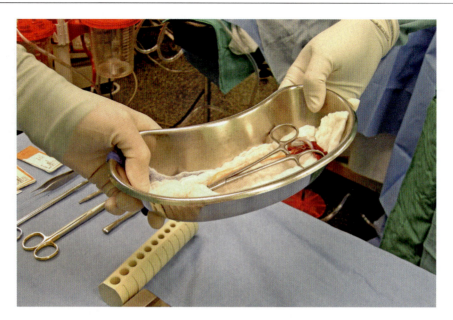

Fig. 4.12 No touch technique

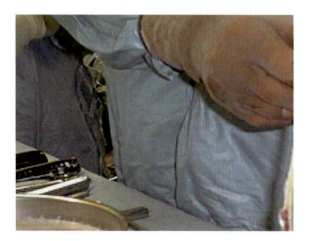

Fig. 4.13 Risk of graft handling

The interference screw used for fixation can also be placed anteriorly to the graft to help correct graft placement by displacing it posteriorly. On the other hand, a tibial tunnel placed in a posterior location may impinge on the PCL in flexion. A posteriorly placed femoral tunnel will be tight in extension but loose in flexion. A trough can be created with the use of a curved rasp to chamfer the back of the notch. Where the femoral back wall is blown out or compromised, a two-incision, outside-in approach can be used to create a second diverging tunnel that allows for interference screw fixation. Another option would be to use an endobutton fixation to allow fixation proximal to the blow out.

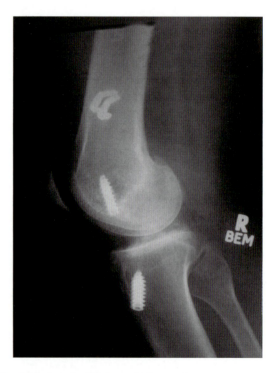

Fig. 4.14 Anterior tibial tunnel placement

Prevention: Tunnel placement remains critical to a successful operation. The stability and longevity of the graft is linked to its anatomical placement in the knee joint. Knowledge of crucial landmarks helps prevent complications related to tunnel placement. On the tibia, consistent landmarks used for ACL reconstruction include the old stump of ACL, 10-15 mm anterior to the PCL, the lateral edge of the medial tibial spine, and the posterior edge of the anterior horn of the lateral meniscus (Figs. 4.15 and 4.16). The guide pin should be placed into the anatomic site of the ACL attachment on the tibia. The size of the ACL varies and the distance anterior to the PCL is, therefore, variable. It is better to think in terms of the anatomic attachment site. Once the guidewire is drilled into the knee, the tip of the protruding wire should be visualized, and the knee should be taken through a range of motion to determine whether it impinges on the notch in full extension before definitive drilling. On the femur, the graft should insert into the posterior wall in the 10 o'clock or 2 o'clock position in right and left knees, respectively.

When drilling the femoral tunnel, it is important to ensure that enough back wall is maintained (2 mm) to prevent "blowing it out." When drilling the femoral tunnel, it is important to see the fringe on the notch and back wall to allow for accurate tunnel placement. The back wall can be visualized by clearing it of soft tissue with a curette prior to drilling the definitive tunnels. Next, the knee should be flexed more than 90°, and a 7 mm offset guide used to ensure that enough of a back wall remains to drill a 10 mm tunnel (Fig. 4.17). Hyperflexion of the knee (Fig. 4.18) when drilling the femoral tunnel through an accessory anteromedial portal is helpful to see the posterior fringe of the femoral wall and accurately place the tunnel (Fig. 4.19).

Before starting the femoral tunnel, a push-pull drill technique should be used to make a footprint and confirm that an adequate back wall remains (Fig. 4.20). Back wall blowout can also be avoided by using a small drill to start (7 mm) and then, using a hand reamer to increase tunnel size in increments of 0.5 mm. It is easier to change tunnel angles slightly with this technique, while obtaining tactile feedback about the integrity of the femoral tunnel.

If the femur is breached distally by less than 5 mm, it can be salvaged by drilling the femoral tunnel more proximally. However, any breach beyond 5 mm makes the use of an interference screw construct unwise. Other fixation and tunneling techniques include the use of an endobutton, nonanatomical or

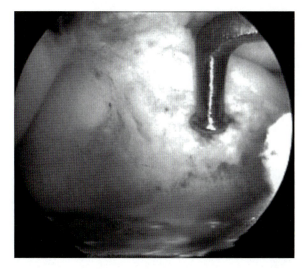

Fig. 4.15 Tibial footprint

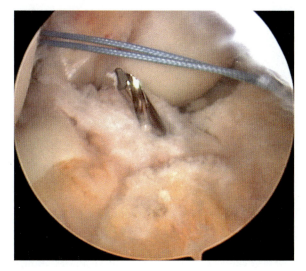

Fig. 4.16 Guide pin in footprint

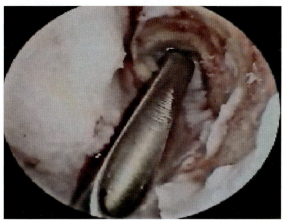

Fig. 4.17 Offset guide to make femoral tunnel

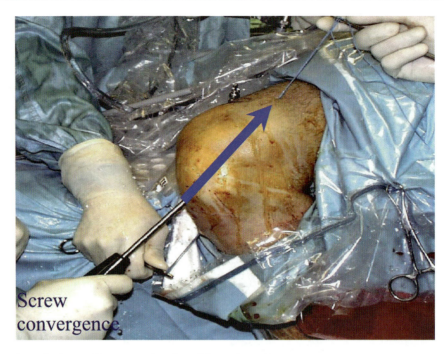

Fig. 4.18 Knee hyperflexion to allow correct location of femoral tunnel

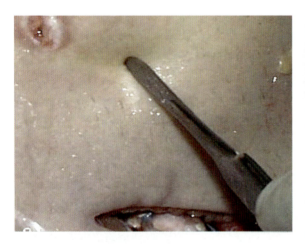

Fig. 4.19 Start point of low anteromedial portal on skin

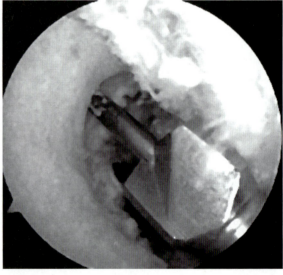

Fig. 4.20 Use of a push–pull drill to make a foot femoral print

over the top placement of the graft, or use of a two-incision approach to create a diverging tunnel.

The back wall blowout (Fig. 4.21) is acceptable when using hamstring grafts with endobutton fixation. But, when using an interference screw fixation, the insertion of the screw anterior to the bone block may push the block out posterior with loss of fixation.

Fine tuning of the position of the guide wire can be done if the push-pull drilling technique is used. If the guide wire is placed too anterior or too posterior, it can be changed before you are committed to drilling the complete tunnel (Fig. 4.22).

External landmarks can also be used when starting the tibial tunnel. The tibial tunnel should start 4-5 cm below the joint line, next to the MCL.

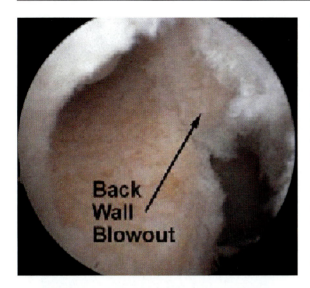

Fig. 4.21 Compromised femoral back wall, the back wall blow out

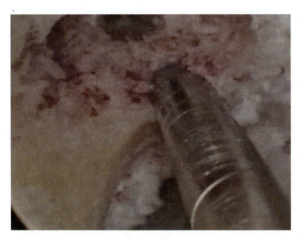

Fig. 4.22 Adjustment of back wall after initial drilling of femoral tunnel – less than 5 mm compromise

The tibial guide should make an angle of less than 70° in the coronal plane.

Problem: Graft passage can be difficult if there is a mismatch between the size of the tunnel and the graft.

Solution: The first step to ensure that the graft passes easily involves clearing any soft tissue that impedes the graft's engagement and entry. If it becomes extremely difficult to pass, then it can be removed and the tunnel dilated, ideally in increments of 0.5 mm. If sutures break during graft passage, the graft can be resutured. If suture strength is a concern, the use of a 20 gauge wire should be considered rather than regular sutures. Also, make sure the passing sutures are through bone, approximately 5 mm from the edge of the plug in a bone tendon bone graft, avoiding soft tissue. Another helpful tip for suture fixation of the bone tendon bone graft is to insert two passing sutures perpendicular to each other. This will reduce the likelihood of cutting both sutures when the screw is inserted. Lubricating the graft with commercially available lubricant and clearing the tunnel entrance is also helpful.

Finally, avoid soaking the graft in saline for too long, as the graft may swell. With a tight fit, the graft can be lacerated during passage. If this occurs, graft integrity should be carefully evaluated. At least 70% of the graft must be intact for it to be functional. The bone plugs in the bone tendon bone graft have different orientations. The tibial bone plug is eccentrically located, while the patella side of the plug is flush with the tendon. This makes the patella tendon more prone to damage/laceration during graft fixation. The tibial plug can be passed in the femur first, to minimize damage to the tendon while the patella plug is placed in the tibia where its fixation to bone is less of a concern.[5,8]

Prevention: Familiarity with instrumentation and ensuring that the equipment is calibrated to obtain consistent measurements will help avoid these problems. Use of sizing guides is crucial and the entire graft should pass through the selected sizing guide to confirm the size. It is not uncommon to hear of a 9 mm graft being impossible to pass through the appropriate sizing guide…only to discover that an upside down # 6 sizing guide was being used! Pay attention!

Problem: *Graft–tunnel length mismatch* is the unplanned discrepancy between the tunnel length and the length of the graft when using a bone patella bone graft (Fig. 4.23).

Solution: If a graft-tunnel mismatch occurs, it can be dealt with in a number of ways. The graft can be advanced farther into the femoral tunnel to shorten its overall length and allow fixation into the tibia. Next, a trough can be made in the tibia and the end of the graft fixed by stapling the graft to the tibia. Finally, the elongated graft (at 13 cm in total length) can be folded over a bone plug on the tendon to reduce its length and allow for distal fixation to bone. Rotation of a graft by up to 540° has been shown to be an effective way of dealing with a graft too long for the tunnel,[9] but this may adversely affect the biomechanical function of the graft. One important but simple tip with hamstring grafts is to always estimate length of the femoral tunnel

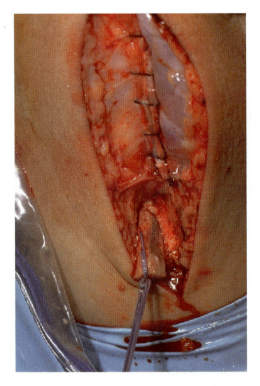

Fig. 4.23 Excessively long graft, extruding through tibial tunnel

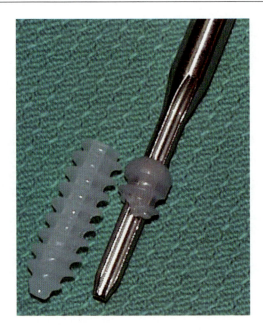

Fig. 4.24 Broken screw

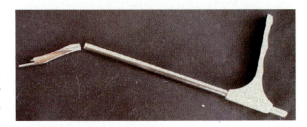

Fig. 4.25 Broken offset guide

by drilling with a 4.5 endobutton drill prior to definitive drilling of the femoral tunnel. This step allows for intraoperative tunnel and/or graft adjustments prior to committing to a particular tunnel.

Prevention: This complication can be prevented by getting an accurate measure of the lengths of the tunnel and graft prior to graft passage. The maximum length of the BTB graft should be 9–10 cm; with 3 cm in the femoral tunnel, 3 cm in the joint, and 4–5 cm in the tibial tunnel. If necessary, the tibial bone plug can be shortened (to a length 15 mm), to allow for fixation of the graft within the tunnel.

Problem: *Breakage of devices* can occur during any stage of the ACL reconstruction and can be prevented with attention to technical detail (Figs. 4.24 and 4.25).

Solution: The interference screws can break during insertion, and if this happens, remove the pieces of the broken screw before inserting a new screw. Complete visualization and special pituitary graspers can be useful in this instance. When reinserting the interference screw, the driver should be completely seated into the screw head and the entrance for the screw should be prepared by notching the entrance to allow for easy engagement of the screw on bone. The notching can be completed by tapping the entrance initially, or using a rangeur to nibble a small piece of the tibial entry site (Fig. 4.26). This step minimizes the risk of breaking the screw or screwdriver, as well. Likewise, the guidewire/K-wire can break in the knee. Again, the key is to visualize the pieces with a scope and remove the pieces atraumatically. At times, over-drilling the remaining wire piece in the tibial tunnel with a 4.5 mm cannulated drill will capture the wire. Once the wire is engaged in the drill bit, it is drilled until it is completely engulfed and removed with the drill bit. In all cases, forceful guidance of a wire when it meets resistance is not advised, as it can result in breakage of the wire. If resistance is met, the wire should be removed or fluoroscopic images obtained to assist with trouble-shooting.

Problem: *Traction sutures break* when passing the bone tendon bone graft.

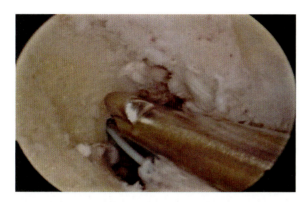

Fig. 4.26 Notching for an entry point of screw insertion

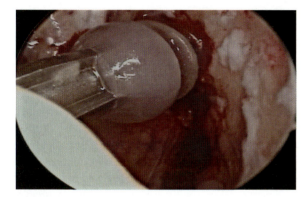

Fig. 4.27 Bio-screw insertion

Solution: If on the femoral side, the graft should be removed and resutured. On the tibial side, the graft can be resutured if it protrudes from the tunnel, or a small hook can be used to apply traction to the graft.

Prevention: Two traction sutures should be placed in the each plug for added security. Also, inserting the sutures in each plug at perpendicular angles to each other minimizes the risk of the screw cutting both sutures. Finally, use of strong suture material, such as fiber wire, is less likely during graft passage.

Problem: *Loose fixation* can adversely affect a technically well-performed operation. Bioabsorbable screws should be sized to allow contact between screw and bone tendon bone graft (Fig. 4.27). In general, the screw size should be not be more than 2 mm smaller that the size of the tunnel when a patella tendon bone graft is used. For example, an 8 mm screw in a 10 mm tunnel.

Where soft tissue grafts are used (hamstrings), the screw size should be 1 mm greater than the graft size. In both cases, a "squeak" can be heard in the final stages of screw insertions as the interference fit between the graft and screw is completed.

Solution: If the graft fixation is tenuous after adequate screw fixation, it is advisable to augment it with a secondary device, such as a staple or button on the tibia. Finally, if bony defects affect fixation of the graft stacking smaller screws or using a screw as a post can be considered. In general, a minimum of 20 mm of overlap between graft and screw is needed for adequate fixation. On the tibial side, fixation of the graft can be augmented with a button, or screw and washer (Fig. 4.28).

Prevention: Being thoroughly familiar with various fixation techniques, such as the endobutton and cross pin, is fundamental. When using the endobutton, it is important to know the tunnel length and allow 10 mm for flipping the button on the anterolateral femur. Marking the graft and watching it pass through the knee via the arthroscope will provide important information about endobutton deployment. Once the endobutton is seated, it can be flipped and confirmation is done with the usual toggling of sutures on each end. Use of different colored sutures is helpful to ensure that each end of the endobutton is positioned on the femur. Toggling the button, visualizing the graft markings and tensioning the graft (and not getting any pistoning) are all very important clinical parameters. If there is concern about the graft's seating, an intraoperative X-ray can locate it. Also, arthroscopic visualization of the suprapatellar pouch can confirm the location of the button. Ultimately, if the button is caught on soft tissues or not fully seated, it may be

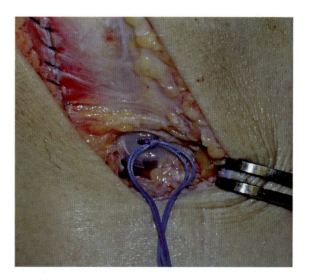

Fig. 4.28 Supplemental fixation with a button

necessary to make a small incision and dissect to the endobutton. At this point, the endobutton may be seated appropriately under direct visualization, or removed and changed.

Problem: The nitinol guide wire or cross pin breaks, or the pin is dislodged.

Solution: When the cross pin breaks or is dislodged, it should be removed by over-drilling to facilitate its removal before another pin or alternate fixation is used. Likewise, breakage of the nitinol guide wire may occur early during implant passage over the wire. When this occurs, the ends of the wire can be retrieved from both medial and lateral sides of the femur. This occurs usually because the graft is not seated proximally enough, or the implant insertion angle is different from the nitinol wire/guide pin insertion angle. The solution is to remove the graft and resize it (for confirmation), and correct the insertion angle of the guidewire and implant. In the case where the graft is seated and secure before wire breakage, an attempt should be made to remove the guidewire but a remnant may remain. Radiologic finding of the wire buried in bone usually does not affect the patient's outcome.

If the targeting drill misses more than twice, then alternate fixation should be sought, as further drilling may lead to stress fractures of the femur. Another tip is that for passage of the graft, 8 mm is needed for the cross pin and the tunnel length must be managed accordingly. Where the cross pin breaks or is dislodged, it should be removed by over drilling to facilitate its removal before another pin or alternate fixation is used.

Prevention: When a device, such as the cross pin, is used as fixation in the femur, a manufacturer's guide should be available to help with trouble shooting during the procedure. Once the femoral tunnel is completed, drilling for the cross pin should be visualized with the arthroscope. This way, central placement of the cross pin within the femoral tunnel is ensured. The targeting sleeve should be secure against bone, and all soft tissue that may interfere with the creation of tunnels should be cleared. Over-tightening of the drill guide on the lateral cortex can cause the drill to skive off the metaphyseal bone of the femur and thus should be avoided.

When using this instrumentation, it is very important to maintain the same flexion angles of the knee throughout the procedure. Any change can affect the trajectory of the implants after each step and lead to difficulty with definitive implantation later in the surgery. Also, soaking the graft will affect its diameter due to swelling. Once this occurs, the cross pins' path may be impeded by the hypertrophied graft. Resizing the tunnel with dilators is prudent if this occurs.

Problem: *Divergent fixation* occurs when the fixation device is more than 15° divergent from tunnel and graft. This significantly reduces the strength of the fixation and eventually impacts on the success of the procedure (Fig. 4.29).

The divergent femoral screw complication occurs when the screw is inserted into the tunnel without sufficient knee flexion. The knee should be flexed up to 120° and not left at 90° during femoral screw insertion.

Prevention: Clear visualization is important when fixation devices are being inserted. In the femur, flexing the knee to 100° or beyond, helps visualize the posterior wall adequately and ensures insertion of the screw in colinear fashion along the graft (Fig. 4.27). In addition, the use of the low anteromedial portal is helpful to get a straight shot into the femur for the tunnel (Fig. 4.19). An angled screwdriver is very helpful for accurate screw fixation to the graft at lesser angles of knee flexion (Fig. 4.31). Guide wires can be used to guide the course of the interference screw and prevent divergence (Fig. 4.30). Commercially available devices, such as centralizers, can be helpful in starting and inserting interference screws. Angled screwdrivers used with guide wires can help place the screw into the tunnel without hyper flexion of the knee (Fig. 4.31).

One should guard against slipping of the graft or pushing the graft into the knee, especially on the tibial side. If this occurs, removal of the screw, retensioning the graft, and reinsertion of the screw is advised. At least 20 mm of the screw should secure the bone or soft tissue graft to allow for secure fixation. To minimize

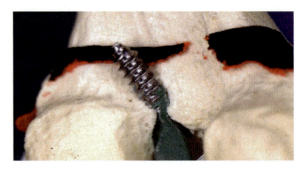

Fig. 4.29 Rear view of a sawbones model with the screw penetrating the back wall of the femoral tunnel

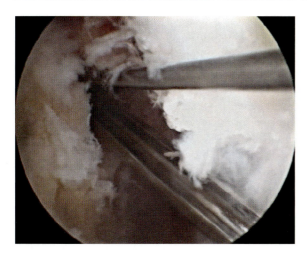

Fig. 4.30 Guide wire for screw insertion

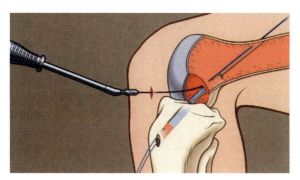

Fig. 4.31 Use of angled screw driver for screw insertion

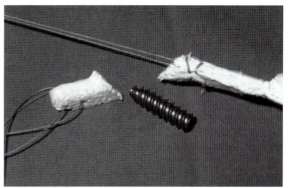

Fig. 4.32 Fracture of graft with the interference screw

graft laceration or abrasion, make sure the screw length does not surpass tunnel length. The surgeon should pay careful attention to tension on the graft during fixation. The fixation should not displace the graft into the knee and constant tension should be maintained on the graft while it is being secured. Although there are several ways to ensure adequate tension on the graft, arthroscopic visualization of the graft is helpful as the knee is moved from full flexion to full extension.

Loss of fixation can also result from fracturing the bone plug during insertion of interference screws (Fig. 4.32). When this complication happens, solutions discussed above (augmentation, soft tissue fixation, suture augmentation) can be considered. If it is difficult to start the insertion of the interference screw, create a notch at the entry point (Fig. 4.27). When using an endobutton as fixation on the femur, sometimes it is not possible to flip or toggle the button. Intraoperative X-rays or fluoroscopy can confirm the location of the button, and also used dynamically to find out where the button's progress is being impeded. If the button is caught on soft tissue in the thigh (muscle and fascia), a firm tug on the distal end of the graft can often settle the button into the femur. If this does not work, and as a last resort, dissect to the button on femur to visualize and seat the button firmly on the femur. Finally, if the button is not flipping because inadequate tunnel depth (confirmed by fluoroscopy), the femoral tunnel can be deepened by a few millimeters to allow the button to flip.

Problem: *The PCL can be lacerated* while drilling tibial and femoral tunnels if attention is not paid to its location.

Solution: In situations where the PCL is damaged, the amount of intact tissue should be examined and decisions made as to how to deal with the injury postoperatively. The decision to reconstruct the PCL will depend on the amount of ligament damage and patient activity level, amongst other factors.

Prevention: Careful technique will avoid this complication. Simple adjustments, such as visualizing the PCL as the drill advances past it, and turning the drill by hand to pass the PCL before power drilling are helpful. Also, instrumentation, such as acorn style drills, will minimize damage to the PCL when drilling through the tibia. Finally, using a probe to pull the PCL away from the drill path is another way to protect it during tunnel placement.

Neurovascular complications can be devastating if not recognized and dealt with immediately.

Solution: If an obvious injury does occur, the procedure should be stopped and appropriate consultations ordered immediately. In the case of a vascular compromise, the tourniquet should be inflated prior to

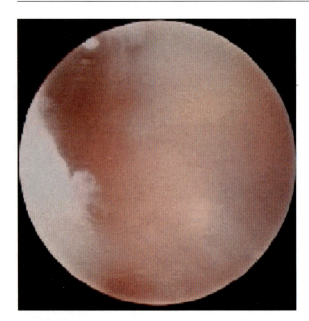

Fig. 4.33 Example of poor visualization, the red out

arrival of the supporting team. The contralateral limb should be prepped and draped as well in case a vascular graft is needed from the other leg.

Prevention: Most difficulties arise from poor arthroscopic visualization and forceful use of equipment (e.g., guide wires). The visualization of the surgical field can be improved with tourniquet use, elevating pump pressure, use of epinephrine in the scope solution, and intraoperative cautery (Fig. 4.33). Careful use of K-wires is important and one should never force a K-wire along its path. When attempting to visualize the back wall of the femur, use a curette to clear soft tissue and minimize risk of injury. While using an arthroscopic burr or shaver, extreme care should be taken to safeguard the posterior neurovascular structures nearby[5] (Fig. 4.2).

Postoperative Factors

Problem: *Infection* of the knee is a serious complication that can occur despite sterile precautions, good technique, and use of perioperative antibiotics.

Solution: Superficial wound infections should be treated with oral antibiotics and followed closely. Deep infections require more aggressive attention. The knee should be irrigated thoroughly and incisions opened and debrided. A current controversy is whether to retain the graft or not. At the present time, our practice is to debride the knee arthroscopically twice and retain the graft, unless it is grossly loose with loss of fixation on either side. If the patient is still symptomatic after a second debridement, the graft is removed and the knee is extensively debrided. Other considerations should include the virulence of the organism and the patients' response to treatment. Upon completion of irrigation and debridement, an infectious diseases consultant should be involved for the use of adjunct antibiotics.

Problem: *Stiffness or arthrofibrosis*, signifying loss of flexion or extension after surgery (Fig. 4.34).

Solution: The key to dealing with this problem starts by evaluating the etiology. Biochemical markers of infection should be obtained to rule out infection. Technical factors, such as tunnel placement, can be assessed radiographically, and advanced imagining (MRI) can also help explain whether a fibroproliferative scar or cyclops lesion is impinging on the graft. This may be the result of an inadequate notchplasty (Fig. 4.35) during the index procedure or an anterior tibial tunnel. The surgeon must determine whether the patient has been faithfully following the physiotherapy regimen. Passive flexion and extension exercises assist in gaining full flexion (Fig. 4.36) and extension (Fig. 4.37). Involving the therapist in the decision making process can resolve many problems. Aggressive passive motion of the patella (Fig. 4.34) should be instituted in

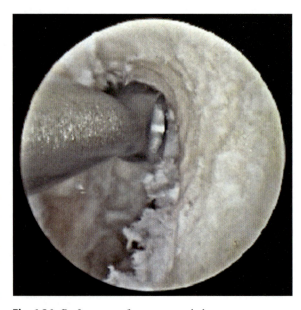

Fig. 4.34 Performance of a proper notchplasty

patients who are showing signs of postoperative stiffness. Arthrofibrosis can be minimized by an extension splint and early range of motion exercises. Finally, medical problems, such as reflex sympathetic dystrophy or infection, should be ruled out as sources of the loss of motion. Where technical errors are the cause, revision surgery should be offered to the patient. Cyclops lesions or adhesions can be treated with an arthroscopic debridement. As a general rule, manipulation to help break up scar tissue is considered if within 6 weeks.[10] But, beyond six weeks, an arthroscopic lysis of adhesions is safer. An adjunct procedure such as a notchplasty can be beneficial if the graft is impinging on the roof of the inter-condylar notch. A small amount of debulking of the graft may also be helpful if done judiciously and in combination with another procedure (e.g., notchplasty). A thermal ablater or small shaver can be used for this procedure. Care should be taken to maintain the functional integrity of the graft before proceeding with a graft debulking procedure. Range of motion and use of a CPM should be encouraged immediately postsurgery, and so pain relief after these procedures is important.

Problem: *Fractures* can occur, more commonly in a patellar tendon bone autograft (Figs. 4.38 and 4.39).

Solution: If recognized early, rigid fixation should be used to treat unstable fractures. A tension band wire through cannulated screws is a secure construct and should allow range of motion exercises and rehabilitation postoperatively surgery.[11] Femoral condyle fractures may also occur if the guide wire is passed through the femur multiple times or if there is excessive pressure on the femur during hyperflexion of the knee. If this occurs, rigid fixation is recommended.

Problem: *Postoperative Instability* is a problem that should be dealt with surgically, but it can in fact arise from technical errors intraoperatively.

Solution/Prevention: Prior to leaving the OR, a Lachman examination and pivot shift test should be performed to ensure the knee is stable. If laxity is noted intraoperatively, the distal fixation should be removed

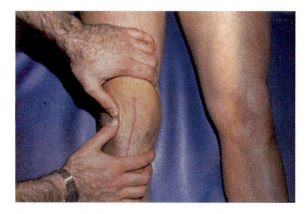

Fig. 4.35 Arthrofibrosis with patellar immobility

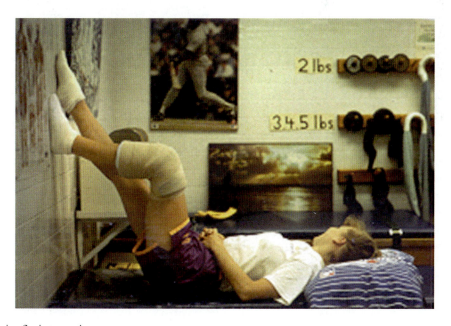

Fig. 4.36 Passive flexion exercises

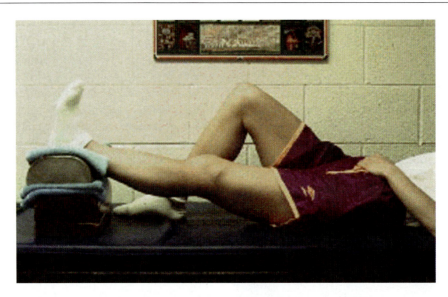

Fig. 4.37 Passive extension exercises with splint

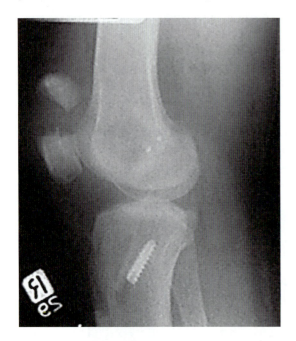

Fig. 4.38 Transverse patellar fracture

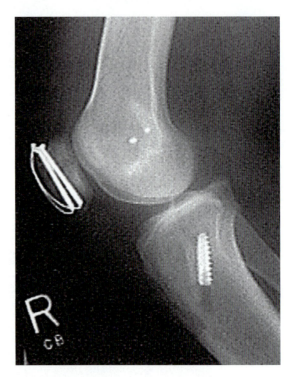

Fig. 4.39 Open reduction and internal fixation of the patellar fracture

and the knee retensioned before reinserting the fixation device. Numerous tensioning devices are available to help with this step. It is our preference to apply tension to the hamstrings graft with a tensioner at 20° of knee flexion. After dialing the tensioner for 50 and 30 N of tension to the semitendinosis and gracilis grafts, respectively, the knee is cycled 10 times (maximum flexion to full extension). The tension on the graft is adjusted until the tensioner remains at 50 and 30 N after cycling. In the bone tendon bone graft, the graft is tensioned at 20° of flexion. A manual Lachman examination should be performed to ensure the knee is stable.

In the late postoperative setting, a new injury should be ruled out, as well as failure of the initial fixation. If laxity is noted early, it is usually a technical error.

If laxity occurs more than 6 months postoperatively, then a reinjury should be suspected. After examining the patient and obtaining advanced imaging, the scenarios that one may encounter include a complete rupture. In the case of a complete rupture, new reconstruction should be pursued as required by the patient's symptoms of instability. But, if a partial rupture is encountered, the surgeon should determine whether the laxity is more dominant in the plane of translation or rotation. A single bundle reconstruction to augment the partial tear can be performed. The anteromedial bundle affects AP stability, while the posterolateral bundle is dominant for rotational stability. Reconstructing the isolated bundle can be completed similar to a primary operation but care must be taken to identify the landmarks needed for correct placement of injured bundle.

Problem: *Tibial tunnel widening* occurs, and becomes apparent postoperatively (Fig. 4.40).

Solution/Prevention: The significance and etiology of tunnel widening are still being debated, in part because of the impact on revision operations. Studies have indicated that there is a relationship between fixation distances to the aperture, with increasing distance correlating with increasing tunnel widening. The main cause of tunnel enlargement appears to be tunnels that are not placed in the anatomic sites. The nonanatomic tunnel is not isometric and more motion of the graft occurs causing a fibrous tissue reaction around the graft in the tunnel. Other factors, such as rehabilitation protocols, type of graft, and fixation devices have also been implicated. The key to operating on cases involving significant tunnel widening is bone stock analysis preoperatively and ensuring alternatives are available, such as synthetic bone grafts.

Problem: Scarring/keloid formation postoperatively can distress the patient greatly despite a technical success (Fig. 4.41).

Solution/Prevention: Prior to surgery, a surgical history including complications should be taken (wound healing, scarring, infections) as this helps to predict similar problems. However, in a case as below, referral to a dermatologist or plastic surgeon would be recommended if the patient is distressed by the appearance of the scar. The treatment options range from topical steroids to scar revision surgery.

Problem: Tunnel blow out in double bundle reconstruction.

Solution: Bone grafting for the compromised tunnel with autogenous bone graft (from the tibial or femoral reamings) is recommended, and then carry on with a single bundle reconstruction. Once the graft is inserted into the noncompromised tunnel, cancellous bone graft should be packed into the defect, tamped into place with any bone tamp. The patient should be nonweight bearing for approximately 8–12 weeks until the graft has been incorporated. The incorporation should be confirmed by X-rays before the reconstruction of the second bundle can be attempted. If the defect in the bone from tunnel confluence is significant and a single bundle reconstruction cannot be completed, then a bone graft procedure takes priority with the ligament reconstruction done after the defects have healed.

Prevention: Taking care to ensure adequate bone bridges of at least 2 mm are maintained between all tunnels is crucial (Figs. 4.42 and 4.43).

Prior to drilling the tunnels, each tunnel site should be marked with electrocautery and an awl to ensure adequate room between tunnels. In addition, when drilling the tibial tunnels, there should be an osseous bridge of at least 1 cm between the drill sites of each tunnel on the tibial cortex. The femoral and tibial tunnel landmarks have been described and are as follows.

The AM tibial tunnel is drilled after localizing the old stump by arthroscopy. Finally, the PL tibial tunnel is in the posterior edge of the triangle located in between the PCL, posterior root of the lateral meniscus, and the AM tunnel (Fig. 4.44).

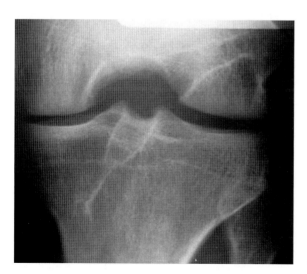

Fig. 4.40 Postoperative tunnel expansion

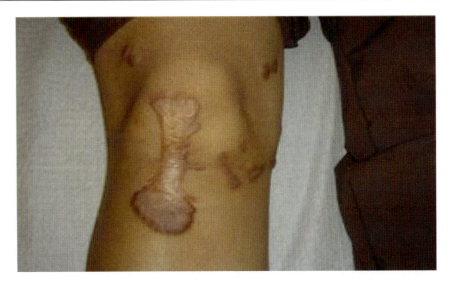

Fig. 4.41 Keloid formation post-BTB graft harvest (photo courtesy of Dr. Jeffrey Halbrecht)

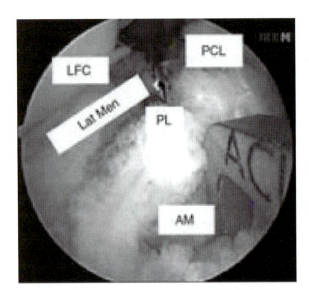

Fig. 4.42 Tibial tunnel placement for a double bundle reconstruction (photo courtesy of Dr. Arturo Almazan)

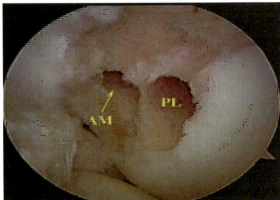

Fig. 4.43 Femoral tunnel placement for double bundle reconstruction (photo courtesy of Dr. Arturo Almazan)

PL (femoral) is located 5–7 mm from the anterolateral cartilage border of the lateral femoral condyle, and 2–3 mm superior to the inferior cartilage border of the lateral femoral condyle. The AM (femoral) tunnel is located 2 posterior to the PL tunnel (Fig. 4.45).

When using the low anteromedial portal to create the anteromedial tunnel on the femur, the drill should not advance beyond a depth of 20 mm. This is because using this portal causes the tunnels to be more distal and at a shallower angle when compared with the trans-tibial tunnel. Also, the cortex on the posterolateral femur is thinner distally and, advancing the drill farther may cause a cortical break through. In the same fashion, when drilling the femoral tunnels trans-tibially, a small drill bit (6 mm) should be used over the guide wire at first. Sequential increase in drill size and use of a hand reamer is safer and would minimize the chances of a blow out. The AM femoral tunnel can be drilled trans-tibially through the PL tibial tunnel. Drilling the tunnel with the 4.5 mm endobutton drill bit will also give an estimate of the total length of the femoral tunnel. Once this distance is known, over drilling through the lateral cortex with the large drill bit can be prevented.

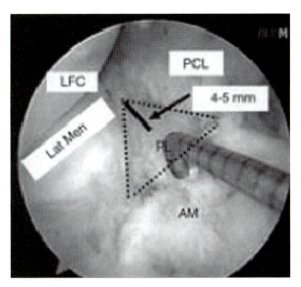

Fig. 4.44 PL tibial tunnel landmarks (photo courtesy of Dr. Arturo Almazan)

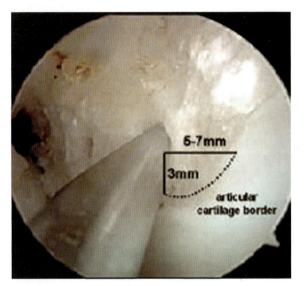

Fig. 4.45 PL femoral tunnel landmarks (photo courtesy of Dr. Arturo Almazan)

Revisions

A thorough knowledge of the cause of the failure of the primary reconstruction is the most important step in pursuing a second reconstructive procedure. All information from the index procedure should be obtained, including operative and rehabilitative notes. Usually failure is the result of technical errors, trauma, biological failure, and patient factors.[12] Once the information from previous operative and postoperative regimens has been obtained, the patient should have a thorough work up. The history should delineate the cause and circumstances of the injury, as well as the chief complaint. Next, the physical examination should assess generalized laxity, gait, alignment, range of motion, and stability of the knee in all planes. Care should be taken to ensure that no injuries, such as posterolateral corner or meniscal injuries, were missed. Next, imaging should assess lower limb alignment and bony and soft tissue in the knee. Plain X-rays reveal alignment, any degenerative processes, hardware and tunnel positioning, as well as bone stock. A CT scan further assesses the bone structure, while an MRI helps assess soft tissue.[13]

The revision procedure should be done only after all pertinent information has been gathered from the patient's history, physical exam, and imaging. Old scar and incisions should be noted, and adequate skin bridges maintained to prevent skin necrosis. Bone graft, several fixation devices, and special instrumentation should be available for the procedure. The surgeon should also be prepared to pursue revision surgery with a two-stage approach, depending on the pathology.[13]

Tunnel analysis is a crucial component for the revision case. Plain X-rays help determine whether there has been tunnel expansion, and serial images help note the progression of expansion. The location of tunnels and the accuracy of their placement can also be determined with radiographs and CT images. Erroneous tunnel placement will require revision with known anatomical landmarks as a guide. Furthermore, the need for bone grafting, additional screw fixation, changing fixation device, and/or staging of bone grafting can also be determined through a complete tunnel analysis. In the case where an errant tunnel was a cause of failure, the path of the new tunnel must be analyzed to see if it will merge with the old tunnel. If the new tunnel has a significant bridge (greater than 2 mm), then the old tunnel with its fixation can be left in situ. However, if the tunnels merge, a bone graft procedure can be completed and the procedure staged. Another option, depending on the extent of the void, is to stack several screws to fill the void with some supplementary bone grafting. If there is doubt about tunnel integrity the safe approach is to bone graft the defects, and return for the definitive procedure after 6–12 weeks.

The process of graft selection depends on the patient's previous graft, the activity level of the patient, the availability of an alternate graft, and the bony or soft tissue deficiencies in the patient's knee. Generally, it is wise to avoid reharvesting a patella autograft on the same knee. Studies have shown that this graft has inferior biomechanical properties compared with the original graft. The use of hamstrings or bone tendon bone grafts from the contralateral knee is an option, but donor site morbidity is a major concern. Allografts have the advantage of no donor site morbidity, smaller incisions, reduced surgical time, and no size limitations. The major concerns with allograft continue to be disease transmission, cost, and graft incorporation.

A variety of instrumentation should be available for use in revision. Removing hardware will require various screw head designs, trephines, curettes, and the easy in easy out screw removal device. Also, flexible guide wires, pituitary graspers, and arthroscopic gouges are helpful. Bone graft or substitutes should be available, as well as screws of differing configurations and sizes. As with any case, the surgeon should be familiar with, and able to improvise using a variety of fixation devices. Prior to going to the OR, obtaining the old operative reports or speaking to the surgeon who did the initial surgery can be helpful in determining the type of hardware used and surgical pitfalls that may affect the revision.

Pediatric ACL

The ACL injuries among skeletal immature patients present different challenges in reconstruction. The ideal management of pediatric ACL injuries is still being debated, but a surgical option aims to stabilize the knee, and minimize further damage to the intraarticular structures. Once a surgical option has been chosen in consultation with parents, the procedure can be undertaken safely with knowledge of a few critical guidelines.

Although several techniques have been described, trans-physeal, extra-articular, or physeal sparing, a well-performed trans-physeal reconstruction can stabilize the knee while minimizing the risks to the patient.

Surgery near an open physis requires an assessment of the patient's level of physical maturity and potential for growth. Advice from a pediatrician regarding expected bone growth will help with the decision about the best time for surgery. For those patients nearing skeletal maturity, surgery can be approached in as with an adult.

Patients who are skeletally immature can also have trans-physeal procedures if certain precautions are taken.[14] A small cross-section of the total physeal surface (less than 5%) should be breached by the tunnels to minimize the risk of growth disturbance. An MRI can help quantify the total surface area of the physis when planning surgery.[15] A more central tibial tunnel with an angle of less than 45° minimizes the risk of angular deformity or compromising the physis of the tibial tubercle. A minimal notchplasty and dissection should occur during surgery to prevent damage to the perichondrial ring. Finally, a soft tissue graft (hamstrings) should be used to minimize damage to the physis.

After surgery, the patient should be followed clinically and radiographically for the following complications: growth arrest, leg length discrepancy, deformities (genu Valgum, genu recurvatum), overgrowth.

References

1. Shelbourne K, Patel D (1995) Timing of surgery in anterior cruciate ligament-injured knees. Knee Surg Sports Traumatol Arthrosc 3(3):148-56
2. Amendola A, Faber K, Willits K et al (1999) Compartment pressure monitoring during anterior cruciate ligament reconstruction. Arthroscopy 15(6):607-12
3. Lubicky J, Cowell H (1998) Wrong site surgery. J Bone Joint Surg Am 80:1398
4. Canale S (2005) Wrong site surgery, a preventable complication. Clin Orthop Relat Res 433:26-9
5. Johnson DH (2004) ACL made simple. Springer, New York, NY
6. Molina M, Nonweiller D, Evans J et al (2000) Contaminated anterior cruciate ligament grafts: The efficacy of 3 sterilization agents. Arthroscopy 16(4):373-8
7. Pasque C, Geib T (2007) Intraoperative anterior cruciate ligament graft contamination. Arthroscopy 23(3):329-31
8. Cain L, Gillogly S, Andrews J (2003) Management of intraoperative complications associated with autogenous patellar tendon graft anterior cruciate ligament reconstruction. Instr Course Lect 52:359-67
9. Verma N, Dennis M, Carreira D et al (2005) Preliminary clinical results of two techniques for addressing graft tunnel mismatch in endoscopic anterior cruciate ligament reconstruction. J Knee Surg 18(3):183-91
10. Petsche T, Hutchinson M (1999) Loss of extension after reconstruction of the anterior cruciate ligament. J Am Acad Orthop Surg 7:119-27
11. Berg E (1996) Management of patella fractures associated with central third bone-patella tendon-bone autograft ACL reconstructions. Arthroscopy 12(6):756-9

12. Kocher M, Steadman R, Briggs K et al (2002) Determinants of patient satisfaction with outcome after anterior cruciate ligament reconstruction. J Bone Joint Surg Am 84:1560-72
13. Bach B (2003) Revision ACL surgery. Arthroscopy 19(10): 14-29
14. Staldelmaier D, Arnoczky S, Dodds J et al (1995) The effect of drilling and soft tissue grafting across open growth plates: A histologic study. Am J Sports Med 23:431-5
15. Larsen M, Garrett W, DeLee J et al (2006) Surgical management of anterior cruciate injuries in patients with open physes. J Am Acad Orthop Surg 14:736-44

Editors' Comments (ACL)

Patella Bone Plug Harvest

Many of the complications associated with harvesting an autologous BPTB graft can be eliminated with the use of a coring reamer to harvest the patella and tibial bone plugs. The editors prefer to utilize an oscillating bone plug harvesting device (Stryker), which cores out a cylindrical plug of bone, avoiding any stress risers, and eliminating risk of damage to the articular surface from osteotomes or inadvertant plunging with a standard microsagital saw. This technique also saves time by creating a smooth cylindrical plug ready for passage rather than a trapezoidal plug obtained with a standard saw that still requires graft trimming.

Back Up Tibial Fixation

A quick and reliable technique to back up the tibial fixation is to use a subcortical suture interlocking anchor, which eliminates the risk of irritation often associated with a proud screw and post. Predrilling with a 3.5 mm drill is necessary prior to inserting the suture interlocking anchor through the thick tibial cortex.

Miscellaneous

It is common at the completion of an ACL reconstruction to find bone fragments and residue from tunnel drilling about the knee, particularly in the popliteal hiatus and posterior compartment. We feel it is important to take time at the completion of the case to carefully irrigate these areas to avoid postoperative effusions and discomfort.

If the sutures holding the tibial portion of the graft are accidentally severed during interference fit fixation (e.g., may occur while tapping the tunnel for a biointerference screw) and there is no exposed tendon or bone the following can be performed. If the tibial tunnel is at least 30 mm, you may consider opening the anterior aspect of the tunnel 5 mm to visualize the graft. If the bone block is located more proximal than 5 mm, the block may be grasped with a sharp crochet hook, retensioned, and an interference screw may be placed. Alternatively, several sutures may be passed arthroscopically with a suture lasso type device at the ACL/tibial aperture junction (akin to a tibial eminence avulsion fracture). The passed sutures may then be regrasped with a suture grasper that can be passed through the tibial tunnel and the graft can be retensioned. The sutures can then be tied over a post. If an additional interference screw is placed confirm arthroscopically that the bone block is not accidentally pushed up into the joint.

Preventing Graft Loosening

The graft should be pretensioned on the back table after preparation, and retensioned again immediately before tibial fixation. This removes any creep from the soft tissue prior to insertion, and limits relaxation of the graft after fixation.

The exact position of the knee during tensioning and tibial fixation is controversial. It is the authors' experience that this position should be customized for the patient. Isometry of the graft should be tested by ranging the knee prior to tibial fixation. If the graft withdraws into the tibial tunnel on extension more than 3 mm, there is either roof impingement or poor isometry. Fixation of the graft in this case should be performed in full extension. If the fixation were to be performed in 20–30° of flexion, there would be excessive tension on the graft postoperatively with extension. Another option to improve isometry in this case would be to consider placing the tibial fixation anterior to the graft to direct it posteriorly and reduce roof impingement.

If there is minimal motion of the graft during range of motion, fixation is usually performed with the knee at 20–30° of flexion to maximize graft stability.

Revision

The most important details to prepare for revision ACL surgery are the ones obtained preoperatively. It is essential to obtain old operative reports to ensure that the correct screwdriver is present. Some manufacturers have changed their screw heads over the years, so check with the rep regarding the year that the original ACL was performed to ensure that the correct instruments will be available. Occasionally, a screw will strip, and will need to be removed by alternative means. We have had success utilizing the Stryker bone plug oscillating saw to core out a femoral screw. Osteotomes or gouges can be used as well, but with more bone damage. Other trephines are also available with commercial hardware removal trays.

We have preferred the use of allograft BPTB for our revisions, since the bone plugs can be prepared to fit any residual defect after hardware removal (size 12–14 or greater). Using this technique, we have rarely found it necessary to bone graft and perform a two stage revision. Achilles tendon allograft can similarly be used as the calcaneal bone block can make up for a large bony defect on the femoral side.

Be prepared to find residual absorbable screw material up to 3 years postimplantation while drilling during a revision. Be sure to remove any particulate matter encountered to prevent an inflammatory reaction and synovitis.

We always have an endobutton available for extracortical fixation during a revision, in case tunnel size or bone quality is compromised in the femoral tunnel.

Historically, revision ACL surgery has been due to poor femoral tunnel placement. Of late, with improved tunnel placement for the femoral tunnel, an argument can be made for performing a double bundle technique as the previously drilled femoral tunnel (anteromedial bundle) may be replaced with an allograft soft tissue construct and a second femoral tunnel (posteromedial bundle) may then be placed at the 9 (right knee) or 3 o'clock (left knee) positions. If one notes that the femoral tunnel is too vertical (12 o'clock position) consider performing the femoral drilling from an accessory anteromedial (AM) portal. Ensure that the knee is flexed at least 110° while drilling.

Chapter 5
Avoiding and Managing Complications in PCL Reconstruction

Shane T. Seroyer and Christopher D. Harner

Top 10 Pearls

- Examination under anesthesia – critical to success of PCL reconstruction; Associated ligamentous injuries must be acknowledged and addressed.
- Tourniquet is not used during PCL reconstruction to allow for instant recognition of arterial injury.
- These cases should not be performed at an ambulatory surgery center. An on-call vascular surgeon should be made aware of the case, and be available should assistance be required.
- Anterior drawer is used to put tension on the ACL to prevent inadvertent debridement and to allow the ease of passage of instruments into the posterior compartment of the knee.
- When performing the anterior drawer, hands should be placed distal to the popliteal fossa to avoid drawing the neurovascular bundle closer to the posterior tibia.
- Preserve the posteromedial bundle and the meniscofemoral ligaments if they are intact.
- When performing double-bundle PCL reconstruction, the anterolateral tunnel is drilled from the lateral tibia to prevent confluence of the tunnels.
- Guidewire/reamer are advanced by power, under fluoroscopy, and stopped at the posterior cortex. The posterior cortex is drilled/reamed by hand.
- Posterolateral corner reconstruction is fixed prior to fixation of the PCL.
- In double-bundle reconstruction, AL bundle is fixed at 90° of flexion and PM bundle is fixed at 30° of flexion. Anterior drawer is applied to fixation of PCL graft.

Introduction and Background

Injury to the posterior cruciate ligament (PCL) occurs at a lower incidence than does injury to the anterior cruciate ligament (ACL). In a prospective analysis of 222 patients presenting to a regional trauma center with acute hemarthrosis of the knee, Fanelli found that the incidence of PCL injury in the cohort was 38%.[1,2] Only 3.5% of the PCL injuries were isolated injuries, emphasizing the need for complete and accurate diagnosis of all associated injuries. The true incidence of PCL injuries is likely underestimated, as many will go undiagnosed due to the often innocuous appearance of isolated PCL injuries. An isolated PCL injury usually occurs after a posteriorly directed force on a flexed knee.[3] The patient often will present with a mild effusion and pain localized to the posterior aspect of the knee. They often can bear weight acutely but do so with a flexed knee gait, thus avoiding terminal extension.[3] There will often be a complaint of pain with deep flexion, squatting, or kneeling.[4] With a low-grade injury the patient often does not complain of instability or mechanical symptoms and is able to continue to compete without recognizing deficit. Historically, grade I and grade II (less than 10 mm posterior translation) PCL injuries have been successfully managed with nonoperative treatment.[3,4] Grade III injuries (>10 mm translation) and combined injuries are usually managed with operative reconstruction of the PCL and associated injuries.

S.T. Seroyer (✉)
University of Pittsburgh Medical Center, 3200 South Water Street, Pittsburgh, PA, 15203, USA
e-mail: serost@upmc.edu

C.D. Harner
Department of Orthopedics, University of Pittsburgh Medical Center, Pittsburgh, Allegheny County, PAennsylvania, USA

The anatomy of the PCL complex is well described, consisting of a much more robust anterolateral (AL) bundle, a posteromedial (PM) bundle, and contribution from one or two meniscofemoral ligaments (MFLs). The AL bundle resists posterior translation of the tibia in flexion, while the PM bundle functions with the knee in positions near extension. Cadaveric studies have shown the importance of the MFLs as secondary stabilizers to posterior tibial translation. At 90° of knee flexion, the MFLs were found to contribute to 28% of the total force resisting posterior translation.[5] The structures of the posterolateral corner have also been demonstrated to provide secondary restraint to posterior translation of the tibia on the femur.[6,7]

Controversy exists, with regard to which portions of the PCL complex should be reconstructed. Historically, reconstruction of the AL bundle alone has been performed. Recent studies have shown that the in situ forces on the PCL may be distributed more evenly between the AL and PM bundles than previously realized.[8] Other recent studies have shown that reconstruction of only the AL bundle with fixation at 90° of flexion may lead to residual posterior translation with the knee near full extension.[9] This has given rise to discussions on the merits of single-bundle reconstruction, single-bundle augmentation, and double-bundle reconstruction of the PCL. Controversy remains as to which technique is most appropriate for which circumstance of injury.

Failure to diagnose and treat associated injuries, most notably to the posterolateral corner, has been implicated as a major cause of failure of PCL reconstruction.[6,10–12] Other intraoperative complications such as tunnel misplacement, improper graft tensioning or fixation, and damage to the popliteal neurovascular bundle can adversely affect outcomes in PCL reconstruction.[6,13–17] In this chapter, we will outline common pitfalls and intraoperative difficulties that may complicate[10,11] the successful reconstruction of the PCL, and provide our strategy to overcome or avoid these situations.

Anesthesia

The choice of anesthesia is made in conjunction with the surgeon, the anesthesiologist, and the patient. Factors including the age of the patient, comorbid medical problems, and the previous anesthesia history of the patient all contribute to the coordinated decision regarding the type of anesthesia selected for the procedure. The anesthesiologist typically chooses either general anesthesia or an epidural anesthetic with concomitant IV sedation. If the anesthesiologist is at all concerned about airway management, general anesthesia is performed. At our center, preoperative femoral and/or sciatic nerve blocks are routinely performed. In addition to intraoperative benefits, the nerve blocks also provide up to 9–12 h of postoperative pain relief. A Foley catheter is placed to help monitor the fluid status during the case. A vascular surgeon should be made aware of the procedure and readily available during any procedure involving the PCL, as unexpected injuries to the neurovascular structures may occur intraoperatively.

Preoperative Evaluation

Imperative in the preoperative evaluation is a thorough documentation of the status of the dorsalis pedis artery, the posterior tibial artery, and the tibial and peroneal nerves. Concomitant posterolateral corner injuries are common, and associated peroneal nerve dysfunction may be present preoperatively. The importance of accurate and detailed documentation of these physical exam findings cannot be overstated. The extremity should be marked in the preoperative holding area by the surgeon, with the assistance of the patient, to ensure the identification of the proper surgical site and extremity. Surgical site marking should be performed using an indelible marker, denoting the word "yes," and including the surgeon's initials. This should be placed in a location visible in the surgical field after operative draping has been performed.

Prior to surgical draping, after induction of anesthesia, a complete and accurate examination of the extremity is essential to the successful execution of surgical reconstruction. This examination should be used to confirm the preoperative suspicion of associated injury complexity. Failure to identify associated injury could render isolated reconstructive efforts of the PCL unsuccessful. Resting position of the tibio-femoral articulation at 90° should be assessed with fluoroscopy, and compared with its position when anterior and posterior drawer have been applied. Lachman examination, pivot shift, and anterior drawer tests should be performed to assess the integrity of the ACL. The examiner must remain cognizant of the ability of the posteriorly subluxed tibia in a PCL injured knee to render the examination techniques of the ACL ambiguous due to abnormal posterior resting position of the tibia. Varus and valgus stress testing of the LCL and the MCL, respectively, should be performed at both 0° and 30°. The dial, or external rotation test, should be performed at 30° and 90° to evaluate the association of a posterolateral corner injury in conjunction with the PCL injury. If external rotation in only increased at 90° one would not be as suspicious of injury to the posterolateral corner, where as an increase in both positions would suggest combined injury to the PCL and PLC. The PCL is examined by performing a posterior drawer test, with the knee at 90°, noting the degree of posterior step off at rest, and with applied force. Comparison of the injured extremity with the uninjured is essential for elucidation of exam findings. Posterior sag test (Godfrey test) and reverse pivot shift may also be performed to assess the integrity of the PCL.

Once the examination under anesthesia is performed and the results are correlated with radiographic and clinical suspicion, the appropriate surgical plan may be determined and appropriate incisions are drawn on the skin to allow for preoperative local anesthetic injection. Due to the frequent occurrence of combined injuries, these incisions may include: posterolateral corner reconstruction, inside-out medial or lateral meniscal repair, and tibial tunnel incisions (single vs. double bundle).

Surface Anatomy and Skin Marking

Standard anatomic landmarks including: the patella, tibial tubercle, Gerdy's tubercle, fibular head, and lateral epicondyle are marked to allow estimation of incision sites for injection (Fig. 5.1). Incisions may change based on the intraoperative findings and the decision to perform a single vs. a double bundle reconstruction. In anticipation of a double-bundle PCL reconstruction, the posterolateral corner incision is marked extending a few centimeters more distal to the standard incision as this extension will allow for approach to the lateral side of the tibia for the placement of the tibial tunnel of the anterolateral bundle. The medial tibial incision (anterolateral bundle in single-bundle reconstruction, posteromedial bundle in double-bundle reconstruction) is approximately 3 cm in length, originating approximately 2 cm distal to the joint line and 2 cm medial to the tibial tubercle on the anteromedial, proximal tibia. A 2-cm incision medial to the medial trochlear surface, within the subvastus interval, is drawn to allow access to the distal femur to tie the PCL graft(s) over a post, as well as for fixation of the femoral end of popliteofibular reconstruction graft. If medial meniscal pathology is suspected, a 3-cm incision posterior to the MCL extending 1 cm above the joint and 2 cm below the joint is drawn, and injected. A posterior medial portal incision is also drawn, but will be made intraoperatively under direct visualization. We also use a superolateral outflow

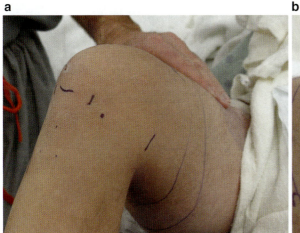
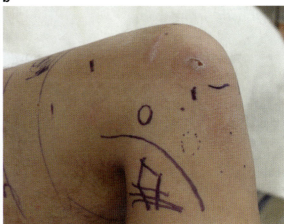

Fig. 5.1 (**a**, **b**) Preoperative skin markings for superolateral outflow; anteromedial, anterolateral, and posteromedial portals; fibular head and peroneal nerve, lateral epicondyle, Gerdy's and tibial tubercle; posterolateral corner incision (AL tibial tunnel for double-bundle reconstruction)

portal, placed just proximal to the superior border of the patella and posterior to the quadriceps tendon. Standard anteromedial and anterolateral arthroscopic portals are marked and injected. All skin planned skin incisions and portals are injected with 0.25% bupivacaine with 1:100,000 epinephrine.

Patient Positioning

The patient is placed in the supine position on the operating room table. Our goal is to have a full, free range of motion of the involved extremity during the procedure with the ability to have the knee statically flexed at 80-90° without any manual assistance. This is accomplished by placing a small gel pad bump under the ipsilateral hip with a post placed on the side of the bed just distal to the greater trochanter; a sterile bump of towels or drapes is wedged between the post and the thigh (Fig. 5.2). The heel is positioned to rest on a 10 lb sandbag that is taped to the bed during the initial positioning. We do not employ the use of a tourniquet during reconstruction of the PCL. Intravenous antibiotics are administered prior to the skin incision. Once the patient has been draped in sterile fashion, the previously described skin incisions are drawn and the dorsalis pedis pulse is once again palpated and marked. The extremity is prepped with alcohol and betadine solutions and draped in a meticulous fashion. The mini c-arm fluoroscopy machine is in the operating suite and draped.

Diagnostic Arthroscopy

The arthroscope is introduced into the knee in standard arthroscopic fashion through the anterolateral portal. The information gained at arthroscopy is used to correlate with the preoperative suspicions based on EUA and MRI findings. Due to the extreme complexity of these cases a thorough, systematic diagnostic arthroscopy is essential to avoid oversights of intra-articular pathology. Gravity inflow is used in conjunction with the superolateral outflow. Extreme care must be exercised in the evaluation and prompt recognition of a compartment syndrome. This is critically important in acute reconstructions as the capsular healing may not be complete enough to maintain joint distention and may allow egress of fluid into the posterior compartment of the leg.

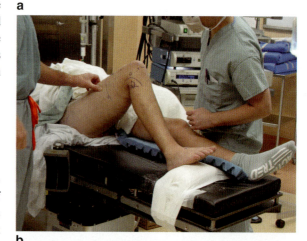

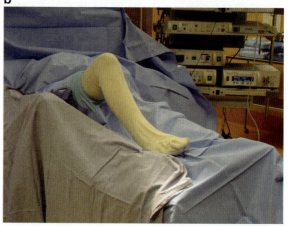

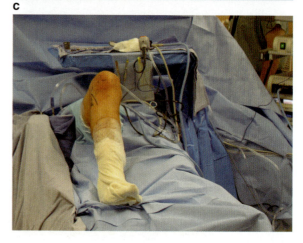

Fig. 5.2 (a-c) Intraoperative positioning, with foot rest and hip post to allow static positioning without manual assistance

The assistant continually palpates the posterior calf to evaluate the fullness of the compartment. If at anytime during the procedure, an increase in the fullness of the compartment raises concern, the arthroscopic technique is abandoned and the remainder of the procedure is performed using open technique. Should this occur, the arthroscope may still be used, at times, in a dry field to allow improved visualization.

All compartments within the knee are thoroughly assessed. The MCL is visualized in the medial compartment, including assessment of the meniscal attachments to the deep MCL. In the lateral compartment the popliteus is inspected for injury.

When evaluating the PCL, special attention is dedicated to elucidating the extent of the pathology to the separate bundles (AL and PM), as well as the presence of and possible damage to the MFLs. The extent of injury to these three separate entities of the PCL complex will help guide the decision on performing a single vs. a double bundle PCL reconstruction. Both the femoral and tibial insertions, as well as the interstitium, of the PCL are examined as injury can occur at any location along the ligament. Interstitial tears of the PCL represent the most common pattern of injury observed.[12] To observe the tibial insertion, a posteromedial portal is established by spinal needle localization, under direct visualization. A 70° arthroscope is placed through the anterolateral portal and advanced through the intracondylar notch adjacent to the medial femoral condyle. Once the arthroscope is in the posterior aspect of the knee, the lens is rotated to allow visualization of the spinal needle entering the knee, just posterior to the medial femoral condyle. Switching the arthroscope and surgical devices between these two portals allows flexibility in the visualization of, and access to, the tibial insertion site of the PCL to allow proper debridement and access to posterior exit site of the tibial tunnel (Fig. 5.3).

Prior to directing our efforts to the PCL reconstruction, we first address any concomitant chondral or meniscal injuries. Due to the young age of most of these patients, we attempt to repair and preserve any injured meniscal tissue possible, affording the patient the greatest chance of success in these complex endeavors. We prefer to repair peripheral meniscal injuries through an inside-out technique. If a repair is needed, sutures will be passed at this junction and tied down directly onto the capsule at the end of the procedure after any reconstructive grafts have been passed and secured. This will prevent undue stress on the meniscal repair as the knee will often be placed in greater than 90° of flexion during the PCL reconstruction.

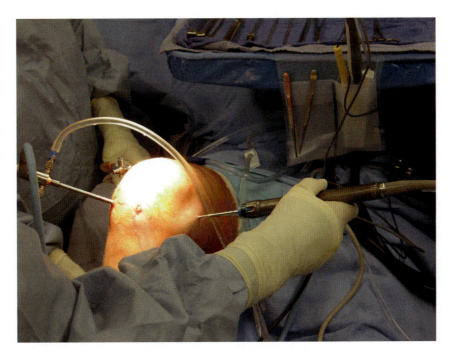

Fig. 5.3 Debridement of PCL tibial origin with full-radius resector in posteromedial portal

PCL Reconstruction

After delineation of the tear pattern of the PCL, arthroscopic debridement is performed (Fig. 5.4). Special care is taken to preserve the PM bundle and the MFL, if they are intact. It is important, while performing this debridement, that an assistant is performing an anterior drawer. This will restore the tibia to its normal position, allowing the ACL to remain tensioned to allow easier delineation of intracondylar structures and prevent from inadvertent debridement of the ACL, or incorrect assessment of its integrity. Performing the drawer will also assist with the ease of passage of the arthroscope and instruments past the ACL and into the posterior aspect of the knee as well as passage of the shuttle sutures and graft. When performing the drawer, it is important that the assistant's hands are placed more distal on the proximal gastrocnemius rather than in the popliteal fossa, which may force the popliteal artery to a position closer in proximity to the posterior tibia and capsule. Drawing the neurovascular bundle closer to the posterior aspect of the tibia increases the likelihood of injury by inadvertent advancement of guidewires, reamers, or during overaggressive debridement of the posterior synovium. A thermal device may be of assistance during debridement of the femoral insertion site, as the geniculate feeders may cause bleeding. After debriding the femoral insertion to provide adequate visualization of the femoral condyle for placement of involved bundle(s) of the tear, attention is turned to the tibial insertion. A PCL curette (Fig. 5.5) is helpful in developing a plane between the native PCL and synovium in the posterior aspect of the knee. Debridement of the synovium in the posterior knee can be achieved with either the full-radius resector in the posteromedial portal and the arthroscope in the anterolateral portal; or by reversing this configuration and placing a 30° arthroscope in the posteromedial portal with the full-radius resector entering the intracondylar notch via the anteromedial portal. Once this plane has been developed, the curette can be used to clear the PCL scar off of its native insertion on the posterior fossa of the tibia (Fig. 5.6). If difficulty arises while passing the curette into the back of the knee, the arthroscope can be placed into the anterolateral portal to allow visualization as the curette enters the posterior knee. Alternatively, with a 70° in the anterolateral portal, the shaver can be inserted in the posteromedial portal and can debride the tibial insertion. The posterior tibial slope needs to be exposed approximately 2–3 cm below the medial joint line to have proper access for tibial tunnel placement. Once the footprint can be adequately visualized, a standard PCL guide can be inserted through the anteromedial portal to assess if the posterior tibia has been adequately exposed distally. The guide is initially set to 50°, but the angle may require adjusting to prevent reaming out the posterior cortex. A draped, sterile mini C-arm is brought in to assess a true lateral projection of the knee. The correct placement of the AL tunnel is located in the distal one-third of the posterior slope of the tibia (Fig. 5.7). This point will be located in the distal-lateral aspect of the footprint. If a double-bundle reconstruction is selected, the AL tibial tunnel will be drilled from the lateral tibia. If a PLC reconstruction is to be performed concomitantly, the lateral incision is made and extended distal and anterior enough to allow exposure to the lateral tibia. In the absence of PLC reconstruction, the AL tibial tunnel of a double-bundle reconstruction is drilled from a point 3–4 cm distal to the joint line. The fascia over the proximal most aspect of the tibialis anterior muscle is incised to expose the tibia. If single-bundle reconstruction is performed, it is drilled from the anterior-medial tibia, 3–4 cm distal to the joint line, halfway between the posterior tibia cortex and the tibial crest. A threaded 3/32 Kirschner wire is drilled under fluoroscopic guidance to 1–2 mm short of the posterior tibial cortex (Fig. 5.8). With the arthroscope in the posteromedial portal, the guidewire is unchucked

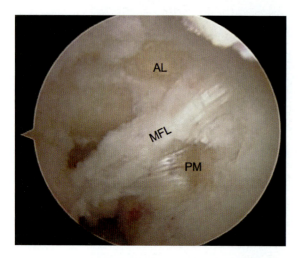

Fig. 5.4 Debridement of femoral insertion of torn AL bundle of PCL, with preservation of meniscofemoral ligament (MFL) and posteromedial (PM) bundle

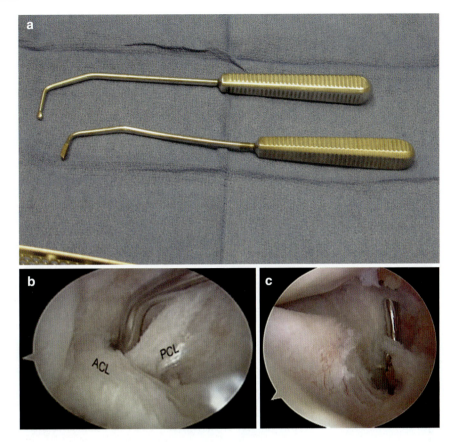

Fig. 5.5 (a) PCL curette and rasp; (b) PCL rasp entering into posterior aspect of knee from anteromedial portal; (c) PCL rasp exposing tibial footprint of PCL, with arthroscope in posteromedial portal

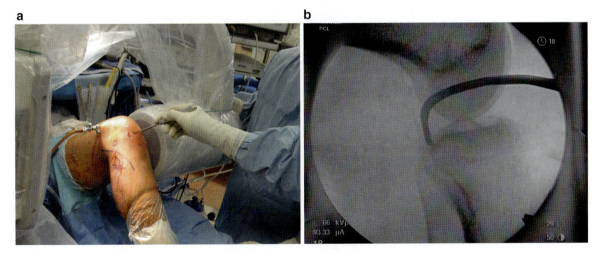

Fig. 5.6 (a) Intraoperative fluoroscopy to ensure adequate distal exposure of the tibial footprint of the PCL. (b) Intraoperative fluoroscopy to confirm proper placement of PCL tibial guide for AL tunnel

from the drill and advanced by hand with the aid of a mallet, under direct visualization, until the guidewire is seen to pierce the cortex. The PCL curette is placed in the posterior knee, in the aforementioned manner, and the tip of the guide wire is cleared of soft tissue for visualization. Prior to reaming, under direct visualization

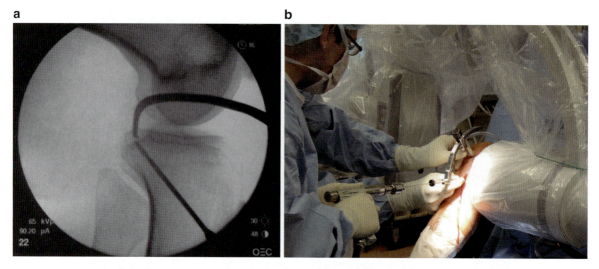

Fig. 5.7 (**a**) Fluoroscopy of AL guidewire. Guide wire is stopped prior to breaching cortex and finished by hand to prevent overpenetration and damage to neurovascular bundle; (**b**) Photograph of AL tunnel being drilled under fluoroscopic guidance

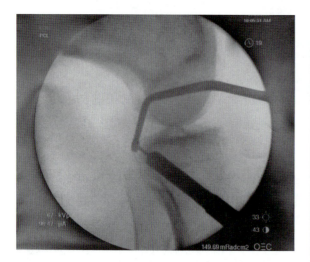

Fig. 5.8 Fluoroscopy of AL tunnel reaming with curette preventing advancement of guidewire

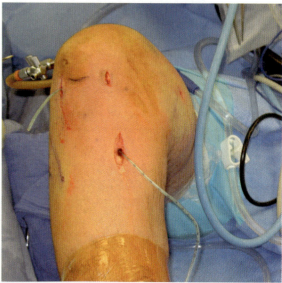

Fig. 5.9 8 French pediatric feeding tube used for suture shuttling

with the arthroscope posteromedially, the curette is placed firmly over the tip of the guide wire to prevent inadvertent advancement of the guidewire. A reamer, 1 mm undersized for final tunnel diameter, is used to ream the tibial tunnel under arthroscopic guidance, until resistance is encountered at the posterior cortex (Fig. 5.9). The reamer is then unchucked from the drill and the posterior cortex is penetrated by hand. The full-radius resector is placed into the tibial tunnel to clean the soft tissue at the aperture of the tunnel and the posterior cortex. The tunnel is then dilated in ½ mm increments to the desired tunnel diameter. In a single-bundle reconstruction, an 11-mm graft is used to reconstruct the anterolateral bundle. In a double-bundle reconstruction, the AL graft is typically 9 mm in diameter and the PM tunnel is typically 7 mm in diameter. If double-bundle reconstruction is performed, the PM tibial tunnel is established in similar fashion to the AL tunnel. A 3/32 guidewire is drilled from the anteromedial tibia to a point proximal and medial to the anterolateral tunnel, within the footprint of the native PCL insertion. Similar to the technique used with preparation of the AL tunnel, the posterior cortex is breeched by hand. A 6-mm compaction drill is used to ream the PM tibial tunnel under arthroscopic visualization with a PCL curette firmly on the guidewire tip to prevent inadvertent advancement. The compaction drill is advanced by hand to perforate the posterior cortex. The tunnel is then dilated by hand, incrementally, with 6 mm, 6.5 mm, and 7 mm dilators. Attention is now focused on establishing the femoral tunnels for the PCL reconstruction, in an anatomical reproduction of native anatomy. The AL femoral tunnel is drilled from the AL portal at the 1 o'clock position on the medial femoral condyle, approximately 5–6 mm off of the articular cartilage. The knee is placed in 130° of flexion to allow for a posterior trajectory of the tunnel, as well as, allowing the tunnel to diverge from the subchondral surface of the medial femoral condyle. In the authors' opinion, drilling this tunnel from outside-to-inside requires drilling/reaming in close proximity and parallel to the subchondral bone, which may be an etiologic factor in the development of postoperative osteonecrosis of the condyle. A 3/32 Kirschner wire is use to establish the location of this tunnel. A compaction drill 1 mm undersized for the final tunnel size (10 mm for single-bundle; 8 mm for double-bundle) is reamed to a depth of 25–30 mm. The tunnel is then dilated by hand in ½-mm increments to its intended size. A 4.5-mm endobutton drill is then used to perforate the cortex of the medial femoral condyle, to allow passage of the endoloop (without endobutton) through the condyle for fixation over a femoral post. If a double-bundle reconstruction is performed, the PM tunnel is then drilled/reamed using identical technique, with the knee in 110° of flexion. The starting point for this tunnel is located at the 3–4 o'clock position approximately 4–5 mm off of the articular cartilage, to allow safe placement of a 7-mm tunnel.

Graft Passage and Fixation

To facilitate graft passage, relay sutures are first placed to lead the graft through the tunnels. Formerly, we made use of a looped 18-gauge wire passed retrograde through the tibial tunnel, into the posterior aspect of the knee and retrieved from the anterolateral portal.

We now employ the use of an 8 French pediatric feeding tube due to its ease of handling and flexibility (Fig. 5.9). It is passed retrograde through the tibial tunnel and retrieved with an arthroscopic grasper placed through the posteromedial portal while visualizing with the scope in the anterolateral portal. The grasper then delivers the tube into the intracondylar notch where it may be grasped by another instrument placed through the anteromedial portal. Once the tube is advanced into the notch, the arthroscope is switched to the anteromedial portal and the feeding tube is then retrieved through the anterolateral portal taking care to pass this above the intermeniscal ligament. A #2 ticron suture is then fed into the lumen of the feeding tube to a distance of several centimeters. The feeding tube is then withdrawn through the tibial tunnel, effectively shuttling the ticron from the anterolateral portal out through the anterolateral tibial tunnel (Fig. 5.10). If performing a double bundle reconstruction, the same steps can be used to establish shuttle sutures for the passage of the PM graft. Of note, the posteromedial lead sutures and grafts should pass from the posterior knee into the notch under the MFLs (if preserved), whereas the AL graft passes over the MFLs. The AL graft is passed first. The ticron suture extending out of the anterolateral portal is tied in overhand fashion around the sutures attached to the tails of the allograft and retrieved out of the tibial tunnel. The femoral end of the graft is doubled over a closed endoloop. In preparation of the graft, a line measured from the looped, femoral end of the allograft to denote the amount of graft to be in the femoral tunnel is marked. This allows for an estimation of the proper positioning of the graft (Fig. 5.11).

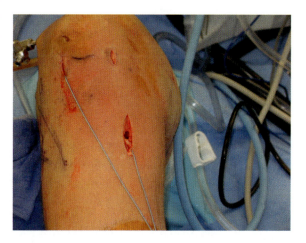

Fig. 5.10 Ticron suture used for graft passage

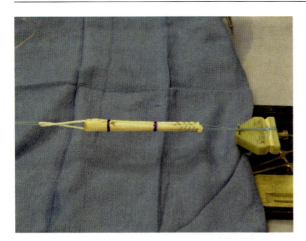

Fig. 5.11 Tibialis anterior allograft used for PCL reconstruction; femoral end with endoloop and marked to ensure maximum amount of graft in tunnel for incorporation

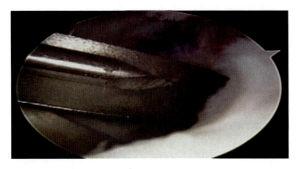

Fig. 5.12 Metal skid used to protect graft from damage from sharp-tipped beath pin during femoral graft passage. Guidewire is advanced under arthroscopic visualization, ensuring containment within skid

At this juncture, the tibial portion of the graft is in the tibial tunnel while the femoral portion remains protruding out of the anterolateral portal. In order to direct the femoral end of the graft into the femoral tunnel, a beath pen must be passed through the femoral tunnel and exiting through the skin to allow suture relay. In order to protect the graft from damage secondary to passage of the sharp-tipped beath pin through the AL portal and intracondylar notch, a dull-tipped metal skid is placed from the AL portal and into the opening of the femoral tunnel with arthroscopic visualization via the anteromedial portal (Fig. 5.12). The beath pin is then passed within the confines of the skid to protect the integrity of the graft. The leading suture of the femoral side of the graft is pulled through the skin of the medial knee and the graft is advanced under visualization into the femoral tunnel. If a double-bundle reconstruction is performed the PM bundle is now passed using similar technique. The skin incision that was marked preoperatively is incised and the vastus medialis obliquus is split in-line with its fibers and the femoral-sided sutures are retrieved through this interval. The graft(s) are fixated with one or two 4.5-mm AO screw(s) and washer(s). The endoloop is tensioned to allow determine proper placement of the postconstruct. In the situation of a double-bundle reconstruction, if the endoloop configuration does not allow one isometric point for the two endoloops, then two separate posts are used.

If a concomitant posterolateral corner injury is present, it is reconstructed at this time. The posterolateral corner reconstruction is tensioned and fixed prior to fixation of the tibial-sided PCL graft(s).

The AL bundle of the PCL graft is tensioned and fixed with the knee in 90° of flexion. A bolster is placed under the tibia, to support its weight against gravity (Fig. 5.13). An anterior drawer is performed prior to fixation, ensuring that the anterior edge of the medial tibial plateau rests approximately 10 mm anterior to the medial femoral condyle. The posteromedial graft is fixated with the knee in 30° of flexion. The anterior drawer force remains constant until both grafts have been adequately tensioned and fixated. It is our preference to provide tibial fixation with 4.5-mm AO screws functioning as a post, however, interference screw fixation may also be utilized as the source of fixation.

Graft Selection and Fixation

Graft selection for PCL reconstruction is multifactorial, and leaves the surgeon with several options. Timing and extent of injury, availability of allograft at the practicing institution, prior history of surgery, and surgeon/patient preference all contribute to graft selection. Autograft choices include patellar tendon, quadriceps tendon, and hamstring tendons. If multiple grafts are needed for a multiligament reconstruction or in case of revision surgery, autograft may be harvested from the contralateral extremity as well. Allograft tissue selection depends on graft availability to the institution from the tissue bank. Achilles tendon allograft has been a

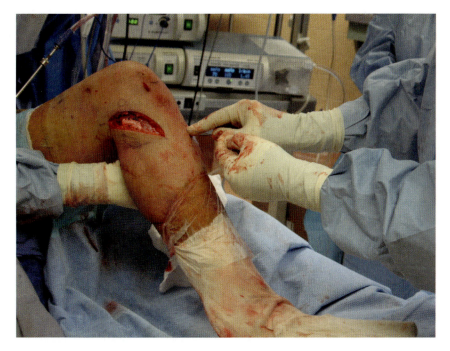

Fig. 5.13 Fixation of AL bundle of PCL reconstruction; Performed at 90° of flexion with anterior drawer

popular selection for PCL reconstruction. Our allograft preference is the tibialis anterior tendon. Integral to the decision of allograft vs. autograft is a detailed discussion with the patient regarding risks and benefits. The autograft allows for better graft incorporation and remodeling, and elimination of risk of disease transmission. We prefer allograft for its decreased surgical time, decreased skin incision and soft-tissue dissection, and decreased donor site morbidity.[18] The patient should also understand the risk assumed with allograft use: increased surgical cost, delay in graft incorporation, and risk of disease transmission.[19]

If performing double-bundle reconstruction, we customarily use a 9-mm AL bundle graft and a 7-mm PM graft. In single-bundle reconstruction, we use an 11-mm graft. To allow for adequate length the graft should be at least 25 mm in length. The graft is doubled over an endoloop, which is used on the femoral side of the graft. The tails of the graft are prepared in standard fashion performing modified Bunnell stitches using #2 ticron. We secure the femoral side of the graft by fixing the endoloop over a post. Tying the sutures over a 4.5-AO screw and washer provides fixation on the tibial side.

Complications

Preventing Intraoperative Complications

PCL injury is often associated with complex injury patterns, and its reconstruction requires astute attention to details. Avoidance of several potential intraoperative and postoperative complications is essential, not only to render the reconstruction successful but also to avoid catastrophic events to the extremity. PCL reconstruction, despite advances in surgical technique, remains one of the more technically challenging operations in orthopedic sports medicine. Abnormal posterior tibial translation, as evidenced by >5 mm translation on KT100 testing at 90° of flexion remains present in 21–33% of cases postoperatively.[6,13,20–22] We employ several intraoperative techniques aimed to avoid possible complications. The most critical complication of PCL reconstruction involves injuring the popliteal artery or the tibial nerve. Other intraoperative complications or difficulties that may arise include: damage to the ACL during debridement of the PCL, increased bleeding due to the vascularity of the PCL, tunnel misplacement, and damage to subchondral surface of the medial femoral condyle leading to osteonecrosis.

Several tactics are utilized to minimize the risk of damaging the neurovascular bundle. Prior to drilling/reaming to establish the tibial tunnel, an interval is developed between the scarred PCL insertion stump and the synovium of the posterior capsule. This will increase the distance between the neurovascular bundle and the posterior tibia.[17] This can be performed using a combination of a PCL curette and a full radius resector. When using the full radius resector, care should be taken to avoid using the teeth of the resector in a posterior direction, as the neurovascular bundle is located just posterior to the capsule. An anterior drawer performed by an assistant, with force applied to the posterior calf, below the level of the proximal tibia to reduce the posteriorly subluxed tibia. It should be emphasized that if the drawer is performed with the assistant's hands in the popliteal fossa, the artery and the nerve may be inadvertently drawn closer to the posterior capsule/tibia rendering it more susceptible to injury. The anterior drawer is also used to increase the distance between the posterior tibia and the popliteal artery and tibial nerve during placement of the guidewire and reaming of the tibial tunnel. When debriding the PCL scar in the intracondylar notch, an anterior drawer will place the ACL under tension to allow easier delineation of the injured PCL tissue. When the ACL appears lax it may be inadvertently damaged during debridement. In addition to use of a full radius resector, use of an electrocautery device for debridement of the PCL near its femoral attachment may be useful, as the geniculate bleeders may cause increased bleeding which can hinder visualization. When debriding the injured PCL, care should be taken to preserve the MFLs and the PM bundle of the PCL, if intact. As mentioned earlier, the MFLs can decrease forces on the reconstructed graft, and an intact native PM bundle may decrease posterior translation in extension.

Once debridement has exposed the tibial insertion of the PCL, we advance the guidewire under fluoroscopic guidance, stopping at the posterior femoral cortex, perforating the cortex by hand, and utilizing direct visualization from the arthroscope in the posteromedial portal. This prevents inadvertent advancement of the guidewire through the posterior capsule, damaging the neurovascular bundle. Since the guidewire may also be unintentionally advanced during reaming, we only ream the tibial when unobstructed visualization (through the posteromedial portal) is permissible and the PCL curette is firmly applied to the guidewire. The posterior cortex of the tibia is perforated with the reamer by hand, under direct visualization. We also periodically check the dorsalis pedis pulse intraoperatively, and again postoperatively to confirm adequate distal blood flow.

In an attempt to prevent damage to the subchondral bone, the knee is flexed to >110° during reaming of the femoral tunnel. This allows a posterior trajectory of the tunnel, away from the subchondral bone of the articular surface of the medial femoral condyle. This also allows for an adequate length of graft in the tunnel for incorporation.

The apertures of all tibial and femoral tunnels are debrided with a full radius resector to ensure that the tunnel has smooth edges. Rough edges may contribute to abrasion and weakening of the graft over time. When passing the femoral end of the graft into its tunnel, we prevent damage to the graft from the sharp-tipped beath pin, by protecting it with a metal skid to guide the beath pin into the femoral tunnel.

Implementation of these techniques, coupled with cautious and well-planned surgical technique, can provide an optimal situation for successful PCL reconstruction.

Recognizing and Dealing with Intraoperative Complications

While meticulous technique to prevent intraoperative complications is more desirable, the surgeon must be prepared to address any intraoperative difficulties which may arise. The most serious of these complications is injury to part of the neurovascular bundle. At our institution when we schedule a PCL reconstruction, we alert the on-call vascular surgeon of our case, and have a number posted on the wall in the operating room so circulating staff can immediately contact the vascular surgeon if a problem should arise. Although damage can occur by over aggressive debridement of the posterior capsule with the full-radius resector, over penetration of a guidewire or reamer through the tibial canal is the most common cause of neurovascular bundle injury. This problem can not only occur as the guidewire is placed, but also result from inadvertent advancement of the guidewire as the reamer is being advanced through the tibia. The surgeon must be hypervigilant to prevent this catastrophic complication from occurring. We do not employ the use of a tourniquet while performing PCL reconstruction. This allows for more rapid recognition of a vascular injury. If a vascular injury does occur, the vascular surgeon should immediately be alerted, and a posterior approach should be undertaken to localize the area of injury. Prompt control of the bleeding is essential. The vascular surgeon undertakes repair of the injury.

Of equally devastating consequence is a missed compartment syndrome. We use gravity inflow and a superolateral outflow portal in attempt to control and minimize intra-articular pressures during the procedure. An assistant intermittently checks the fullness of the posterior compartment of the leg. If at any time during the procedure, fullness and pressure is noted to increase, the arthroscopic portion of the procedure is abandoned in favor of an open approach. The arthroscope may still be used on occasion, in a dry field, to allow for increased visualization and magnification. Should a compartment syndrome be a suspect, a standard posteromedial incision should be made and the superficial and deep posterior compartments should be released. Several factors can increase the likelihood of developing a compartment syndrome. In acute reconstructions (less than 2 weeks from injury), a capsular injury may not have sufficiently healed to maintain capsular distention and may lead to extravasation of fluid into the posterior calf.[12] Capsular breach may also be iatrogenic, resulting from overaggressive debridement of the posterior capsule.

Post-reconstructive exam, including range-of-motion and anterior/posterior stability testing, should be performed to assess for improper tensioning of the PCL (Fig. 5.14). This exam should be performed prior to surgical closure. If an abnormality is detected at this time, revision fixation may be performed to correct the issue.

Postoperative Complications

Postoperative complications of PCL reconstruction may include clinical failure of the graft, commonly evidenced by persistent posterior subluxation or instability of the knee, or loss of motion.[6,10] Standard postoperative surgical complications including infection and venous thromboembolism are always a concern. Preoperative and postoperative antibiotics are given, coupled with routine

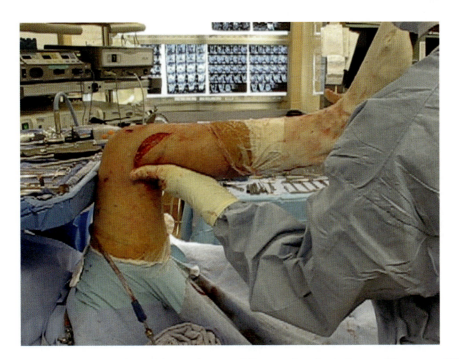

Fig. 5.14 Post-reconstructive examination of knee prior to wound closure to ensure proper tensioning of ligaments, with full range-of-motion, and restored ligament stability

clinical evaluation of surgical incisions, in an attempt to decrease the incidence of infection. In high-risk patients, with a past history of blood clot or a known clotting disorder, postoperative thromboembolic prophylaxis is provided. The younger age and mobility, coupled with crutch weight bearing postoperatively, generally act to decrease the likelihood of thromboembolic events in this patient population.

Loss of motion after PCL reconstruction usually is manifested as a loss of flexion.[10,11] Reported causes include suprapatellar adhesion, improper tunnel placement, or graft positioning/tensioning. Suprapatellar adhesions may occur more commonly if quadriceps tendon autograft is harvested for the reconstruction. Meticulous surgical techniques are required to ensure proper graft and tunnel positioning and tensioning. Use of the synovator/burr to debride and smooth the edges of the tibial and the femoral tunnel can minimize the abrasion of the grafts, which may lead to weakening or rupture.

Proper tunnel placement is also instrumental to the longevity of the graft and overall success of PCL reconstruction. In their review, Noyes et al. found that tibial tunnel misplacement most commonly occurred in a position proximal to the anatomical tibial insertion. This led to the graft assuming a more vertical position, thus decreasing the ability to resist posterior translation.[6] They also found that femoral tunnels were often placed more posterior to the anatomic insertion leading to increased posterior translation in flexion.[6]

The postoperative protocol is also important in preventing suboptimal clinical results. Early weight-bearing in flexion or early open-chain hamstring exercises can lead to persistent posterior tibial subluxation due to stretching of the graft from early eccentric pull of the hamstring on the PCL graft. We address this by keeping the patient locked in a knee brace in full extension for the first 4 weeks. Open-chain hamstring exercises are prohibited for 3 months and the knee brace is not unlocked for gait training until good quadriceps function is demonstrated.

Revision PCL Surgery

Failure of PCL surgery remains an enigmatic problem with a lack of abundant literature or historical data to guide the surgeon in his/her approach to this complex issue. The patient may subjectively complain of stiffness, instability, and loss of motion or pain. Objectively there may be clinical evidence of laxity, loss of motion, or radiographic evidence of progressive degenerative arthritis.[6] It is a very complex and challenging situation, which should be approached with caution by even the most experienced of surgeons.

A discussion of merit on revision PCL surgery is much too complex for inclusion in this chapter. Etiologies of the failure of the primary reconstruction are often multifactorial and include surgical error, lack of biologic incorporation of graft material, or trauma to the reconstructed graft. As previously mentioned, failure to recognize and treat combined injuries, errors in tunnel placement, or graft tensioning and fixation are all surgeon-derived variables that may lead to failure and require the need for revision PCL surgery.[6] Trauma to the graft in the form of early aggressive rehabilitation, particularly flexion weight-bearing or frank trauma to the knee can lead to loosening of or outright failure of the graft.

Essential to the successful undertaking of revision PCL reconstruction is the proper elucidation of the mode of failure of the primary reconstruction. Without addressing the cause of the failure (i.e., missed combined injury or limb malalignment) a simple repeat PCL reconstruction likely will result in identical results. A thorough physical examination including gait analysis (varus thrust) along with appropriate ancillary examinations will assist in the ability to discover the mode of failure. Imaging should be used for the evaluation of varus or sagittal tibial slope malalignment, tibial subluxation, tunnel misplacement or widening, or any associated articular cartilage or meniscal pathology.

Revision PCL surgery is a salvage operation and patients should be made aware that results are not to be expected to parallel those of primary surgery. The etiology of the failure will dictate the surgeons' approach to the revision. Novel techniques including single vs. double-staged operations, combined high tibial osteotomy, and tibial inlay techniques may be required to circumvent situations that may make the revision difficult or high-risk for recurrent failure. Misplaced or widened tunnels often require staged bone-grafting procedures prior to revision reconstruction. Varus or sagittal plane malalignment may require a uni or biplanar high tibial osteotomy to reduce postoperative forces on the PCL or posterolateral corner. Indwelling hardware in the tibial that is difficult to remove may require the surgeon to utilize a tibial inlay technique for the reconstruction. As with primary reconstruction single vs. double-bundle reconstruction of the PCL depends on the extent of injury to the PCL complex.

Immediate Postoperative Care

Standard wound closure is performed, and nonadherent dressings, sterile gauze, and bias stockinette are applied. Prior to emergence from anesthesia, the patient is placed in a hinged knee brace locked in full extension. The patient is admitted overnight for observation with anticipated discharge the following morning. Postoperative thromboprophylaxis is reserved for high-risk patients with prior history of blood clots, or known clotting disorder.

Postoperative Rehabilitation

The immediate goals postoperatively are to protect healing structures/incisions, to maximize quadriceps firing, and to restore full passive extension.

The brace remains locked in full extension for the first 4 postoperative weeks. Isometric quadriceps exercises, with the knee in extension, are permitted during this time period. Passive flexion, limited to 90°, begins at postoperative week 4, with special attention from the physical therapist to apply anterior force on the proximal tibia to prevent posterior tibial subluxation during motion. Active flexion is prohibited for the first 6 weeks postoperatively, to prevent posterior subluxation of the tibia as result of eccentric pull of the hamstring muscles. Passive- and active-assisted range-of-motion exercises are initiated at 6 weeks, with gradual increases in range-of-motion limits. Open-chain quadriceps exercises, within range-of-motion limits of 60–75°, are allowed after 4 weeks. Closed-chain hamstring exercises are allowed at 6 weeks postoperatively. Open-chain hamstring exercises are prohibited in the first 3 months to prevent posterior tibial subluxation and undue tension on the PCL graft.

Partial crutch weight-bearing is progressed as tolerated over the first 4 weeks. If a posterolateral corner repair is performed, however, partial weight bearing in the brace is continued for 12 weeks. The brace is unlocked for gait training once good quadriceps control is regained. Sedentary work may be resumed around 4 weeks postoperatively; whereas heavy labor is prohibited for the first 6–9 months. Running may be resumed at 6 months, and return to sports is typically allowed between 9 and 12 months.

References

1. Fanelli G (1993) Posterior cruciate ligament injuries in trauma patients. Arthroscopy 9(3):291-4
2. Fanelli G, Edson C (1995) Posterior cruciate ligament injuries in trauma patients: Part II. Arthroscopy 11(5):526-9
3. Shelbourne K, O'shea J (1999) Natural history of nonoperatively treated posterior cruciate ligament injuries. Sports Med Arthrosc Rev 7:235-42
4. Petrigliano F, McAllister D (2006) Isolated posterior cruciate ligament injuries of the knee. Sports Med Arthrosc Rev 14(4):206-12
5. Gupte C, Bull A, Thomas R et al (2003) The meniscofemoral ligaments: secondary restraints to the posterior drawer. Analysis of anteroposterior and rotary laxity in the intact and posterior-cruciate-deficient knee. J Bone Joint Surg 85(5):765-73
6. Noyes F, Barber-Westin S (2005) Posterior cruciate ligament revision reconstruction, part 1: causes of surgical failure in 52 consecutive operations. Am J Sports Med 33(5):646-54
7. Markolf K, Graves B, Sigward S et al (2007) Popliteus bypass and popliteofibular ligament reconstructions reduce posterior tibial translations and forces in a posterior cruciate ligament graft. Arthroscopy 23(5):482-7
8. Fox R, Harner C, Sakane M et al (1998) Determination of the in situ forces in the human posterior cruciate ligament using robotic technology. A cadaveric study. Am J Sports Med 26(3):395-401
9. Harner C, Janaushek M, Ma C et al (2000) The effect of knee flexion angle and application of an anterior tibial load at the time of graft fixation on the biomechanics of a posterior cruciate ligament-reconstructed knee. Am J Sports Med 28(4):460-5
10. Fanelli G, Monahan T (1999) Complications of posterior cruciate ligament reconstruction. Sports Med Arthrosc Rev 7:296-302
11. Fanelli G (2004) Complications in posterior cruciate ligament reconstruction. Sports Med Arthrosc Rev 12(3):196-201
12. Chhabra A, Kline A, Harner C (2006) Single-bundle versus double-bundle posterior cruciate ligament reconstruction: scientific rationale and surgical technique. Instr Course Lect 55:497-507
13. Harner C, Waltrip R, Bennett C et al (2004) Surgical management of knee dislocations. J Bone Joint Surg Am 86-A(2):262-73
14. Matava M, Sethi N, Totty W (2000) Proximity of the posterior cruciate ligament insertion to the popliteal artery as a

function of the knee flexion angle: implications for posterior cruciate ligament reconstruction. Arthroscopy 16(8): 796-804
15. Makino A, Costa-Paz M, Aponte-Tinao L et al (2005) Popliteal artery laceration during arthroscopic posterior cruciate ligament reconstruction. Arthroscopy 21(11):1396
16. Cohen S, Boyd L, Miller M (2004) Vascular risk associated with posterior cruciate ligament reconstruction using the arthroscopic transtibial tunnel technique. J Knee Surg 17(4):211-3
17. Ahn J, Wang J, Lee S et al (2007) Increasing the distance between the posterior cruciate ligament and the popliteal neurovascular bundle by a limited posterior capsular release during arthroscopic transtibial posterior cruciate ligament reconstruction: a cadaveric angiographic study. Am J Sports Med 35(5):787-92
18. Shapiro M, Freedman E (1995) Allograft reconstruction of the anterior and posterior cruciate ligaments after traumatic knee dislocation. Am J Sports Med 23(5):580-7
19. Jackson D, Corsetti J, Simon T (1996) Biologic incorporation of allograft anterior cruciate ligament replacements. Clin Orthop Relat Res Mar(324):126-33
20. Mariani P, Adriani E, Santori N et al (1997) Arthroscopic posterior cruciate ligament reconstruction with bone-tendon-bone patellar graft. Knee Surg Sports Traumatol Arthrosc 5:239-44
21. L'Insalata J, Harner C (1996) Treatment of acute and chronic posterior cruciate ligament deficiency. New approaches. Am J Knee Surg 9(4):185-93
22. Chen C, Chen W, Shih C (2000) Arthroscopic double-bundled posterior cruciate ligament reconstruction with quadriceps tendon-patellar bone autograft. Arthroscopy 16(7):780-2

Editors' Comments (PCL)

When evaluating for PCL insufficiency, evaluate the knee for associated ACL, LCL, posterolateral, and/or MCL insufficiency. While the posterolateral corner is often involved do not miss an associated MCL injury. Clinical exam is often more helpful than the MRI in determining these associated injuries.

To avoid the ill effects of the "killer turn" when performing transtibial PCL reconstruction, consider aperture fixation of the bone block or tendon construct with an interference screw under direct visualization from the posteromedial portal. The interference screw may be backed up on the anterior tibial cortex with a post and screw or a suture interference anchor. Lessen the effects of the "killer turn" and ease the passage of the graft with gortex smoothers (Smith & Nephew).

The inlay PCL technique can be used in a revision setting. When utilizing an autologous BPTB graft, drill and tap the 3.2-mm hole in the bone block prior to inlay fixation on the posterior tibia. Do not pass a bone block >20 mm in length for the femoral socket as this will make the passage more challenging from posterior to anterior and retrieval in the intercondylar notch.

Chapter 6
Avoiding and Managing Complications of Collateral Ligament Surgery of the Knee

Leon E. Paulos and Kirk Mendez

Top 10 Pearls

- Prior to repairing a severe knee ligament injury, it is important that the surgeon understands the relationships of normal anatomic structures and their landmarks, as well as the pattern of injuries that can be expected.
- During the initial exposure of a badly damaged knee, it is helpful to first identify and protect the normal structures and landmarks and then proceed to accomplish an anatomic (isometric) repair of each damaged structure. No primary restraints should be ignored unless other more urgent medical problems take priority.
- Restoration of the deep components of the medial collateral ligament (MCL) and lateral collateral ligament (LCL) and their related capsular structures are important to a successful outcome for reconstruction or revision of chronic varus or valgus patholaxity.
- Always attempt to restore the posterior oblique ligament (POL)-medial meniscus brake-stop mechanism. Restore the torn capsular attachments to any remaining meniscus rim or, if there is no rim, consider a meniscus transplant.
- Depending on swelling, motion, and pain try to repair or reconstruct grade IV MCL and LCL injuries simultaneously with the cruciate repair(s) within the first 5-7 days (golden period) after injury. Begin immediate postoperative range of motion with the aid of a continuous passive motion (CPM) device.
- Always attempt to repair or reconstruct the superficial MCL (sMCL) and LCL and associated posteromedial and posterolateral structures anatomically. This includes an isometric repair, which can be better accomplished by understanding Burmester's curves. The sMCL should never be shortened or placed in the anterior third of the tibial shaft (Fig. 6.1). Be prepared to not only correct all relevant patholaxities, but also native hyperlaxity of secondary restraints in recalcitrant cases.
- Sutures should usually be used in association with metal fixation of ligament tissues, rather than staples or washers by themselves.
- Chronic ligament instability reconstructions or revisions will generally fail in the setting of moderate to severe concomitant varus or valgus mechanical malalignment.
- Immediate passive range of motion and quadriceps activation are the keys to preventing arthrofibrosis. If the knee must be immobilized, place it in a position that results in the highest tension on the ligament that has been repaired or reconstructed.
- The use of crutches with limited weight bearing may or may not be necessary to protect a ligament reconstruction, but it is imperative to protect the cartilage surfaces for a knee that is swollen and erythematic.[1]

L.E. Paulos (✉)
1040 Gulf Breeze Parkway, Suite 203, Gulf Breeze, FL 32561
e-mail: lonniepaulos@sbcglobal.net

K. Mendez
Private Practice, Orthopedic Specialist of Nevada, Las Vegas, NVevada, USA

Introduction and Background

The difficulty and complication rate associated with multiligament injuries of the knee are significantly higher than those found with isolated ligament ruptures.[2] Aware of

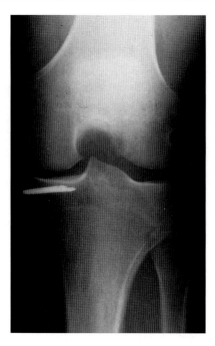

Fig. 6.1 Anteroposterior radiograph showing an MCL staple used to fix the sMCL and dMCL simultaneously near the joint line

this fact, many surgeons will tend to treat only the associated cruciate injury in hopes that the other damaged primary and secondary restraints will heal. Many times, as will be discussed, this is an appropriate course of treatment. However, depending on the severity of the ligament injury, the specific combination of ligaments injured, and other associated preexisting factors (such as native hyperlaxity, hostile mechanical axis, or chondral and meniscus damage), the surgeon has to be prepared to repair, reconstruct, and rehabilitate a knee with damage to multiple primary restraints.

Historically, surgery to repair multiple ligaments has been complicated by recurrent laxity, motion loss, skin loss, and a higher infection rate.[3,4] If the treating surgeon is to avoid these problems, it is imperative that a sound understanding exists of normal knee anatomy, biomechanics, injury patterns, postoperative pain control, and rehabilitation modalities.

MCL Injuries

The most common knee injuries occur in various degrees to the medial-side structures. Injuries range from a grade I sprain of the MCL to combined injuries involving the MCL, medial meniscus, posteromedial corner, anterior cruciate ligament (ACL), or posterior cruciate ligament (PCL). The MCL is the most frequently injured ligament of the knee.[5,6] The vast majority of MCL injuries usually heal without the need for surgical intervention; however, chronic medial laxity can develop and require surgical treatment as do some acute, combined injuries.[7–10]

Anatomy

The capsuloligamentous structures of the medial knee are a sleeve of tissues that can be divided into thirds (Fig. 6.2). The anterior third consists of the capsule, anterior third of the meniscus, and the longitudinal medial patellar retinaculum. These structures contribute relatively little to the stability of the knee.[11]

The middle third includes the sMCL and deep MCL (dMCL), as well as the midportion of the medial meniscus. The anterior portion of the sMCL has no attachment to the meniscus; however, the posterior sMCL has oblique fibers that run into the posteromedial structures of the knee. The dMCL firmly attaches to the medial meniscus.

The posterior third of the medial knee is known as the posteromedial corner (Fig. 6.3).[12] This region consists of the posteromedial meniscus horn, POL, capsule, and semimembranosus muscle. The POL arises from the adductor tubercle and has three distal attachments (Fig. 6.4). The semimembranosus muscle actively controls the posteromedial corner where its five arms insert. These tissues act as both dynamic and static stabilizers.[10]

The sMCL is the main structure to resist valgus loading. This structure averages 11 cm in length and 1.5 cm in width. The sMCL is attached proximally to the medial femoral epicondyle, just anterior to the adductor tubercle, and distally 4-6 cm below the joint line beneath the pes anserinus insertion. Deep to the MCL is the medial capsular ligament (also called the deep MCL), which is divided into the meniscotibial and meniscofemoral fibers. The POL originates just posterior to the superficial MCL and inserts just below the joint line.

Warren and Marshall described the three layer concept of the medial knee.[13] Layer 1 includes the sartorius fascia. Layer 2 consists of the superficial MCL, the POL,

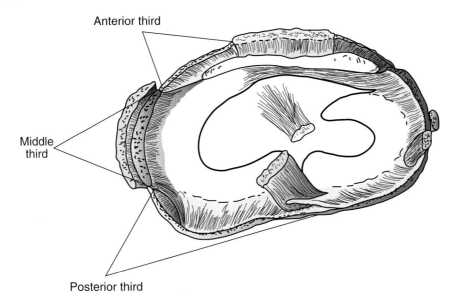

Fig. 6.2 Cross-section of the medial side of the knee

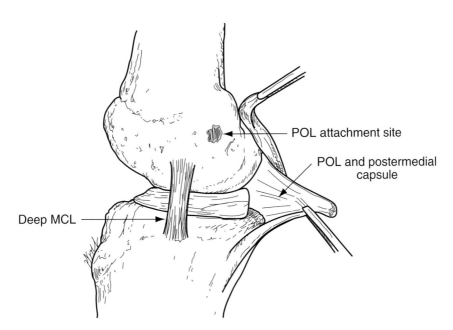

Fig. 6.3 Note the attachment sites of the various structures of the medial side of the knee. *POL* posterior oblique ligament

and the semimembranous. The gracilis and semitendinosus tendons are located between layers 1 and 2. Layer 3 consists of the deep MCL and the posteromedial capsule. It is the authors' opinion that the POL is intimately associated with the posterior capsule and should be included in layer 3.

The three static stabilizers of the medial knee are sMCL, dMCL, and posterior POL (Figs. 6.5 and 6.6). The dynamic support of the medial knee is provided by the quadriceps, the pes anserinus, and the various attachment sites of the semimembranosus muscle. Muller[12] refers to the posteromedial knee as

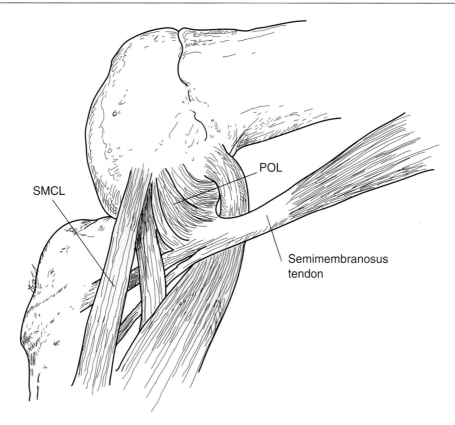

Fig. 6.4 Posteromedial corner of the knee. Note the attachment of the posterior oblique ligament (POL) relative to the superficial medial collateral ligament (SMCL)

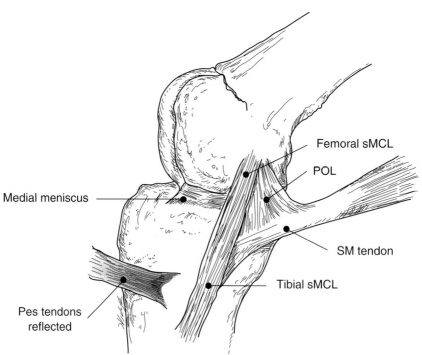

Fig. 6.5 Note that no fibers of the sMCL attach anterior to the mid-tibial shaft

6 Avoiding and Managing Complications of Collateral Ligament Surgery of the Knee

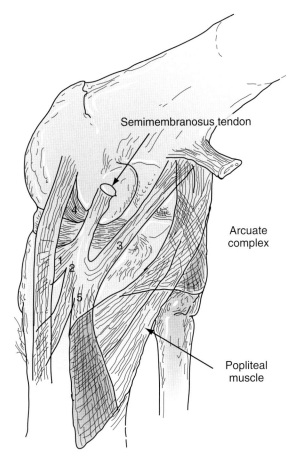

1 Pars reflexa
2 Direct insertion
3 Oblique popliteal ligament
4 Insertion that blends with the POL
5 Insertion that blends with the popliteal fascia

Fig. 6.6 The posteromedial knee showing the five arms of the semimembranosus tendon

the semimembranosus corner, which provides dynamic resistance to valgus and rotatory stresses placed on the knee (Fig. 6.6).

Biomechanics

Numerous studies have confirmed that the sMCL is the primary restraint to valgus loading of the knee.[12–14] The three functional units of the medial knee are the anterior fibers of the sMCL, dMCL, and POL. The anterior (4-5 mm) fibers of the sMCL are the primary restraint to abduction and external rotatory loads on the medial side of the knee.[13] In a cadaveric study, no significant valgus or rotation occurred when the superficial anterior fibers were left intact.[13]

Grood et al.[14] reported that the sMCL provided 78% of medial stability with the knee at 25° at flexion. The dMCL accounted for only 4% at 25° of flexion. Likewise, the POL accounted for only 4% at this flexion angle. The deep MCL tightens in flexion and relaxes in full extension.[15] Gardiner demonstrated that the anterior portion of the MCL has a relatively constant strain throughout the range of knee motion.[16]

The POL functions to resist valgus stress mainly when the knee is in full extension. When the knee is in flexion, the POL is relaxed and the anterior aspect lies beneath the posterior portion of the MCL. To function in flexion, the semimembranosus must dynamize this structure. The pull of the semimembranosus also pulls the meniscus posterior and prevents entrapment.[17]

The pes anserinus inserts just anterior to the MCL and directly overlies it (Fig. 6.7). This structure dynamically reinforces the ligament and stabilizes the medial knee. Depending on the amount of knee flexion, 40% of the MCL and almost the entire POL are covered by the pes anserinus. In addition to the ligament protecting function in extension, the pes anserinus also acts synergistically with the MCL in flexion, where it resists external rotation.[12]

The posteromedial knee acts as a brake-stop to prevent anterior tibial translation in an ACL-deficient knee.

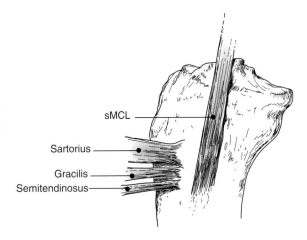

Fig. 6.7 The pes anserinus inserts just anterior to the sMCL and plays an important role in resisting external rotation with the knee in flexion

When the ACL is disrupted, posterior displacement of the femur wedges the posteromedial meniscus horn between the tibial plateau and the femoral condyle, which restrains the tibia from further displacement (Figs. 6.8 and 6.9). Without the meniscus, contributions to the stability of the posteromedial corner are seriously compromised.[18] The importance of the posteromedial meniscus cannot be overstated since it redirects forces received and consequently functions as a brake-stop to limit anterior tibial translation in the ACL-deficient knee.[12,18] The POL is intimately attached to the posterior horn of the medial meniscus and acts in a synergistical manner to improve this brake-stop function.

The Burmester Curve

The Burmester curve, although not completely accurate, represents a useful model for understanding isometry of the collateral ligaments as they follow an approximate circular path during knee motion. As described by Menschik in 1974,[19] the Burmester curve is named after the German mathematician Burmester, who in 1888 published the textbook of Kinematics. The curve is important with regard to the sites of ligament insertions in the knee. The ligaments insert at the sites predicted by the theory. The MCL attachment on the tibia follows a

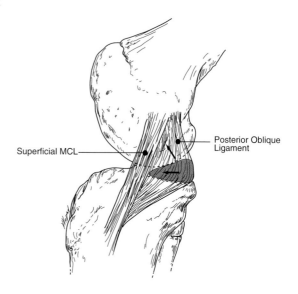

Fig. 6.9 Force vector created when the tibia subluxes anteriorly after an ACL tear is resisted by an opposite force vector created through the attachment of the posterior oblique ligament to the posterior horn of the medial meniscus

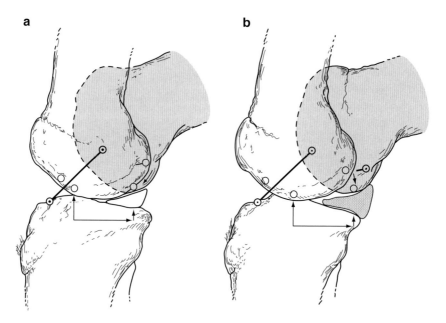

Fig. 6.8 (**a**) The function of the intact ACL. (**b**) Loss of ACL function leads to excessive femoral rolling, resulting in an abnormal posterior shift of the femoral contact point on both the medial and lateral sides. The posterior horns of the menisci are severely stressed as they act to brake this rolling movement

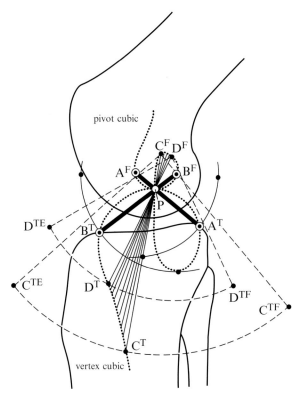

Fig. 6.10 The Burmester curve (Reprinted with permission from Muller[12])

circular path as shown in Fig. 6.10, representing a constant distance during flexion and extension.[12]

Understanding the Burmester curve is important as one can appreciate that shifting the ligament insertion just 1 cm anteriorly or superiorly dramatically alters ligament length with knee motion. If placed in this nonanatomic position, the ligament is stretched 16.7% and will constrain the knee, or the repair will fail. Note that the sMCL is located on the middle-posterior third of the tibia, not the anterior third. No fibers of the sMCL attach anterior to the mid tibial shaft.

Injury Classification and Examination

Typically, a history of a valgus force applied laterally to the upper leg or lower thigh with the foot planted is elicited. Reports suggest that most injuries to the MCL are located near the femoral origin. Grade I and II injuries may occur with noncontact twisting injuries in sports such as soccer, basketball, or skiing. Significant tears (grade III) are much more likely the result of a contact or high speed injury, or a fall from a height.

The capsular tissues have been shown to tear by an interstitial mechanism and provide some resistance even when the sMCL is torn.[14] The authors agree with Hughston that the capsular tissues are the "first line of defense" and restrain forces before the sMCL. Once the primary restraint is torn, the secondary restraints limit further joint space opening.

"First Line of Defense" vs. Primary Restraint

At lower loads and smaller joint openings, the dMCL protects the knee and functions in concert with the primary restraints. With a valgus stress, all restraints incur the load simultaneously but deform at varying amounts based on the knee flexion angle, fiber orientation, and rotation.

On the basis of cadaver studies, passive stabilizers have been divided into primary and secondary restraints. Because a structure is called a primary restraint does not necessarily imply that it resists the applied force first or even encounters it independently. The phrases "first line of defense" and primary restraint are not synonymous. Primary restraints provide the major resistance to a particular stress, whereas the structure or structures that undergo the initial stress or failure are the "first line of defense." For example, the sMCL acts as the primary restraint at 30° of flexion, whereas the "first line of defense" at all angles of flexion consists of the sMCL, POL, dMCL, posteromedial capsule, and medial meniscus.[20,21]

Hughston et al.[11] described anteromedial rotatory instability (AMRI) as an abnormal excess opening of the medial joint space in abduction at 30° of knee flexion, with a simultaneous anteromedial rotatory subluxation of the medial tibial condyle on the central axis of the intact PCL. This instability pattern is attributed to injuries of the POL and the five arms of the semimembranosus insertion. However, only physiologic anterior tibial translation will occur if the ACL is intact. Thus, for moderate to severe AMRI to occur, the ACL must be compromised.

Physical Examination

Patients with medial-sided knee injuries have varying degrees of pain, swelling, and loss of motion. Accurate localization of the injury can be obtained in nearly 70% of the cases with tenderness to palpation and localized swelling.[11]

The patient must be relaxed for an accurate examination to be conducted. The contralateral knee should always be used as a control. Abduction stress testing is performed at varying degrees of knee flexion. To examine the stability of the sMCL, a valgus force is applied to the knee flexed at 30° with the foot in external rotation (Fig. 6.11).

A valgus stress is also applied at 0° of flexion, which tests the integrity of the POL and PCL. Valgus laxity at both flexion angles indicates injury to the MCL and POL, and likely the cruciate ligaments. If the knee is stable to valgus stress at full extension, the POL is likely intact. Concomitant ACL injuries occur in up to 78% of patients with grade III MCL injuries and 100% of those with grade IV injuries. Appropriate provocative testing should be performed for these injuries.[20] A complete and thorough examination of the knee is done to rule out other injuries.

Laxity is graded according to the amount of joint opening as described by Hughston.[22] The classification system grades the amount of joint openings as 1+ (3–5 mm), 2+ (6–10 mm), and 3+ (>10 mm).

The severity system classifies MCL injuries into three grades. Grade I involves a few fibers resulting in localized tenderness, but no instability is present. Grade II injuries involve tearing of more fibers, but still no instability exists. A grade III tear comprises complete disruption of the ligament, with varying grades of instability. In addition, we classify a grade IV injury as one which has >15 mm of opening and laxity to both rotatory and valgus loads. This injury occurs with a tear of the sMCL in conjunction with tears of the POL, ACL/PCL, posteromedial capsule, and medial meniscus. Sometimes, a grade IV injury is seen at arthroscopy with the sMCL entrapped in the medial compartment (Fig. 6.12). A grade IV injury nearly always requires operative treatment.

During the physical examination, grade I and II injuries have definite endpoints. Grade III tears have a soft endpoint, or no endpoint to a valgus stress. It should be noted that in isolated grade III tears, the endpoint in the valgus-stressed knee at 30° of flexion represents the intact ACL, although the endpoint is encountered beyond

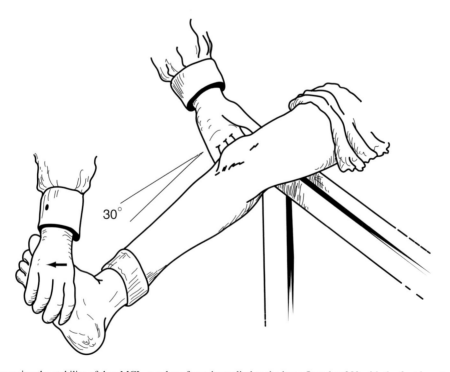

Fig. 6.11 To examine the stability of the sMCL, a valgus force is applied to the knee flexed at 30° with the foot in external rotation

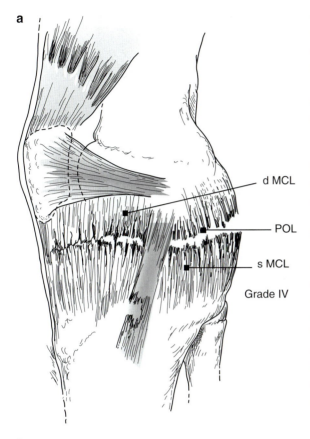

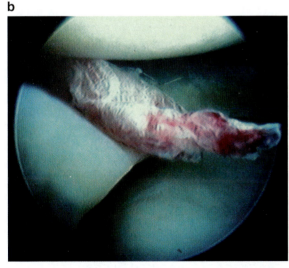

Fig. 6.12 (a) Grade IV MCL injury. (b) Arthroscopic view of tissue from MCL ligament tear laying intra-articularly over the medial meniscus

the normal medial opening as determined by comparison to the contralateral, uninjured knee. A grade IV injury has medial opening greater than that of a grade III injury with no end point, as well as external rotation of the tibia when valgus stress is applied.[23] A "suck sign" may be present, which represents the skin being pulled into the joint line opening, creating an indentation.

For a brief period of time following injury, a patient may be relatively pain-free even if the MCL is completely torn. Hughston et al.[11] reported that sometimes a complete disruption occurs "without significant pain, effusion, or disability for walking." In addition, the hemarthrosis that occurs with a concomitant ACL tear may be absent due to extravasation of blood from a medial capsular tear.

Increased laxity to abduction stress testing in 30° of knee flexion, coupled with anterior rotatory subluxation of the medial tibial plateau on the medial femoral condyle, helps diagnose AMRI. The rotatory component may be better appreciated by applying a rotatory stress while holding the limb on the plantar surface of the foot instead of the distal leg during abduction. The 90° anterior drawer test with the foot held in external rotation (Slocum(20) test) also evaluates AMRI. This is also a good test to determine whether loss of the medial brake-stop has occurred with a peripheral tear or significant intrasubstance tear of the medial meniscus and POL.

Evaluation of all adolescents with suspected medial-sided injuries should include stress radiographs to exclude injuries of the physeal plate.

Treatment of Isolated Tears

Very high success rates have been reported in the nonoperative treatment of grade I and grade II MCL sprains.[24,25] The MCL is an extracapsular structure and has demonstrated an ability to heal when the torn ends are closely apposed.[7,24,26–28] The majority of grade I and II lesions heal in 2-6 weeks using a brace and protected range of motion.[24,29] Treatment consists of a brief period of immobilization and protected weight bearing. Isometric exercises are performed within a few days of injury and then progressive resistance exercises are initiated. Although studies indicate that a slight amount of residual laxity remains in some patients, it is of no functional significance.[30] Studies have also demonstrated a low incidence of reinjury during the athletic season following the injury.[31]

Treatment of isolated grade III tears is less controversial than in the past, with nonoperative treatment being

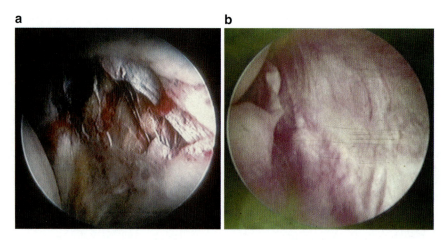

Fig. 6.13 Arthroscopic view using 70° scope inserted through the intercondylar notch and rotated medial to observe the posterior oblique ligament and posterior horn of the medial meniscus. (**a**) Completely torn POL in midsubstance. (**b**) Detachment of POL and capsule from posterior horn of medial meniscus

standard. The importance of excluding any associated injuries is paramount. In 1974, Ellsasser et al.[24] reported equally satisfactory results in professional football players treated conservatively as opposed to those treated surgically. The players returned to football between 3 and 8 weeks. These authors emphasized the importance of a repeat examination within 10 days and confirmation of a good endpoint on valgus stress testing.

Kannus and Jarvinen[32] reported that isolated grade III tears of the MCL had poor long-term results when treated nonoperatively. Early surgical repair was recommended. This study was cited as evidence that grade III tears of the MCL should be treated operatively; however, moderate to severe anterior instability due to ACL rupture was reported in the majority of the knees in this study, none of which received an ACL reconstruction.

Indelicato et al.[30] compared surgical and nonsurgical treatment of patients with isolated Grade III MCL injuries. Good to excellent results were reported in 14 of 16 operative cases and in 18 of 20 nonoperative cases. The patients treated nonoperatively spent significantly less time in rehabilitation.

Jones et al.[27] reported that 22 of 24 high school football players were able to return to sports an average time of 34 days following conservative treatment. These patients were placed in a knee brace that applied a varus stress the first week after the injury.

It is the authors' experience that a valgus mechanical axis may exaggerate functional disability, especially in female patients. Valgus-aligned patients require a longer period of crutch use and should be warned of the possible development of chronic instability. Factors that decrease the chances of successful nonoperative treatment include valgus alignment, associated cruciate ligament injury, and injury to the dMCL or POL (Fig. 6.13).[22,33,34]

Our recommended treatment of isolated, acute injuries is nonoperative. A brief period of immobilization is followed by protected range of motion in a hinged knee brace. Whenever possible, the patient is placed in a varus-producing knee brace. A brief period of limited weight bearing with crutches is used in individuals with a valgus mechanical axis. Crutches are discontinued when patients are able to walk without a limp. Patients are progressed from closed kinetic chain to open kinetic chain exercises with progressive resistance. Athletes are allowed to return to play when strength is 90% of the uninjured knee and the patient is able to participate in sport specific agility drills pain-free. A brace is worn for the rest of the season, but discontinued the following year.

Treatment of Combined Grade III MCL/ACL Injuries

There is no consensus regarding treatment of combined ACL and grade III MCL injuries. In the young active patient, 90% of all knee ligament injuries involve the ACL, MCL, or both of these structures.[6] Some authors have recommended surgical reconstruction of the ACL only.[29,35-38] Others have stated that operative MCL repair and nonoperative treatment of the ACL lead to good results.[33,39,40] Lundberg et al.[41] reported in a 10-year comparison study of isolated and combined MCL/ACL ruptures that patients with combined MCL injuries had more reinjuries and repeat surgeries that those with an isolated MCL injury. However, the Lysholm knee scores and activity levels were similar in both groups.

To determine whether the MCL should be repaired, some authors advocate an examination of valgus stability after the ACL has been reconstructed. Indelicato[28] prefers to assess valgus stability with the knee in full extension or slight flexion and if 2+ or 3+ laxity is found. Then primary repair of the MCL and POL is performed. Groff and Harner[42] recommend considering a MCL repair if the knee demonstrates laxity at full extension after ACL reconstruction. Shelbourne recommends nonoperative treatment of the MCL in combined ACL/MCL injuries, regardless of the severity of the MCL injury.[43] Jacobson and Chi[44] recommend initial nonoperative treatment of the MCL in all combined ACL/MCL injuries for 4-6 weeks, with a repeat examination to determine whether reconstruction is needed.

It is the authors' opinion that the need for medial repair should be determined prior to ACL reconstruction. Testing the need for medial repair after the ACL reconstruction gives a false sense of stability and leads to overtensioning the ACL graft to stabilize the knee at the time of surgery. Furthermore, subsequent secondary restraint patholaxity can contribute to ACL failure after reconstruction.[45,46]

Our approach to treating a combined ACL/grade III MCL injury is to allow the patient to regain motion and strength and allow swelling to subside. The importance of achieving full motion prior to surgery cannot be overemphasized, as numerous studies reported stiffness as a complication of combined ACL/MCL surgery.[47,48] After a sufficient time period to regain motion (usually 3 weeks), the knee is again examined and patients without an endpoint to valgus testing are scheduled for medial repair/reconstruction. It is very rare for a patient to require a MCL repair with a grade III MCL and combined ACL injury.

In patients with grade IV MCL/ACL injuries, surgery is performed as soon as possible. We do not wait until full knee motion is regained. This approach allows the ACL reconstruction to act as an internal splint to help protect the MCL repair during healing. Again, the diagnosis is confirmed with 3+ laxity to valgus testing, as well as a positive Slocum test. Ideally, surgery is performed within 5-7 days of the injury. Immediate and full range of motion is then begun, often with the use of a CPM.

Whenever medial meniscus pathology is seen in conjunction with an ACL injury, an MCL or posteromedial complex injury should be strongly suspected.

In addition to grade IV injuries with intra-articular entrapment, other situations in which a medial-sided repair may be performed with a combined MCL/ACL injury include the following:

1. Medial meniscus peripheral tear: reattach the POL and repair the MCL and meniscus after the knee has been visualized with the arthroscope.
2. If the MCL is torn at the tibial attachment site, it is visualized at the time of ACL reconstruction (Fig. 6.14).
3. In a patient with traumatic patellar dislocation requiring medial patellofemoral ligament reconstruction/repair.
4. Large bony avulsion of sMCL.
5. Valgus laxity at 0° of flexion in a knee with significant valgus malalignment.

Surgical Treatment

The general principals of acute repair of the medial-sided knee structures are as follows:

1. Understand the tear pattern so that the anatomy can be properly restored.

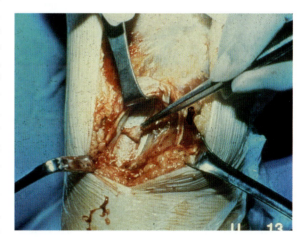

Fig. 6.14 Avulsed distal attachment of MCL exposed at time of hamstring tendon harvest for ACL reconstruction

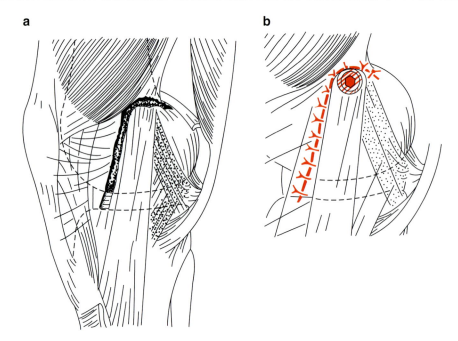

Fig. 6.15 The proximal global avulsion of both the MCL and POL. (**a**) This is the most easily repaired and most prognostically favorable of the combined medial ligamentous injuries. (**b**) Both ligaments can be reattached in mechanically ideal fashion with a screw and toothed washer. The remainder of the tear is repaired with approximating sutures (Reprinted with permission from Muller[12])

2. Perform an anatomic and isometric repair.
3. Use sutures with or without hardware for strong, but compliant fixation.

The authors agree with LaPrade et al.[49] that understanding specific structures and their attachment sites is important to subsequent repairs or reconstructions. However, knowledge of the "layers" of the medial knee structures is vital for atraumatic surgical exposure.

With grade IV MCL injuries, understanding the injury patterns on the medial side of the knee is important for proper restoration of function. Muller[12] describes several injury patterns, which will briefly be reviewed.

Proximal Avulsion of Both MCL and POL

With this tear pattern, the femur usually has a bare area where the ligament has been avulsed. This tear pattern is usually associated with a valgus/flexion, external rotation mechanism, and a concomitant ACL tear. Repair of this injury is ideal with sutures as well as a screw and ligament washer after the bone has been prepared (Fig. 6.15). Initially, sutures are tied at 20° of knee flexion and then the screw is inserted with the knee in full extension.

Vertical Tear Through the Semimembranosus Corner

This tear is caused by excessive external rotation. ACL rupture is the rule with this injury and AMRI is present. It is important that the sutures are placed so that the POL is advanced in an anteroinferior direction along the Burmester curve, so that it can glide beneath the sMCL. The sMCL is repaired as well (Fig. 6.16).

Y-Shaped Tear

The Y-shaped tear is not uncommon. The surgeon should recognize all three limbs of the tear because

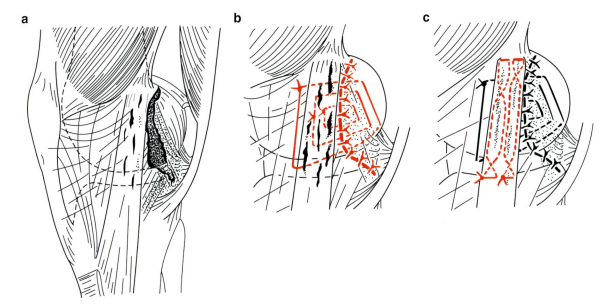

Fig. 6.16 The vertical tear. (**a**) This tear through the semimembranosus corner, shown here with a typical associated injury of the MCL, reminds us that the tears discussed so far are almost always accompanied by lesions of the MCL. It is not unusual for third degree injuries of the deep layer to be accompanied by first or second degree lesions of the MCL. (**b**) The tension suture pulls the semimembranosus corner anteriorly beneath the MCL. Often as additional tension suture must be placed to exert tension in a more anteroinferior direction. (**c**) Following repair of the deep layer, the MCL is repaired, here with the Bunnell suture technique (Reprinted with permission from Muller[12])

stability cannot be restored unless all three limbs are addressed. A meniscus injury should be suspected with this tear pattern. The angle of the suture placement should restore the function of the POL consistent with Burmester curves (Fig. 6.17).

Zigzag Tear

Tears running in a zigzag fashion across the capsuloligamentous structures are more difficult to assess (Fig. 6.18). The tabs are often tangled and separated from one another. The tears may extend across the meniscus to involve the meniscotibial fibers.

Diagonal Tears

These tear patterns are probably the easiest to recognize, as they represent detachment of the entire posterior capsular plate (Figs. 6.19 and 6.20).

Surgical Treatment

A thorough examination under anesthesia is performed to rule out associated injuries as well as to assess patellar stability. Particular interest is given to the outcome of the Slocum test (90° anterior drawer with the foot in external rotation), as this identifies knees in which the medial brake-stop is nonfunctional.

A low pressure, diagnostic arthroscopy is performed and the 70° scope is passed through the notch to visualize the posterior compartment and integrity of the meniscus horn. We believe that severe capsular disruption is not a contraindication to diagnostic arthroscopy. In these patients, a pump is not used to force fluid into the knee. Simple gravity irrigation is implemented instead.

A straight incision is made on the medial side of the knee from the medial femoral epicondyle to the medial proximal tibia. Care is taken to avoid damage to the infrapatellar branch of the saphenous nerve. The sartorial and crural fascia are incised. The sMCL, dMCL, and POL are identified. As a rule, the deepest structures are repaired first. Repair of the dMCL is the "key" to a

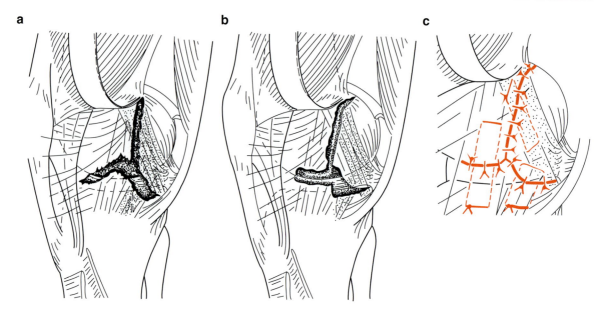

Fig. 6.17 The Y-shaped tear. (**a**, **b**) One limb of this tear may run horizontally and thus involve the peripheral meniscal attachment with no damage to the meniscus itself. (**c**) Technique of suture repair for this type of Y tear (Reprinted with permission from Muller[12])

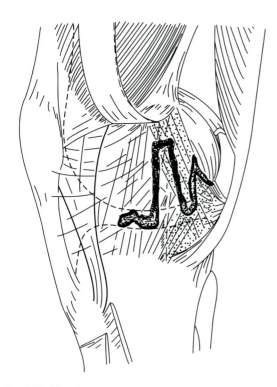

Fig. 6.18 The zigzag tear. Use legend from Fig. 215 (Reprinted with permission from Muller[12])

successful outcome and the use of suture anchors allows anatomic restoration (Fig. 6.21). In addition, it is important to recreate the dynamic function of the meniscus brake-stop by placing sutures through the POL and tying them with the knee in extension after POL repair and advancement.

If an interstitial tear of the sMCL is present, it is reinforced with an autograft or allograft to allow early knee motion. When augmenting an interstitial tear of the sMCL, we always perform a meticulous anatomic repair using a small Dacron type suture. No tissues are excised and all fibers are attached to bone or to each other using multiple vertical sutures. Dacron encourages tissue in-growth and is very nonreactive.

After the suture repair is completed, the augmentation tissue is laid within the sMCL fibers and attached with Dacron sutures. Anatomic tibial and femoral fixation occurs via bone-anchors with a screw and ligament washer back-up. We always try to reestablish the brake-stop mechanism and repair the medial meniscus or its rim whenever possible. In general, with a severe injury (grade IV) to the medial side of the knee combined with an ACL tear, a hamstring autograft is not used as a graft source. The pes insertion acts synergistically with the sMCL and ACL and. Therefore, should be preserved to maintain these relationships, as well as enhance revascularization.

Isometric repair of the sMCL is performed consistent with Burmester's curve and insuring that the tissue repaired reveals normal tension throughout the range of motion.

6 Avoiding and Managing Complications of Collateral Ligament Surgery of the Knee

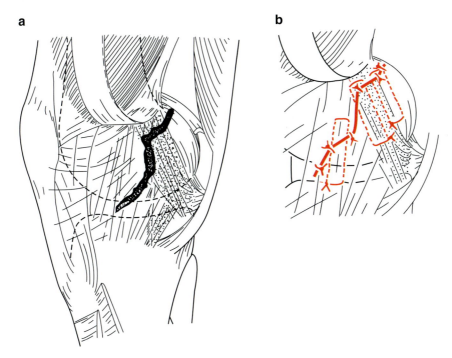

Fig. 6.19 The posterosuperior-to-anteroinferior diagonal tear. (**a**) This tear of the deep layer and POL is frequently observed in complex medial ligamentous injuries. (**b**) Technique of suture repair (Reprinted with permission from Muller[12])

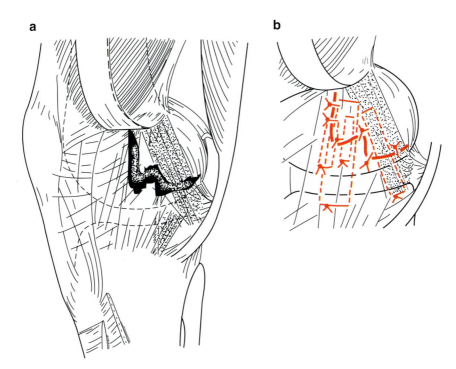

Fig. 6.20 The anterosuperior-to-posteroinferior diagonal tear. (**a**) A common form limited to the femoromeniscal fibers. (**b**) Repair with overlapping tension sutures in the most severely stretched portions of the ligament (Reprinted with permission from Muller[12])

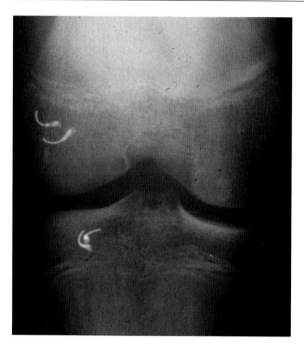

Fig. 6.21 Radiograph demonstrating anatomic placement of bone anchors used for repair of deep MCL

If the sMCL tibial attachment is avulsed, it is reattached at its attachment site with suture anchors, with or without a ligament washer and bone screw, while the knee is held in 20–30° of flexion. A slight varus stress is also applied when the sutures are tied. Caution is exercised not to shorten the ligament or transpose its attachment anterior on the tibial shaft.

Chronic Instability

Chronic medial laxity is uncommon, but can be debilitating. Chronic medial knee injuries are often associated with other ligament injuries, as well as a valgus mechanical axis, which needs to be simultaneously corrected. The patient may present with failed ACL, PCL, or combined ligament reconstructions. Valgus alignment may be noted on radiographs and physical examination. In patients with previous failed surgery and valgus knee alignment, a varus-producing osteotomy is performed at the same time as a medial reconstruction. Surgical goals for reconstruction of chronic medial laxity are as follows (in order of importance):

1. *Establish neutral to slight (1–2°) varus mechanical alignment.* If valgus alignment is greater than 10°, a distal femoral varus-producing osteotomy is performed. With smaller amounts of valgus malalignment, a proximal lateral opening or medial closing wedge high tibial osteotomy can be performed. An opening lateral wedge will tend to tighten posterolateral tissues and further support the medial reconstruction. The importance of acceptable mechanical alignment cannot be overstated since a medial-sided repair may fail in the setting of a valgus mechanical axis.

2. *Restore the brake-stop mechanism.* Any peripheral meniscus tears are repaired with Ethibond sutures passed through zone specific cannulae using an inside-out technique. A patient with <50% residual medial meniscus and continued medial instability is a candidate for a meniscus transplant. The transplant is performed at the same time as the MCL reconstruction.

3. *Restore the dMCL restraint.* If necessary, all remaining tissues of the sMCL and dMCL can be converted to use for restoration of the dMCL. If the tissue is of poor quality, then it is augmented with a healthy autograft from the fibers of the sMCL or semimembranosus if necessary. After dMCL reconstruction, and with the knee near full extension, the POL is advanced to its proper position and the medial meniscus sutures are tied (Fig. 6.22).

4. *Restore patellar stability* using medial retinaculum and the medial patellofemoral ligament for anatomic repair. A portion of the adductor or quadriceps tendon may also be used if necessary.

5. *Reestablish the sMCL* using direct repair, or augmentation (Fig. 6.23) with a patellar tendon, hamstring, or Achilles tendon allograft. Strong fixation is provided by incorporating a bone block at the femoral attachment. A hamstring allograft is secured with interference screws and supplemented with heavy suture fixation on the lateral femoral cortex. Fixation on the tibial side is accomplished with anchors. A ligament screw and washer may be used as a well for reinforcement. However, if the only available graft is too short to anatomically replace the sMCL, then suture fixation is safer than rigid metal fixation.

Postoperative Care

The patient is initially immobilized for a period of 1–2 weeks. The knee is protected with a varus-producing

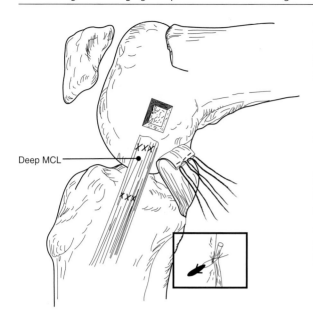

Fig. 6.22 Reconstruction of deep MCL. All available tissue, including the sMCL, is used to reconstruct this dMCL using bone/suture anchors

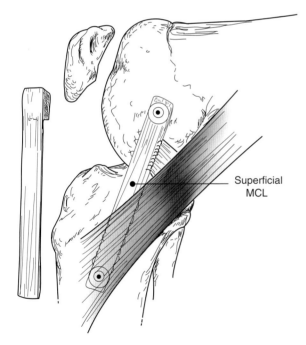

Fig. 6.23 Superficial MCL reconstruction using patellar tendon allograft. The POL is further secured to the sMCL near its femoral attachment

hinged knee brace, locked at 0° of flexion. Straight leg raises are permitted as soon as pain allows. The importance of obtaining full extension is stressed to the patient. Toe-touch weight bearing is allowed the first 2 weeks and progressed to full by 6 weeks. A strengthening program with progressive resistive exercises is then initiated. Patients usually achieve independent recovery by 12 weeks and return to activities by 9-12 months.

Lateral Collateral Ligament Injuries

Isolated injuries of the LCL are relatively rare.[50] LCL injury is often combined with other ligamentous injury of the posterolateral corner and cruciate ligaments. A brief overview of the LCL anatomy and biomechanics, as well as diagnosis and treatment of isolated LCL injuries, will follow.

Anatomy and Biomechanics

The extra-articular LCL is attached proximally to the lateral femoral epicondyle and inserts on the fibular head. The LCL is oriented slightly posterior and lateral as it extends from its femoral attachment to its fibular attachment. As the ligament courses distally, its more medial fibers insert into a groove at the lateral edge of the fibular head, 1 cm anterior to its apex (Fig. 6.24). The LCL is intimately associated with the short and long head of the biceps femoris. The LCL's length at 90° of knee flexion is significantly less than at 0° of knee flexion.

The lateral side of the knee can be divided into three distinct layers. Layer 1 consists of the iliotibial band (ITB) and biceps femoris tendon. Layer 2 consists of the quadriceps retinaculum and the lateral patellofemoral ligament. Layer 3 consists of the LCL, fabellofibular ligament, popliteofibular ligament (PFL), popliteus muscle and tendon, and the arcuate complex.[51]

The LCL is the primary restraint to varus stress of the knee and reinforces the lateral capsule.[52,53] Grood and coworkers[14] demonstrated that the LCL provided 55% of the total restraint to varus stress at 5° of flexion and 69% of the restraint at 25° of flexion. With increasing flexion, the lateral capsule provided less resistance. Gollehon and associates[54] demonstrated that cutting the LCL as well as the popliteus complex brought about a significant increase in external tibial rotation. A force of 750 N is required to cause failure of the LCL.[52]

Sidles et al.[55] evaluated the isometry of the lateral side of the knee. This study demonstrated that the anterior

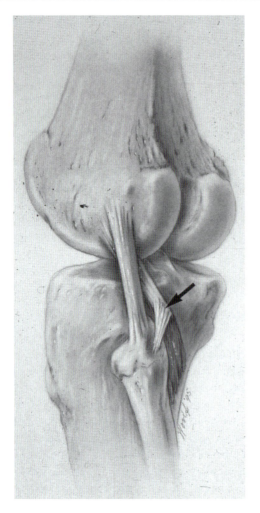

Fig. 6.24 Attachments of LCL. The *arrow* points out the popliteofibular ligament

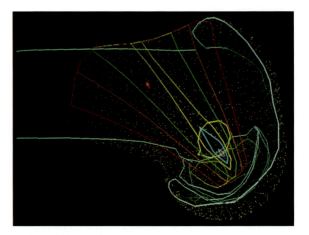

Fig. 6.25 Data points for analysis of isometric behavior of tissue attached near the lateral epicondyle of the femur. *Blue* indicates most isometric position, *yellow* indicates acceptable isometric position

and posterior fibular head is reciprocally isometric to the anterior and posterior areas of the lateral femoral epicondyle through a functional range of motion (Fig. 6.25).

On the lateral side of the knee, stability in extension is for the most part passive while stability in flexion is chiefly active. The principle of dynamic stabilization of the knee predominates with the biceps and semitendinosus/semimembranosus motor groups. Since a greater amount of motion occurs on the lateral side compared with the medial side of the knee, the purely passive lateral ligamentous structures are not as rigid as those on the medial side. The LCL relaxes during flexion and considerable internal or external rotation is required for this ligament to be torn. The principle dynamic stabilizers on the lateral side are the lateral gastrocnemius, the popliteus muscle and tendon, the biceps femoris, and the ITB.

Without a doubt, greater variability is encountered on the lateral side of the knee as it relates to anatomy and biomechanics. Significant contributions to varus stability will differ between the lateral capsule, LCL, and ITB from patient to patient. This fact helps explain why some patients incur a Segound fracture with a torn ACL, while others do not.[56] In addition, a patient's knee patholaxity is actually exacerbated when the ITB has been used as a graft substitute and then subsequently fails. For this reason, great caution and meticulous repair must be exercised when using or repairing the ITB during surgery.

Examination

The integrity of the LCL is tested at 0° of flexion by applying a varus stress to the knee. Again, laxity is graded as 1+, 2+, and 3+ as described by Hughston. Likewise, the severity of LCL injuries are graded as grade I, II, and III.

A grade IV injury similar to the medial side may be present and is often associated with a peroneal nerve injury and is always associated with an ACL and/or PCL tear. A grade IV injury represents injury to the LCL as well as the posterolateral structures and cruciate complex.

Treatment

Isolated tears of the LCL are usually treated conservatively. Treatment is similar to that of isolated injuries of the MCL, with use of a brace and progressive strengthening exercises. Again, caution and awareness is required that a varus mechanical alignment may complicate the outcome of this seemingly simple injury.

Surgical Treatment

Surgical treatment is considered when the patient has failed nonoperative management or has a bony avulsion of the LCL. Another indication is a grade III LCL with a concomitant ACL injury in a varus-aligned knee.

Acute avulsions may be secured with a screw and washer or by tension band technique. Our preferred method of reconstruction for grade II or III posterolateral rotatory instability (PLRI) is the "figure-eight" reconstruction as described by Larson and Belfie[57] (Fig. 6.26). Graft material usually consists of a semitendinosus autograft or allograft. A curvilinear incision is made just anterior to the fibular head. The peroneal nerve is identified and a limited neuroplasty is carried out. A 5 mm cannulated reamer is passed through the proximal fibula from an anterior-to-posterior direction. The tunnel is approximately 2 cm from the most proximal tip of the fibula. The lateral femoral epicondyle is palpated and the ITB is incised. Two Beath needles are passed just anterior and posterior to the lateral epicondyle. An appropriate sized reamer is drilled to a depth of 30 mm. A 22–24 cm graft is crisscrossed and passed under the ITB and knee capsule. Fixation is provided with interference screws and the graft is tensioned with the knee in 30° of flexion and neutral rotation.

Noyes and Barber-Westin described another technique for LCL reconstruction.[58] An 8 mm wide bone-patellar tendon-bone graft (autograft or allograft) is used to replace the LCL. A straight incision is made over the lateral joint line. Skin flaps are mobilized and an incision along the posterior border of the ITB is made. A tunnel at the proximal fibular attachment site is made over a guide pin. The tunnel diameter matches that of the graft, usually 8–10 mm. The graft is gently tapped into the fibular tunnel and secured with an interference screw or two cortical screws. A guide pin is used to drill the femoral tunnel at an angle of 30°. The tunnel drilled matches the size of the graft. Sutures are place to pull the graft through the femoral tunnel and

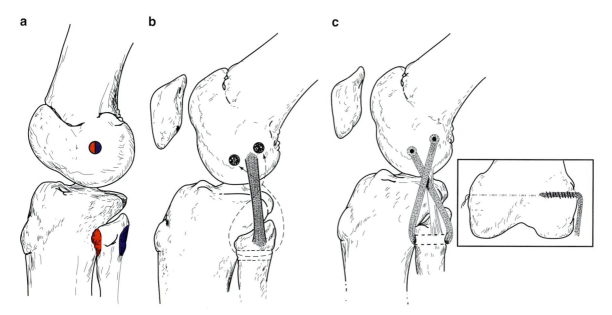

Fig. 6.26 (a) The area anterior to the lateral epicondyle (LCL attachment) is most isometric to the area on the posterior fibular head. The posterior area of the epicondyle is most isometric to the area on the anterior fibular head. (b, c) Larson's "Figure of 8" reconstruction using a soft tissue graft (Reprinted with permission from Roger Larson, personal communication)

the graft is tensioned at 30° of knee flexion using an interference screw (Fig. 6.27).

In the case of severe Grade III varus laxity, or chronic reconstruction of grade III PLRI injuries, our procedure of choice is to use a "split-tailed" Achilles tendon allograft. The senior author developed and has used this procedure since 1983. An entire Achilles tendon is used. The bone block is shaped to a dimension of 20-mm long by 20-mm wide by 10-mm thick. The block is predrilled in the center with a 5 mm drill. An Achilles tendon is split and each arm rolled and sutured to form fusiform grafts that are approximately 6 mm in diameter and 15–20 cm long (Fig. 6.28a). A matching bone segment is resected from the lateral femoral condyle at the level of, and including, the lateral epicondyle. The Achilles bone block is then secured in the defect to the lateral femoral condyle using a 40 mm cancellous bone screw and washer (Fig. 6.28b). Two drill holes are made distally. One courses through the fibular head approximately 2 cm from the tip, and the second passes through the proximal tibia from posterior-to-anterior. The posterior tibial landmark is the posterior tibial tubercle and the anterior landmark is Gerdy's tubercle.

The anterior Achilles limb is passed under the ITB and knee capsule to emerge near the posterior tibial tubercle. It is then passed around a 1 cm tendinous portion of the lateral gastrocnemius muscle near its femoral attachment, and then back into the tibia tunnel to emerge anteriorly near Gerdy's tubercle. The nonisometric condition of this limb is partially compensated for by including a portion of the lateral gastrocnemius muscle.

The posterior Achilles limb passes over the inferior arm and is then passed through the fibular drill hole from posterior-to-anterior. Caution is necessary to avoid a fibular tunnel blowout by drilling too close to the tip of the fibular head. If this occurs, then suture anchors deployed in the proximal fibular cortex can be used to secure the graft. Both arms are secured in their respective tunnels using interference screw fixation with knee at 30° of flexion and neutral rotation. The tails of the graft arms are further secured using a ligament staple or screw and ligament washer (Fig. 6.28c).

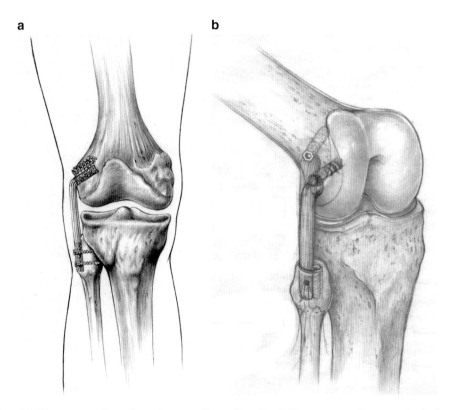

Fig. 6.27 Noyes' LCL reconstruction using a bone-patellar tendon-bone autograft or allograft (Reprinted with permission from Frank Noyes, personal communication)

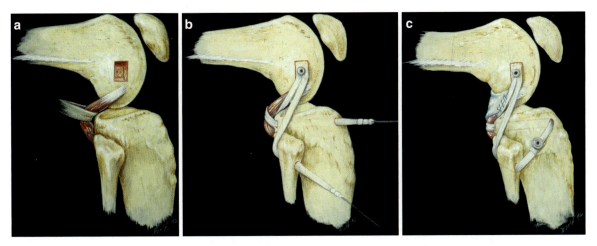

Fig. 6.28 (**a**) Resected bone block from LCL attachment on the lateral femoral condyle. (**b**) Achilles tendon bone block is secured to the femur using 40 mm cancellous bone screw and both arms of the scissor-tail graft are in place. Note the posterior graft also encircles a portion of the lateral gastrocnemius head so as to dampen the nonisometric effects of motion. (**c**) Grafts in place and secured

Postoperative Care

The knee is immobilized in 20° of flexion for 3 weeks in a locked, hinged knee brace. Patellar mobilizations as well as straight leg raises are begun immediately postoperatively. The importance of regaining full extension is stressed to the patient. Active and passive knee motion is initiated at the third week along with quadriceps strengthening. No active knee flexion is allowed until the 12th week. Whenever possible, a brace that places a valgus stress is used. The addition of the exercise bike to the rehabilitation program begins in the nineth postoperative week.

Hints for Avoiding Knee Motion Problems

1. Do not operate on a knee that is warm, swollen, and painful.
2. Do not initiate or exacerbate pain through forceful physical therapy or manipulation.
3. Do not manipulate a knee that is swollen, painful, and warm, with a quadriceps lag and poor quadriceps contraction. The corollary is true. When a patient fails to progress in therapy and their return of motion plateaus, a manipulation is safe at any time as long as the knee is not excessively warm, painful, or swollen.
4. Patella entrapment indicates the requirement of anti-inflammatory medications including oral steroids, the cessation of forceful physical therapy, and the initiation of self-activated quadriceps exercises.
5. An adverse mechanical axis ultimately trumps all soft tissue reconstructions regardless of surgical technique, tissue strength, or quality of fixation.
6. Lack of postoperative extension is exceedingly difficult for both the patient and surgeon. Lack of flexion is an easier opponent. Always immobilize in extension, work on quadriceps strength and extension as a priority. Do not avoid short arch quadriceps exercises.
7. A stiff knee will loosen over time and not tighten (as many believe) as long as pain is avoided, muscles are strengthened, anatomic and isometric ligament surgery is performed, and the patient is not over-or under-rehabilitating.
8. Too-loose of a knee is preferable to a knee that is too tight.

References

1. Green D, Noble P, Bocell J Jr et al (2006) Effect of early full weight-bearing after joint injury on inflammation and cartilage degradation. J Bone Joint Surg Am 88(10):2201-9
2. Paulos L, Rosenberg T, Drawbert J et al (1987) Infrapatellar contracture syndrome. An unrecognized cause of knee stiffness with patella entrapment and patella infera. Am J Sports Med 15(4):331-41

3. Paulos L, Wnorowski D, Greenwald A (1994) Infrapatellar contracture syndrome. Diagnosis, treatment, and long-term followup. Am J Sports Med 22(4):440-9
4. Noyes F, Barber-Westin S, Albright J (2006) An analysis of the causes of failure in 57 consecutive posterolateral operative procedures. Am J Sports Med 34(9):1419-30
5. LeRoy C, Saunders J, Bost F et al (1944) Injuries to the ligaments of the knee joint. J Bone Joint Surg 26-A(3):503-21
6. Miyasaka K, Daniel D, Stone M (1991) The incidence of knee ligament injuries in the general population. Am J Knee Surg 4:3-8
7. Indelicato P (1983) Non-operative treatment of complete tears of the medial collateral ligament of the knee. J Bone Joint Surg 65A(3):323-9
8. Yoshiya S, Kuroda R, Mizuno K et al (2005) Medial collateral ligament reconstruction using autogenous hamstring tendons: technique and results in initial cases. Am J Sports Med 33(9):1380-5
9. Halinen J, Lindahl J, Hirvensalo E et al (2006) Operative and nonoperative treatments of medial collateral ligament rupture with early anterior cruciate ligament reconstruction: a prospective randomized study. Am J Sports Med 34(7):1134-40
10. Sims W, Jacobson K (2004) The posteromedial corner of the knee: medial-sided injury patterns revisited. Am J Sports Med 32(2):337-45
11. Hughston J, Andrews J, Cross M et al (1976) Classification of knee ligament instabilities. Part I. The medial compartment and cruciate ligaments. J Bone Joint Surg 58A(2):159-72
12. Muller W (1983) The Knee: Form, Function and Ligament Reconstruction. Springer-Verlag, New York, NY
13. Warren L, Marshall J, Girgis F (1974) The prime static stabilizer of the medial side of the knee. J Bone Joint Surg Am 56(4):665-74
14. Grood E, Noyes F, Butler D et al (1981) Ligamentous and capsular restraints preventing straight medial and lateral laxity in intact human cadaver knees. J Bone Joint Surg Am 63(8):1257-69
15. Mains D, Andrews J, Stonecipher T (1977) Medial and anterior-posterior ligament stability of the human knee, measured with a stress apparatus. Am J Sports Med 5(4):144-53
16. Gardiner J, Weiss J, Rosenberg T (2001) Strain in the human medial collateral ligament during valgus loading of the knee. Clin Orthop Relat Res 391:266-74
17. Hughston J, Eilers A (1973) The role of the posterior oblique ligament in repairs of acute medial (collateral) ligament tears of the knee. J Bone Joint Surg Am 55(5):923-40
18. Levy I, Torzilli P, Warren R (1982) The effect of medial meniscectomy on anterior-posterior motion of the knee. J Bone Joint Surg Am 64(6):883-8
19. Menschik A (1974) Mechanics of the knee-joint. 1 (author's transl). Z Orthop Ihre Grenzgeb 112(3):481-95
20. Slocum D, Larson R (1968) Rotatory instability of the knee. Its pathogenesis and a clinical test to demonstrate its presence. J Bone Joint Surg Am 50(2):211-25
21. Kennedy J, Fowler P (1971) Medial and anterior instability of the knee. An anatomical and clinical study using stress machines. J Bone Joint Surg 53A(7):1257-70
22. Hughston J (1994) The importance of the posterior oblique ligament in repairs of acute tears of the medial ligaments in knees with and without an associated rupture of the anterior cruciate ligament. Results of long-term follow-up. J Bone Joint Surg Am 76(9):1328-44
23. Paulos L, Rosenberg T, Parker R (1987) The medial knee ligaments: Pathomechanics and surgical repair with emphasis on the external-rotation pivot-shift test. Techn Orthop 2(2):37-46
24. Ellsasser J, Reynolds F, Omohundro J (1974) The nonoperative treatment of collateral ligament injuries of the knee in professional football players. An analysis of seventy-four injuries treated non-operatively and twenty-four injuries treated surgically. J Bone Joint Surg Am 56(6):1185-90
25. Ginsburg J, Ellsasser J (1978) Problem areas in the diagnosis and treatment of ligament injuries of the knee. Clin Orthop Relat Res 132:201-5
26. Kannus P (1988) Long-term results of conservatively treated medial collateral ligament injuries of the knee joint. Clin Orthop Relat Res 226:103-12
27. Jones R, Henley M, Francis P (1986) Nonoperative management of isolated grade III collateral ligament injury in high school football players. Clin Orthop Relat Res 213:137-40
28. Indelicato P (1995) Isolated medial collateral ligament injuries in the knee. J Am Acad Orthop Surg 3(1):9-14
29. Fetto J, Marshall J (1978) Medial collateral ligament injuries of the knee: A rationale for treatment. Clin Orthop Relat Res 132:206-18
30. Indelicato P, Hermansdorfer J, Huegel M (1990) Nonoperative management of complete tears of the medial collateral ligament of the knee in intercollegiate football players. Clin Orthop Relat Res 256:174-7
31. Derscheid G, Garrick J (1981) Medial collateral ligament injuries in football. Nonoperative management of grade I and grade II sprains. Am J Sports Med 9(6):365-8
32. Kannus P, Jarvinen M (1987) Long-term prognosis of non-operatively treated acute knee distortions having primary hemarthrosis without clinical instability. Am J Sports Med 15(2):138-43
33. Frolke J, Oskam J, Vierhout P (1998) Primary reconstruction of the medial collateral ligament in combined injury of the medial collateral and anterior cruciate ligaments. Short-term results. Knee Surg Sports Traumatol Arthrosc 6(2):103-6
34. CAmon J, Saha S (1994) Management of medial collateral ligament laxity. Orthop Clin North Am 25(3):527-32
35. Andersson C, Gillquist J (1992) Treatment of acute isolated and combined ruptures of the anterior cruciate ligament. A long-term follow-up study. Am J Sports Med 20(1):7-12
36. Hillard-Sembell D, Daniel D, Stone M et al (1996) Combined injuries of the anterior cruciate and medial collateral ligaments of the knee. Effect of treatment on stability and function of the joint. J Bone Joint Surg 78A(2):169-76
37. Millett P, Pennock A, Sterett W et al (2004) Early ACL reconstruction in combined ACL-MCL injuries. J Knee Surg 17(2):94-8
38. Noyes F, Barber-Westin S (1995) The treatment of acute combined ruptures of the anterior cruciate and medial ligaments of the knee. Am J Sports Med 23(4):380-9
39. Hughston J, Barrett G (1983) Acute anteromedial rotatory instability. Long-term results of surgical repair. J Bone Joint Surg 65A(2):145-53

40. Shirakura K, Terauchi M, Katayama M et al (2000) The management of medial ligament tears in patients with combined anterior cruciate and medial ligament lesions. Int Orthop 24(2):108-11
41. Lundberg M, Messner K (1996) Long-term prognosis of isolated partial medial collateral ligament ruptures. A ten-year clinical and radiographic evaluation of a prospectively observed group of patients. Am J Sports Med 24(2):160-3
42. Groff Y, Harner C (2003) Medial collateral ligament reconstruction. In: Jackson DW (ed) Master Techniques in Orthopaedic Surgery Reconstructive Knee Surgery, Second edth edn. Lippincott Williams & Wilkins, Philadelphia, pp 193-208
43. Shelbourne K, Patel D (1995) Management of combined injuries of the anterior cruciate and medial collateral ligaments. J Bone Joint Surg 77A:800-6
44. Jacobson K, Chi F (2006) Evaluation and treatment of medial collateral ligament and medial-sided injuries of the knee. Sports Med Arthrosc 14(2):58-66
45. Jaureguito J, Paulos L (1996) Why grafts fail. Clin Orthop Relat Res 325:25-41
46. Shapiro M, Markolf K, Finerman G et al (1991) The effect of section of the medial collateral ligament on force generated in the anterior cruciate ligament. J Bone Joint Surg 73A(2):248-56
47. Petersen W, Laprell H (1999) Combined injuries of the medial collateral ligament and the anterior cruciate ligament. Early ACL reconstruction versus late ACL reconstruction. Arch Orthop Trauma Surg 119(5-6):258-62
48. Harner C, Irrgang J, Paul J et al (1992) Loss of motion after anterior cruciate ligament reconstruction. Am J Sports Med 20:499-506
49. LaPrade R, Engebretsen A, Ly T et al (2007) The anatomy of the medial part of the knee. J Bone Joint Surg Am 89(9):2000-10
50. Grood E, Stowers S, Noyes F (1988) Limits of movement in the human knee. Effect of sectioning the posterior cruciate ligament and posterolateral structures. J Bone Joint Surg Am 70(1):88-97
51. Seebacher J, Inglis A, Marshall J et al (1982) The structure of the posterolateral aspect of the knee. J Bone Joint Surg 64A:536-41
52. Maynard M, Deng X, Wickiewicz T et al (1996) The popliteofibular ligament. Rediscovery of a key element in posterolateral stability. Am J Sports Med 24(3):311-6
53. DeLee J, Riley M, Rockwood C Jr (1983) Acute straight lateral instability of the knee. Am J Sports Med 11(6):404-11
54. Gollehon D, Torzilli P, Warren R (1987) The role of the posterolateral and cruciate ligaments in the stability of the human knee. A biomechanical study. J Bone Joint Surg Am 69(2):233-42
55. Sidles J, Larson R, Garbini J et al (1988) Ligament length relationship in the moving knee. J Orthop Res 6(4):593-610
56. Segond P (1879) Reserches cliniques et experimentales sure es epachernents sanquins de genou par entarse. Progres Med 7:297
57. Larson R, Belfie D (2003) Lateral collateral ligament reconstruction utilizing semitendinosus tendon. Tech in Knee Surg 2(3):190-9
58. Noyes F, Barber-Westin S (2007) Posterolateral knee reconstruction with an anatomical bone-patellar tendon-bone reconstruction of the fibular collateral ligament. Am J Sports Med 35(2):259-73

Editors' Comments (Collateral Ligaments)

Should a screw and post fail at the femoral origin of the MCL consider drilling a tunnel at the level of the medial femoral epicondyle. The tunnel diameter should match the graft size and drilled to a depth of 20–25 mm. A beath pin can then be driven across in a medial to lateral direction and an interference screw that matches the graft size or one size larger should be used. The graft can be tensioned at the femoral side following initial tibial sided fixation. Ensure that the tibial side is affixed at least 7 cm distal to the medial joint line so as not to capture the knee.

If the LCL graft breaks through the fibular head tunnel proximally consider fixing the graft into the fibular head with an interference screw with the graft directed distally into the medullary canal. This should be secured prior to fixation on the femoral side.

For MCL injuries, it is often possible to advance the native tissue and achieve stability without using a graft. An incision is made posterior to the sMCL between the sMCL and the POL; an elevator is used to undermine the attachment site between the sMCL and the epicondylar attachment and a traction suture is used to tension the sMCL and advance it proximally. Fixation of the tensioned ligament is performed with a spiked soft tissue screw and washer, while holding the leg in varus, flexion and internal rotation. We prefer a 17 mm hubcap washer for MCL fixation and a 6.5 mm cancellous screw

When perfoming a MCL procedure at the same sitting as a hamstring harvest for ACL reconstruction, plan ahead to use an incision that will be useful for both procedures, as there is a risk for skin necrosis with a very narrow skin bridge between the two incisions.

When performing a LCL/PL reconstruction, hold the leg in internal rotation and valgus when tightening the graft.

Consider prebending your postop locked hinged knee brace slightly into varus for MCL reconstruction and a valgus prebend for LCL reconstruction. This will help unload your repair.

Be careful with tight bandages or braces postoperatively for LCL reconstruction since this may contribute to risk for peroneal nerve injury. Protect the nerve during surgery, document intact function of the peroneal nerve in the recovery room, and loosen the brace and bandages at first signs of postoperative nerve impairment.

Undiagnosed AMRI as well as PLRI are occasional causes for persistent instability complaints following otherwise successful ACL surgery. Examine all "failed" ACL cases for these instability patterns.

We prefer to protect all collateral ligament surgeries with nonweight bearing for 4-6 weeks since load bearing will likely place a displacement load on the repair/reconstruction. Range of motion is allowed with the hinged brace still in place, but unlocked to further prevent any inadvertent stress to the repair.

Chapter 7
Avoiding and Managing Complications in Osteotomies of the Knee

David A. Vasconcellos, J. Robert Giffin, and Annunziato Amendola

Top 10 Pearls

- Patient selection and compliance during the postoperative rehabilitation is critical to achieving a successful outcome with osteotomy surgery. A trial of an unloader knee brace prior to performing the operation may be beneficial in helping to predict pain relief following the procedure.
- Careful preoperative planning using full-length weight-bearing radiographs (hips to ankles) can help to avoid problems with over- or undercorrection of the deformity.
- Address typical varus deformities on the tibial side, and valgus deformities on the femoral side. However, patients with small (<7.5°) valgus deformities and neutral or varus alignment of the contralateral knee can be more easily addressed on the tibial side.
- Understand the anatomy and place the retractors subperiosteally adjacent to the bone to prevent neurovascular injury.
- Exact positioning of the guide/guide pin is critical. Placement of the osteotomy too close to the joint can contribute to an intra-articular fracture. Do not come any closer than 15 mm to the joint surface with either opening or closing wedge osteotomy.
- Avoid an osteotomy that is too oblique, especially for large corrections, as this causes instability: maintain a 15–20° angle cut for better opposition and stability.
- Cautious performance of the osteotomy and taking fluoroscopic images will help to ensure that the osteotomy is in the appropriate location and heading in the correct direction. Knowing the length of the osteotomy, how far the osteotomes are engaged in the bone, and using fluoroscopic imaging will help to avoid penetrating the opposite cortex and creating an unstable osteotomy.
- When performing an opening wedge osteotomy, an intact posterior/posterolateral cortex is the most common reason for the osteotomy not to open. Place an osteotome centrally to open the site, and then work the cortex with a narrow osteotome.
- For a high tibial osteotomy, be aware of how plate placement influences the posterior tibial slope. To avoid inadvertent changes of the slope in the sagittal plane, the osteotomy gap should narrow from back to front. The anterior tibial gap should be one-half of the posteromedial gap. The tendency with a closing wedge osteotomy is to remove more bone anteriorly, thus decreasing the slope.
- Individualize rehabilitation. For more stable osteotomies (closing wedge, smaller opening wedge) the rehabilitation can be more aggressive than large or unstable corrections.

D.A. Vasconcellos
Department of Orthopedics and Rehabilitation, University of Iowa Hospitals and Clinics, 200 Hawkins Drive, Iowa City, IA, 52442, USA
e-mail: davevasco@gmail.com

J.R. Giffin
Department of Orthopedic Surgery, University of Western Ontario, London, OntarioN, Canada

A. Amendola (✉)
Department of Orthopedics and Rehabilitation, University of Iowa Hospitals and Clinics, Iowa City, IAowa, USA
e-mail: ned-amendola@uiowa.edu

Introduction and Background

Osteotomies around the knee are technically demanding surgical procedures requiring careful preoperative planning and precise surgical technique. When procedures

Table 7.1 Knee osteotomy complications

	Isolated procedure (N=44)	Combined procedure (N=35)	All procedures (N=79)	All % comp
Major complications				
Intra-articular fracture	1	1	2	2.5%
Compartment syndrome	1	0	1	1.3%
Deep infection	1	0	1	1.3%
Exostosis	1	1	2	2.5%
Hardware failure	3	1	4	5.1%
Correction failure	1	1	2	2.5%
Contracture	2	2	4	5.1%
Neuroma	0	1	1	1.3%
Nonunion	0	0	0	0.0%
Total	10	7	17	21.5%
Minor complications				
Superficial infection	6	2	8	10.1%
Painful hardware	3	6	9	11.4%
Delayed union	3	0	3	3.8%
Hematoma	4	0	4	5.1%
Anterior knee pain	10	4	14	17.7%
Pes anserinus pain	1	1	2	2.5%
Total	27	13	40	50.6%

do not go as planned, it is important that the surgeon recognizes the problem and/or complication and has an appropriate course of action to rectify the situation. In this chapter, the complications associated with both high tibial osteotomies and distal femoral osteotomies of the knee will be reviewed. Strategies for prevention and management of these complications will be discussed.

High tibial osteotomy (HTO) and distal femoral osteotomy (DFO) are both widely accepted treatment options for young, active patients with symptomatic medial or lateral compartment gonarthrosis that is associated with a varus or valgus malaligned lower extremity. Realignment surgery may also performed in conjunction with other surgical procedures aimed at addressing concomitant ligamentous instability, meniscal deficiency, patellar maltracking, and chondral defects. Failure to recognize and/or address an underlying malalignment problem may lead to premature failure of other reconstructive surgical procedures about the knee due to mechanical overload.

In a recent review at the University of Iowa, the overall incidence of major complications following knee osteotomy surgery was 18%. Twenty nine percent of the patients had minor complications. However, it was interesting to note that the complication rate was not statistically different between patients undergoing isolated realignment surgery vs. combined procedures, or with HTO compared with DFO. The most common major complication in this cohort of patients was failure of hardware 5% (Table 7.1).[1] Out of 79 cases, there were two cases of intra-articular fracture (2.5%), and failure of proper correction in two cases (2.5%). This complication rate seems to be consistent with other studies published in the literature.

Several studies report on the incidence of complications with osteotomies. In one series of 24 distal femoral varus osteotomies that were followed long term, the authors report five complications in four patients which includes one patient with stiffness requiring manipulation, one with superficial wound infection resolving with intravenous antibiotics, and one with pulmonary embolus. One patient had failure of fixation which was revised and then suffered a fracture proximal to the plate leading to a second revision to a total knee arthroplasty (TKA) with a long-stemmed component.[2] Another study of 30 patients with distal femoral osteotomies had one case of nonunion treated with iliac crest bone grafting, and no cases of stiffness which was related to their early rehab program. They had several cases of screw breakage which did not affect healing at the osteotomy site.[3]

The risk of intra-articular fracture has been reported to be as high as 11% with opening wedge HTO[4] and 10–20% with lateral closing wedge HTO.[5]

Undercorrection or overcorrection of deformities may be more common than we think. Marti reports that only about half of the patients in their series having an opening wedge had the desired amount of coronal correction restoring the desired position of the mechanical axis.

Thirty-one percent were undercorrected and 19% were overcorrected.[6] This issue is of particular importance for sagittal (cruciate) instability of the knee, to prevent aggravating existing ACL or PCL laxity.

The risk of infection after osteotomy is low. The risk is higher for techniques that employ external fixation. Pins entering the joint capsule around the knee theoretically may contaminate the joint with a simple pin tract infection. Superficial infection is a common complication when performing a HTO using a dynamic axial external fixator. Superficial infection is reported to occur in 37–50% of cases.[7,8] Most of these superficial infections were controlled with antibiotics and pin care. Failure secondary to osteomyelitis of the proximal tibia was reported in one patient at a rate of 1.3%.[8] A large series of 308 open-wedge osteotomies using a hemicallotasis technique reported a 51% incidence of pin tract infections of which 96% were minor and responded to antibiotic treatment and pin site care. The other 4% required an irrigation and debridement. This series reported one case of septic arthritis.[9]

It is that important that our joint preserving procedures or the complications that may come with them do not complicate future salvage options. TKA may be performed as a salvage operation for failed osteotomy surgery. However, revision osteotomy surgery should be considered in the young patient, where arthroplasty is not a viable option. Deep infection is one of the worst complications that could complicate future arthroplasty by increasing the risk for infection of implants. This must especially be considered in osteotomy techniques employing external fixation where the risk of superficial infection and possibly deep infection may be higher. HTOs are thought to make exposure for subsequent arthroplasty more difficult. Some authors suggest that TKA after DFO is more difficult secondary to scarring, while other authors suggest that a prior DFO to correct valgus alignment may make TKA easier to perform because it makes soft tissue balancing easier and patellar tracking better compared to a TKA performed in a valgus knee.[2] The results of TKA after both HTO and DFO are divided.[10,11]

Functional Anatomy at Risk

Popliteal artery
Tibial nerve
Peroneal nerve
Posterior tibial nerve
Saphenous nerve
Articular cartilage

Complications

Undercorrection and Overcorrection

Failure to accurately correct the deformity can occur for a variety of reasons. Improper preoperative planning, failed technical execution, and patient noncompliance during postoperative rehabilitation are all possible reasons that the surgeon may not achieve the desired correction when performing osteotomy surgery (Fig. 7.1a, b). Undercorrection of the deformity will not effectively shift weight away from the affected compartment and may result in a poor outcome and possible recurrence of the patient's deformity. However, excessive overcorrection is also not tolerated well by patients, especially patients with excessive ligamentous laxity or collateral instability, and may lead to early failure as well (Fig. 7.2a, b). Revision surgery is required to correct the coronal malalignment and re-establish the proper mechanical alignment.

Typical varus deformities are addressed on the tibial side, and valgus deformities on the femoral side. However, patients with small valgus deformities (<7.5°) and neutral or varus alignment of the contralateral knee can be more easily addressed on the tibial side. Attempting to correct a large valgus deformity on the tibial side can lead to joint line obliquity (Fig. 7.3).

Proper preoperative planning is the first key to obtaining the correct alignment. Planning begins with obtaining appropriate radiographs to assess limb deformity. Bilateral AP weight-bearing radiographs in full extension, bilateral PA weight-bearing radiographs at 45° of flexion, lateral, and skyline films should be obtained to assess the condition of the knee. A full-length standing AP radiograph of the entire lower extremity, centered at the knee, provides a comprehensive analysis of limb alignment.[12] Radiographs taken in the supine position may underestimate deformity and required correction, while single limb standing views may overestimate the deformity and correction especially in patients with ligamentous instability.[13] The mechanical axis is a straight line drawn from the center of the hip to the center of the ankle and shows where

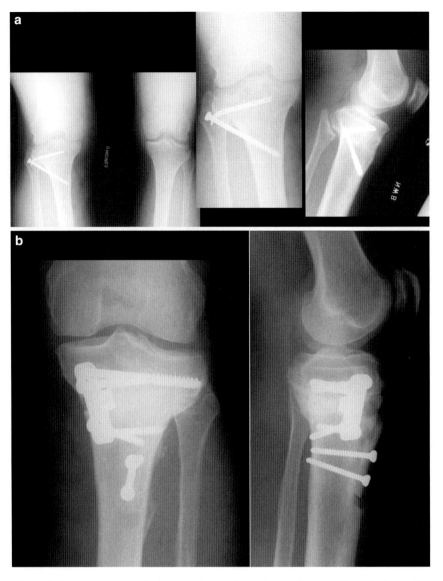

Fig. 7.1 (**a**) AP radiograph demonstrates coronal overcorrection of a lateral closing wedge HTO into excessive valgus and hyperextension. There is poor fixation of the osteotomy with a 1/3 tubular plate and screw. Lateral radiograph shows a hyperextension deformity (decreased tibial slope). (**b**) Biplanar opening wedge osteotomy with tibial tubercle osteotomy to correct the malalignment

the weight passes through the knee joint. The valgus producing HTO is planned to place the weight-bearing line to fall at a selected position approximately 62.5% across the width of the tibial plateau from medial to lateral, which generally corresponds to the tip of the lateral tibial spine. For varus producing distal femoral osteotomies, this is corrected to the medial tibial spine (62.5% from lateral to medial). The contribution of excessive soft tissue laxity or collateral ligament injury should be evaluated and considered during correction calculations to avoid excessive overcorrection.[14,15]

It can be very difficult to accurately assess limb alignment in the operating room. Careful preoperative planning from quality full-length double standing radiographs is essential to achieving acceptable postoperative correction. Visual inspection of the alignment of the lower extremity from the foot of the operating table by experienced surgeons also helps to achieve the

7 Avoiding and Managing Complications in Osteotomies of the Knee

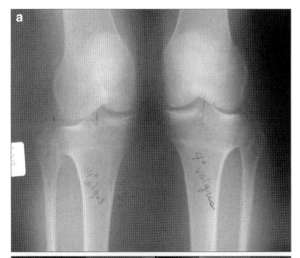

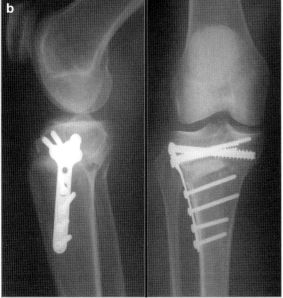

Fig. 7.2 (**a**) Radiographs after bilateral closing wedge HTOs with overcorrection of right knee into excessive valgus. (**b**) Revision with a lateral opening wedge high tibial osteotomy

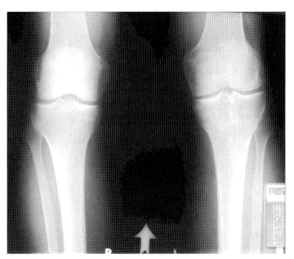

Fig. 7.3 The left knee had a previous opening wedge tibial osteotomy for valgus malalignment. The large correction created an oblique joint line

desired correction. The surgeon also needs to appreciate how axial rotation of the extremity will change the appearance of the leg in the coronal plane.[16]

Intraoperative fluoroscopy with the use of the electrocautery cord can be a useful tool for assessing lower limb alignment. The method is less reliable in patients who are obese or have pathologic laxity of the knee joint. The fluoroscopic method involves extending a taut electrocautery cord from the center of the hip to the center of the ankle and represents the mechanical axis of the limb. An AP image of the knee is obtained, and the alignment of the cord in relation to the center of the knee is used to assess correction. The method shows a strong correlation with standing AP lower extremity films.[17] However, this technique is potentially subject to parallax error from the fluoroscopic beam and altering the rotation of the extremity during measurement can lead to pitfalls.

The surgeon can also place axial weight-bearing against the foot with the knee at 10° of flexion to ensure that there is closure of both the medial and the lateral knee joint compartments under fluoroscopy. Another option is to use the large c-arm with a radiolucent table to visualize the hip, knee, and ankle joints. An alignment rod is then used intraoperatively both before and after correction.

Closing wedge HTO has the inherent difficulty of removing a precisely sized wedge of bone. The surgeon must take into account several factors such as the saw blade thickness and the compression of the cancellous bone. The surgeon must also realize that the distal portion of the osteotomy invaginates into the proximal cancellous piece easily if not cautious. Technical error when performing the closing wedge can easily lead to either overcorrection or undercorrection of the deformity.

Opening wedge osteotomy deals with some of the pitfalls from closing wedge, but does present with some of its own disadvantages. The opening wedge, with one bone cut, allows for easier adjustment and control of the angle of correction intraoperatively.

For distal femoral osteotomies either an opening wedge or closing wedge osteotomy may be performed. The correction for the opening wedge DFO is also easy to adjust similar to that of the HTO. The commonly utilized closing wedge DFO technique utilizes a blade-plate. The blade portion of the 90° bladeplate is placed parallel to the joint line, which ensures correction to 0° of varus. A minimal amount of bone needs to be removed for the closing wedge, because as the plate is applied to the shaft the diaphyseal spike of bone is compressed into the cancellous metaphyseal bone achieving the proper amount of correction with the joint line perpendicular to the femoral shaft.[18]

Wang suggests that after a medial closing wedge DFO that there can be a loss of position of the blade-plate in patients with osteopenia leading to coronal malalignment. In several cases they had to take their blade-plate out, bend it to correct for varus deformity, and then reinsert it. Currently, they recommend a wedge of cortical bone from the osteotomy site be placed in the slot between the blade and the medial femoral condyle. They have not had to revise any of their patients in this clinical situation after using this technique. They also suggest the addition of a derotation screw that transfixes the medial cortex of the proximal fragment obliquely to the lateral cortex of the distal fragment after osteosynthesis. It is placed either through or outside the plate and is intended to provide additional rotational stability for the early rehabilitation program.[19] We do not have any experience with these techniques.

Patella Baja

Lateral closing wedge HTO has been associated with a high incidence of postoperative patella baja.[20] An association exists between patella baja and anterior knee pain. It also may make converting to TKA more technically difficult. The patella baja is not a result of the change in bony architecture after a lateral closing wedge HTO, but is from the contracture of the infra patellar tissue and tendon itself. These findings were often in the setting of cast immobilization following HTO. Rigid internal fixation allows for early aggressive postoperative motion that may help to minimize scarring and shortening of the patellar tendon that can occur following HTO.[21,22]

Changes in the bony structure of the tibia induced by HTO affect patellar height. Lateral closing wedge osteotomy increases patellar height, while medial opening wedge osteotomy performed above the tibial tubercle lowers patellar height by raising the joint line. This usually happens in the absence of any shortening of the patellar tendon. A 64% incidence of patella baja has been reported with opening wedge HTO.[23] Other studies suggest that patellar height is not significantly affected when proper attention is given to maintaining the proper tibial slope. When the tibial slope is properly maintained there is little change in the anterior gap at the osteotomy site and therefore little change in the patellar height.[24]

Appropriate technique, correction, and rigid internal fixation allows for aggressive physical therapy to obtain range of motion and decrease the risk of arthrofibrosis. If coronal alignment correction is the goal of the procedure, pay close attention to maintaining the proper tibial slope to avoid bony impingement or alteration of patellar height.

Fracture – Unstable Hinge

Propagation of the osteotomy through the opposite cortex during osteotomy is undesirable because it creates an unstable hinge (Fig. 7.4). This creates translational

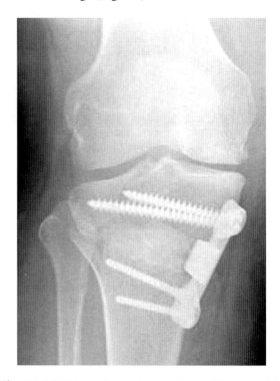

Fig. 7.4 Medial opening wedge osteotomy with an unstable lateral hinge. Note fracture through the lateral tibial cortex

instability and may affect the ability of the fixation technique to afford the desired stability. This is not as critical with closing wedge osteotomies. The proximal fragment gets destabilized and if not addressed can potentially lead to malunion, nonunion, or hardware failure. It is important to recognize this problem intraoperatively and to have a strategy to reduce and stabilize the fragment.

To prevent this problem, a calibrated guide pin can be used to assess the length of the osteotomy. Knowing the length of the osteotomy as well as the depth of penetration of the osteotomes should help avoid placing the osteotomes too far. Second, periodic checks of the osteotomy should be made under fluoroscopy to avoid penetration of the opposite cortex. The osteotome should be inserted to about 1 cm away from the opposite cortex. It is important to take time on this step to avoid subsequent problems.

If you do penetrate the opposite cortex and have an unstable hinge, there are several options. It is important that the fixation device is strong enough to provide the additional stability necessary in this situation. For HTOs or DFOs the opposite side can be approached, and then staples (Fig. 7.5), a 1/3 tubular plate (Fig. 7.6), or a figure of 8 plate can be applied to recreate the hinge. The fixation can then be carried out as originally planned. A second strategy would be to obtain a good reduction of the fragment, pin it in place if necessary, and then apply a more substantial fixation device, i.e., a sturdier plate on the medial or lateral side depending on the type of osteotomy. Consideration could be given to using a locking type of plate, a femoral plate on the tibia, or a standard proximal tibia or distal femoral AO plate. As long as the reduction is obtained before applying the plate, a locking plate alone may help stabilize the fragment without the need for double-sided plating.

For closing wedge osteotomies instability of the fragment is less problematic. The fragment should be reduced taking care to assess the translation and the

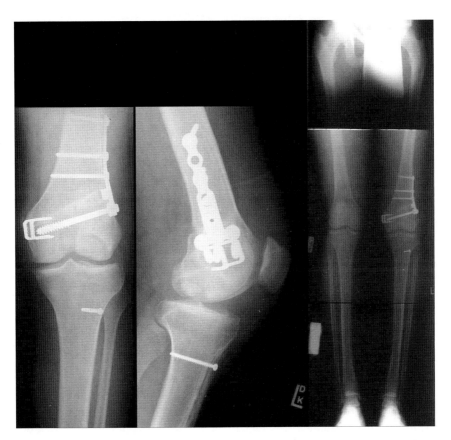

Fig. 7.5 Radiographs following a distal femoral lateral opening wedge osteotomy complicated by fracture of the medial cortex. The unstable hinge was stabilized by the application of two Richards staples placed on the medial side. The long leg film shows reestablishment of good alignment

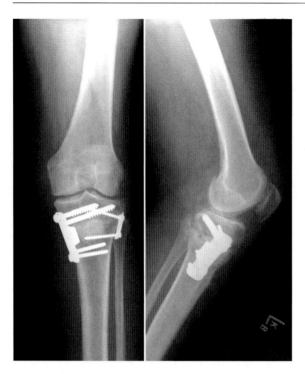

Fig. 7.6 Medial opening wedge osteotomy with an unstable hinge that was stabilized with a three hole 1/3 tubular plate on the lateral side

rotation of the fragment. Hardware can then be usually applied in the standard fashion, although delayed unions and nonunions have been described with closing wedge osteotomies as well. Staples have traditionally been utilized in the literature, but it seems plating closing wedges laterally provides greater stability.

Intra-articular Fracture

Intra-articular fracture during osteotomy is a severe complication given the potential for creating an intra-articular step-off within the knee joint. The risk is usually due to the guide pin being positioned too close to the joint, leaving too little metaphyseal cancellous bone between the osteotomy and the joint surface. It also may be from failure to completely interrupt the posterior or the anterior cortex.[25]

For an opening wedge osteotomy, taking a meticulous approach to completely make all the osteotomy cuts, before attempting to open the osteotomy, is essential. First, a calibrated guide pin is placed along the intended path of the osteotomy and acts as a guide for performing the osteotomy. This serves not only to give an approximate length of the osteotomy, but also to protect the osteotomes from migration toward the joint and create an intra-articular fracture. The microsagittal saw is then used to start the osteotomy by making a cortical cut on the side of the pin away from the joint. The pin protects the instruments from straying too close to the joint. This is then followed by a wide, thin, flexible AO osteotome systematically working across the bone from anterior to posterior. As much of the osteotomy as possible should be done with the thin osteotomes. The solid, broad, but thin osteotomes are then used to complete the osteotomy. Our early experience, intra-articular fractures were caused by using thicker, traditional osteotomes. Intermittent fluoroscopic images are used to check to make sure that the osteotomy does not proceed too far and that it stays on the intended path. The bevel of the osteotome is always placed away from the joint with the flat edge right up against the guidepin. The 1-cm rule is followed – 1 cm of cortex is left intact on the opposite cortex to act as a hinge, and the osteotomy should stop at a very minimum of 1 cm (preferably 1.5 cm) away from the joint line (some authors even say no closer than 2 cm). Creating a fragment too thin will create a higher chance of propagating an intra-articular fracture. A useful technique to ensure completeness of the osteotomy is to place a broad osteotome centrally to open the osteotomy slightly, and then work with a long, thin osteotome along the anterior and the posterior cortices. The mobility of the osteotomy is checked by gently manipulating the leg. Ensure that the osteotomy is mobile and opens slightly before proceeding with the wedge osteotome. If the osteotomy seems incomplete, then check again with the narrow osteotomes anteriorly and posteriorly. "Stacking osteotomes" can also be used to encourage mobility in the osteotomy. A tapered calibrated osteotome is then engaged in the osteotomy site. The tapered osteotome is kept in line with the osteotomy and then is slowly advanced (roughly 5 mm/min) to allow for gradual opening of the osteotomy. Gradual opening or closing of the osteotomy allows for stress relaxation of the intact far cortex to occur. Any forceful completion or opening of the osteotomy should be avoided.

For a closing wedge osteotomy, an angular cutting guide can be used or a specific-size wedge can be removed. Our preferred technique is to remove the outer cortex and a large portion of the wedge with saw cuts, then remove the opposite half with a combination or curettes, rongeurs, and osteotomes before closing the osteotomy. Using a spinal rongeur under direct vision to remove the posterior cortex is very safe and ensures completion of the osteotomy before closing. Otherwise, there is a significant risk for intra-articular fracture. It is important to check the position of the retractors to ensure soft tissue protection and to cut the anterior and the posterior cortices fully to within 1 cm of the opposite cortex.

If an intra-articular fracture does occur, then several factors must be taken into account. The type of osteotomy, whether the osteotomy is complete or not, and whether the fracture is displaced or nondisplaced are all considerations. Usually these fractures are not displaced if the fracture is recognized as soon as it happens. If the intra-articular fragment is displaced, priority must be given to reestablishment of the joint surface. The joint is reduced and then fixed with multiple screws. If the osteotomy is not completed, then the intra-articular fracture is fixed with multiple screws and if the osteotomy is completed, then standard fixation is applied avoiding the previously placed screws. If there is a nondisplaced fracture in a closing wedge osteotomy and the osteotomy is completed and closed, standard fixation can be applied since the fracture is stable. Consideration should be given to placing screws across the fracture but is not mandatory. In the other scenarios with a nondisplaced fracture, the situation is unstable and the potential for displacement exists. Screws should be placed across the fracture to prevent displacement. In an opening wedge, the fragment is not supported well and potentially unstable so screws should be placed, the osteotomy finished if it is not, and then fixation applied. Screws should also be placed across a nondisplaced fracture for a closing wedge when the osteotomy is not yet completed. After fixation of the fragment is obtained, the osteotomy can then be completed, closed, and fixation applied decreasing the risk for displacing the fragment. For tibial osteotomies, the screws should be placed from the lateral side to obtain good purchase in the bigger medial fragment, as well as avoid potential injury to the peroneal nerve.

Intra-articular fractures that occur with an opening wedge osteotomy are usually not displaced. However, the proximal fragment should be fixed with multiple rafter screws placed from the lateral side under the joint surface (Fig. 7.7). After the fracture is stabilized, the osteotomy can be resumed, being careful to avoid the screws.

Closing wedge osteotomies usually cause a "steeple type" of fracture deformity of the proximal tibia. This

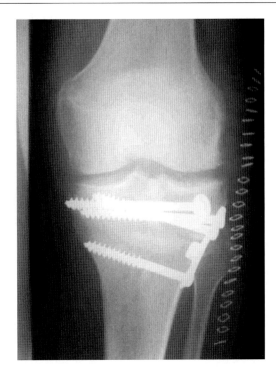

Fig. 7.7 Lateral opening wedge HTO complicated by a nondisplaced intra-articular fracture during surgery. Two screws across the tibial plateau were used to stabilize the fracture

usually occurs as you are trying to close the osteotomy site, before the osteotomy is completed. In the case of intra-articular fracture, the joint should be reduced, and screws placed across the proximal fragment from the lateral side. The osteotomy will need to be finished on the opposite side. When mobility is obtained, the osteotomy is then closed and standard fixation is applied.

Alteration in Sagittal Slope

When performing a HTO, utilizing any technique, inadvertent alterations in the sagittal slope can occur. The normal posterior tibial slope is 0-10°. The tendency with closing wedge osteotomy is to close the osteotomy anteriorly more than posteriorly, thus decreasing the slope (Fig. 7.8). The tendency is the opposite with the opening wedge HTO, where opening the wedge more anteriorly than posteriorly often occurs because the surgeon is working on the anteromedial tibia, and not medial to lateral, which is more difficult.

With opening wedge osteotomy, one needs to pay attention to the slope and any alteration can be avoided.

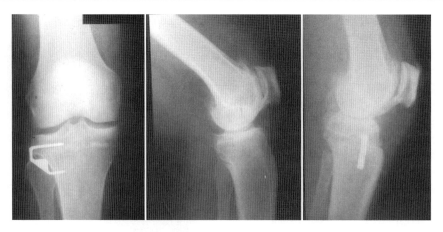

Fig. 7.8 Closing wedge HTO with resection of the proximal fibula and fixation with a single Richards staple complicated by a decrease in the tibial slope. AP view shows excellent coronal correction. Comparison of the preoperative and postoperative lateral radiographs demonstrates a decrease in the tibial slope

The line of the osteotomy should parallel the posterior slope and not run strictly perpendicular to the shaft in the sagittal plane. Since the tibia is triangular in cross section with apex anterior, the size of the wedge opening anteriorly at the tubercle should be less than that of the posteromedial corner to avoid changing the tibial slope. A general rule is that the anterior tibial gap should be one-half of the posteromedial gap. If the gap is anteriorly equal to the gap at the posteromedial corner, the posterior slope of the tibia will be inadvertently increased. A gap error of a single millimeter will result in approximately 2° of change in the posterior tibial slope.[26] The sagittal slope can be deliberately altered in instability patterns to decrease tibial translations and assist with knee stability. A decreased posterior tibial slope will decrease anterior tibial translation in the presence of anterior cruciate ligament (ACL) deficiency. In the posterior cruciate ligament (PCL) deficient knee, increasing the tibial slope can be beneficial by increasing anterior tibial translation.[27,28]

The slope is adjusted by the type of plate used and its positioning. Placing the knee in full extension or hyperextension when applying fixation will allow closure of the gap anteriorly. A tapered Arthrex plate placed at the posteromedial corner of the tibia helps avoid inadvertent changes to the tibial slope and prevents overcorrection in the coronal plane that may occur when the plate is placed more anteriorly.

If a change in the tibial slope is detected intraoperatively, the positioning of the plate should first be assessed. Opening wedge HTO tends to inadvertently increase posterior tibial slope.[6] The most common mistake is that the plate is placed too far anterior causing an increase in the posterior tibial slope. The plate can be adjusted to sit more posteriorly. Consideration can be given to using a tapered plate if one is not already being used.

With closing wedge osteotomy, the most common alteration is to decrease the posterior slope because there is more bone resected anteriorly, or the wedge is not closed posteriorly because the fibula is preventing the osteotomy to close. Many techniques have been described to prevent the latter: incise the tib fib joint to allow mobility, resect the proximal tib fib joint (Coventry), resect the proximal fibula, or perform a fibular osteotomy distally (Maquet, Kettlecamp). All these procedures put the peroneal nerve at risk; so many surgeons try to avoid doing anything to the proximal fibula, thus commonly leading to decreased slope. Therefore following a closing wedge osteotomy, one must ensure the osteotomy is closed posteriorly with fluoroscopy in order to maintain the proper sagittal alignment.

If a change in the tibial slope is detected postoperatively it is generally an issue if it prevents full knee extension because of increased slope, or if it accentuates a cruciate instability pattern. Pathologic changes in the slope requiring corrective osteotomy may present with ligament deficiency and instability or the inability to regain full extension. The fixed flexion contracture and impingement can also cause anterior knee pain.

Attention must also be given to the sagittal alignment in a DFO (Fig. 7.9). The osteotomy must be oriented

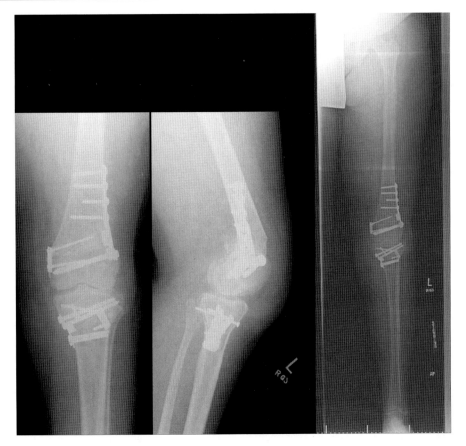

Fig. 7.9 Double osteotomy of the femur and tibia complicated by sagittal plane malalignment of the distal femur. The AP radiograph demonstrates evidence of an unstable osteotomy. This was corrected with additional medial fixation. The unstable osteotomy allowed flexion to occur at the femoral osteotomy site as seen on the lateral radiograph

in the sagittal plane perpendicular to the longitudinal axis of the femur. This allows the long arm of the plate to remain completely in contact with the bone in the center of the diaphysis. The spacer tooth of the Arthrex plate forms a right angle with the plate. If the osteotomy cut in the sagittal plane is oblique the plate will not conform to the femoral shaft. This can potentially lead to screw or plate failure, collapse of the osteotomy, malunion, or nonunion.[25] Instability at the osteotomy site can lead to potential malalignment in all planes and needs to be carefully addressed intraoperatively.

Vascular Injury

Injury to the popliteal artery is an extremely rare complication but has been reported in the literature. Several studies confirm that the popliteal artery lies very close to the posterior cortex of the proximal tibia and is in danger if a saw or osteotome strays from the bone. The popliteal artery lies from 4 to 11 mm from the posterior tibial cortex with the knee in full extension. In addition, the popliteal artery does not reliably move away from the tibia with knee flexion.[29] This been confirmed with MRI.[30]

The posterior retractor must be placed immediately adjacent to the tibia to protect the popliteal artery. The osteotomes should be directed in the medial and lateral direction, and avoid going posterior. Opening the osteotomy up with an osteotome centrally and then working the back cortex with a narrow osteotome should allow for better feel that the osteotome is staying along the posterior cortex.

When performing a DFO, a posterior Homan retractor should be utilized and the leg should remain gently flexed to protect the artery, however, knee position may not change the proximity of the artery.

Generally, the tourniquet is inflated for the procedure, but certainly can be done without a tourniquet if there are any concerns about vascularity. After the tourniquet is released if profuse arterial bleeding is encountered a vascular injury is suspected. Further detailed evaluation is necessary and a vascular surgeon may be consulted. With stability of the osteotomy, the knee can be manipulated and positioned for optimal visualization as desired by the surgeon.

Nerve Injury

The peroneal nerve is the structure at most risk. It can be injured directly or indirectly. Direct injury can be with a saw, knife, pin, screw, or other surgical instrument at the time of surgery. Indirect injury can occur from a compressive dressing, or postoperative compartment syndrome. The dome tibial osteotomy has been associated with injury to the posterior tibial nerve.[31]

Nerve injury after opening wedge HTO has been reported in up to 15% of patients in some reports,[32] but most series demonstrate the nerve injury after opening wedge osteotomy appears to be extremely rare.

Use of a fibular osteotomy, common with a lateral closing wedge HTO, has been linked to peroneal nerve injury. The highest risk region for damage to the motor branches of the peroneal nerve is 30 mm distal to the fibular head; At 68–153 mm distal to the fibular head it is again at risk. Osteotomy in the vicinity of the head of the fibula is associated with a higher rate of peroneal nerve palsy than fibular osteotomy performed more than 15 cm distal to the head of the fibula. The superficial peroneal nerve is at risk with more distal osteotomies.[33]

When doing any sort of fibular osteotomy, understanding the anatomy of the peroneal nerve is a prerequisite, and it should be protected through the entire case.

When performing a medial opening wedge HTO, there is no need to perform a fibular osteotomy. However, there is still a potential for peroneal nerve deficits.[32] Some deficits have been related to increased pressure in the anterior compartment.

If there is a peroneal nerve deficit, then the decision must be made whether the cause is likely stems from a neuropraxia or neurotmesis. If it is possible that the nerve may have been severed, then it should be surgically explored and repaired. If neuropraxia is suspected, then the patient should be closely monitored. A patient should be placed in an AFO until return of peroneal motor function to prevent ankle contracture. EMGs and nerve conduction studies should be performed at 4–6 weeks to look for evidence of reinnervation. If return is unlikely, consideration can be given to a posterior tibialis tendon transfer to provide dorsiflexion and eversion of the foot.

Compartment Syndrome

Compartment syndrome is a rare but serious problem. This has been documented and associated with closing wedge osteotomy, with the lateral approach and bleeding into the anterolateral compartment. Early diagnosis and treatment are essential. If the patient exhibits pain out of proportion to the physical examination postoperatively and pain with passive motion of the foot and toes, the diagnosis should be made and then the appropriate treatment should be instituted. Generally these patient's are postoperatively medicated and examination may not be clear. If there is any suspicion, then compartment pressures should be measured. If elevated, the patient should be emergently taken for surgical decompression. Because of the potential for epidural anesthesia or nerve blocks to mask the symptoms of a compartment syndrome, close observation and routine neurovascular checks are essential in the postoperative period.

Infection

The incidence of deep infection after osteotomy is 0–4%.[34] Superficial infections are common with techniques involving the use of an external fixator. Pin tract infections have been reported in as many as 25–50% of these patients.[8] Pin tract infections are typically superficial and respond well to pin care and oral antibiotics. Deep infections require debridement and long-term IV antibiotics for at least 6 weeks. Many patients having an osteotomy will need joint replacement in the future. It is important to avoid infection so that the risk of infection with future joint replacement is minimized.

Preoperative antibiotics should be administered within 1 h of the surgical procedure. It is recommended to continue antibiotics in the hospital for the next 16-24 h. Meticulous attention to sterile technique should be carried out. Any pin tract infection should be addressed promptly. Any deep infection after osteotomy should be treated in accordance with the principles used to treat an infected fracture – to achieve bone union and eradicate the infection.

Delayed Union/Malunion

Nonunion is uncommon after closing wedge osteotomy because of opposed cancellous surfaces. It is more common after an opening wedge osteotomy, where healing must traverse a space filled with bone graft or bone graft substitute (Fig. 7.10a, b). Large angular corrections are a concern with this technique partly due to the risk of nonunion. If the angular correction is greater than 20°, one should consider correcting the angular deformity using an external fixation frame and distraction osteogenesis.

If there is no evidence of bony union at 3 months, consideration should be given to repeat bone grafting to stimulate healing. The use of autograft bone should be considered. Patient risk factors for nonunion include tobacco use and diabetes. Large corrections may be a relative contraindication in this patient population.

Failure of Fixation

The cause of failure of fixation is multifactorial. It can be related to a lack of the necessary stability required for an osteotomy, especially in the case of an unstable one. If a plate is not applied properly it may lead to either loss of fixation points or may cause malalignment (Fig. 7.11). A race occurs between the healing of the osteotomy site and hardware failure due to repetitive stresses. If the osteotomy site does not heal, continued stress and micromotion will lead to hardware failure. Patient factors that effect bone healing may play a role. Patient compliance is certainly an issue, as early weight-bearing may not be tolerated by the construct. Poor bone density or quality may make the purchase of screws poor and lead to screw cutout.

To optimize fixation in cancellous bone, we recommend using fully threaded cancellous screws to maximize screw purchase. If fixation of screws is tentative, attempts should be made to redirect the screws to obtain better purchase or replace the screws with a larger sized screw. If good fixation is still unattainable, usually a result of poor bone quality, then conversion to a locked construct or a blade plate is recommended. A larger or longer plate with more points of fixation can be used. If the construct is felt to have borderline fixation, consideration could be given to applying a second small plate to augment stability. In the very rare case that fixation was still problematic; a ringed external fixator could be applied.

When failure of fixation does occur postoperatively, revision plating and bone grafting will need to be performed. A more rigid construct with autograft bone grafting is usually incorporated to optimize healing (Fig. 7.12a, b).

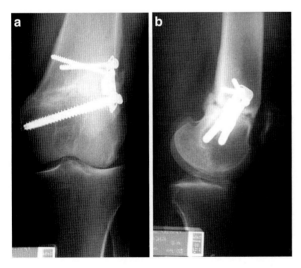

Fig. 7.10 (**a**) AP and (**b**) Lateral of a nonunion after distal femoral lateral opening wedge osteotomy. The tibial Puddhu plate that was utilized provided inadequate fixation

Symptomatic/Retained Hardware

Hardware becomes symptomatic in a small percentage of patients, and in these cases hardware can be removed. Hardware does not need to be routinely removed.

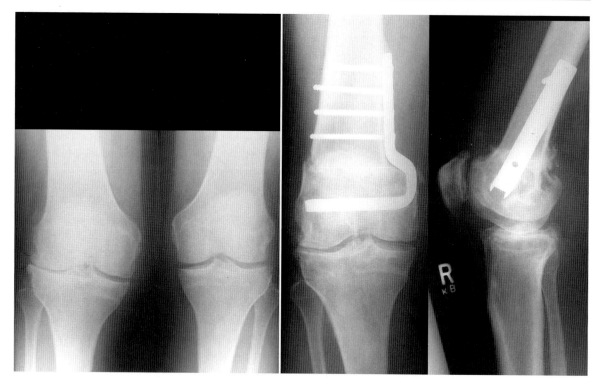

Fig. 7.11 Preoperative radiographs show wear of the lateral compartment with valgus alignment. Realignment was performed with a medial closing wedge osteotomy with a blade plate. The lateral post-op radiograph demonstrates a common problem that occurs with plate application when the blade is not placed perpendicular to the axis of the femur where the proximal plate lies off of the femoral shaft. This can potentially lead to a loss of fixation proximally. If the blade is not perpendicular to the femur and the plate is fit to the shaft the distal fragment can rotate leading to sagittal plane malalignment

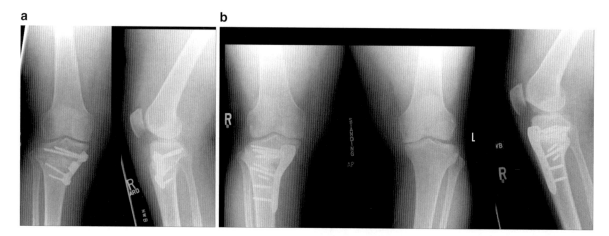

Fig. 7.12 (**a**) Nonunion and failure of fixation after a medial opening wedge high tibial osteotomy. A break in the lateral cortex intraoperatively created a step deformity and an unstable osteotomy without adequate fixation. (**b**) This was revised with a medial tibial locking plate and repeat bone grafting

Hardware can be removed either prior to undergoing TKA, or at the time of arthroplasty.

Stiffness/Arthrofibrosis

Stiffness occasionally does occur after osteotomy. We expect full return to preoperative knee range of motion at 6–8 weeks post-op. If the patient does not regain full range of motion with aggressive physical therapy by this time, consideration should be given to performing a manipulation under anesthesia. If patient lacks full extension, then structural reasons need to be ruled out. Sometimes there is a bumper osteophyte that was not resected that can block full extension. In this case, the patient will need an arthroscopy, and the bumper osteophyte should be burred down. The knee range of motion should then be reassessed and manipulation performed if needed. Close attention should be given to the tibial slope on radiographs. An inadvertent increase in the posterior tibial slope leads to the inability to regain full extension. In this case, manipulation under anesthesia should not be performed. Patients may present with a painful knee that they cannot fully extend. The treatment in this case would require either revision of fixation or an anterior closing wedge osteotomy to correct the posterior tibial slope.

Complications of Combined HTO and ACL Reconstruction

A combined HTO/ACL reconstruction can have all the potential complications already discussed, but has some additional considerations that are important. Preoperative planning begins with the decision to perform a staged vs. a combined procedure.[35–37] If the problem is pain with medial compartment overload in a patient with chronic ACL deficiency, an unloading osteotomy is indicated. In this case, an ACL reconstruction can be performed later if necessary. In the younger and more active patient with instability and malalignment, one may consider a combined procedure. In addition, one needs to determine the amount of correction required, the type of osteotomy that is going to be performed, and the type of ACL surgery.

Most importantly, in any scenario with ACL instability, particular attention needs to be directed at the sagittal plane or altering the tibial slope. This must be taken into account along with the coronal correction of the osteotomy. It is imperative to try to reduce the slope in these cases to help the ACL instability. In the case of PCL instability, one may try to increase the slope slightly to improve the posterior sag.

ACL deficiency is helped by decreasing the tibial slope (Fig. 7.13a-g). It is important to decrease the tibial slope to decrease anterior tibial translation in the ACL-deficient knee. It is especially important to not allow an increase in the tibial slope to occur as is the tendency with an opening wedge HTO as this would accentuate the ACL deficiency and could lead to graft failure and continued instability. However, with this in mind, performing an opening wedge HTO allows more controlled biplanar corrections. At the time of fixation, a bump is placed under the leg to hyperextend the knee and to close the osteotomy anteriorly. The osteotomy is fixed with the plate posteromedially. A tapered plate can help facilitate closing of the osteotomy anteriorly. Fixation can be added anteriorly with a staple or 2-hole plate to create a stable anterior hinge.

If the ACL reconstruction is performed first, the tibial tunnel can be a stress riser for the HTO. The ACL tibial tunnel can also be disrupted with the osteotomy. Strategies for prevention of these complications are important. Preserving knee range of motion is important with a concurrent ACL reconstruction, so early range-of-motion exercises are crucial postoperatively.

We prefer to perform the HTO first in order to prevent a stress riser from the tibial tunnel. This also avoids the potential disruption of the tibial tunnel with the osteotomy. The tibial tunnel is drilled with the tunnel located just above the osteotomy site anteromedially. The osteotomy should be performed distally and obliquely to allow drilling of the tibial tunnel above the osteotomy site. The plate and screws for the osteotomy should be placed as posteriorly as possible to allow room for the tibial tunnel. The position of the tunnels for the ACL is crucial and should not be compromised. Fixation on the tibial side is usually with an interference screw. Retroscrew fixation from within the joint may be of value in this situation. Secondary fixation can be obtained below the level of the osteotomy site if necessary.[38,39]

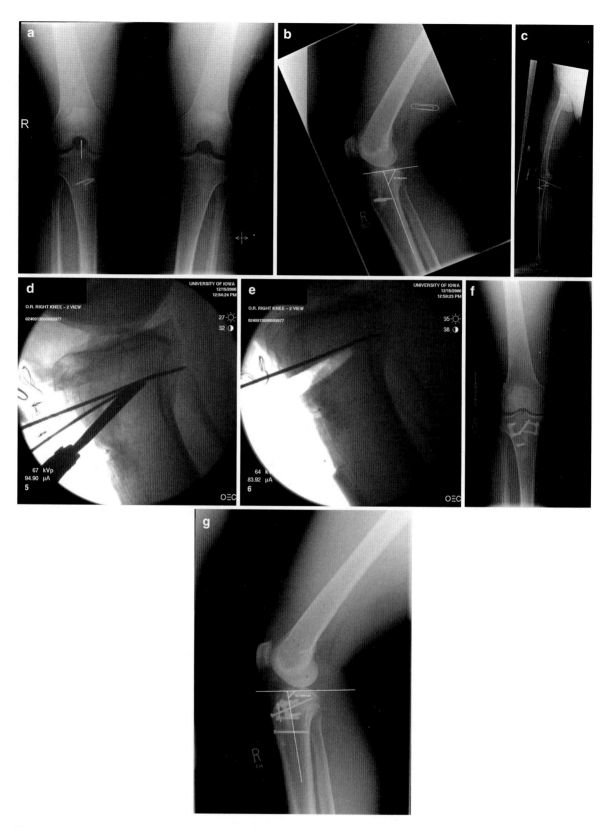

Fig. 7.13 (**a-g**) Case of a patient with two failed ACL surgeries and increased tibial slope. Coronal alignment measured with the long standing film is normal. The mechanical axis is marked on the AP radiograph (**a**). The lateral radiograph shows a 21° tibial slope (**b**). The long leg lateral view (**c**), which more accurately assesses alignment, shows a 23° tibial slope. A tibial tubercle osteotomy and an anterior closing wedge osteotomy are performed. Guide pins are placed as guides for the osteotomy (**d**), and the bone wedge is removed (**e**). Postoperative radiographs (**f**, **g**) show fixation of the osteotomy with two figure of eight plates anteriorly. The tibial tubercle is fixed with two screws. The lateral radiograph shows correction of the tibial slope to 8°

Understanding all of these principles is prerequisite to avoiding complications with both the osteotomy and the ACL reconstruction.

References

1. Willey M, Wolf B, Kocaglu B et al (submitted for publication) Complications associated with realignment osteotomy of the knee performed simultaneously with additional reconstructive procedures. University of Iowa Hospitals and Clinics, Iowa City, IA
2. Finkelstein J, Gross A, Davis A (1996) Varus osteotomy of the distal part of the femur. A survivorship analysis. J Bone Joint Surg Am 78(9):1348-52
3. Wang J, Hsu C (2005) Distal femoral varus osteotomy for osteoarthritis of the knee. J Bone Joint Surg Am 87(1):127-33
4. Hernigou P, Medevielle D, Debeyre J et al (1987) Proximal tibial osteotomy for osteoarthritis with varus deformity. A ten to thirteen-year follow-up study. J Bone Joint Surg Am 69(3):332-54
5. Matthews L, Goldstein S, Malvitz T et al (1988) Proximal tibial osteotomy. Factors that influence the duration of satisfactory function. Clin Orthop Relat Res Apr(229):193-200
6. Marti C, Gautier E, Wachtl S et al (2004) Accuracy of frontal and sagittal plane correction in open-wedge high tibial osteotomy. Arthroscopy 20(4):366-72
7. Fowler J, Gie G, Maceachern A (1991) Upper tibial valgus osteotomy using a dynamic external fixator. J Bone Joint Surg Br 73(4):690-1
8. Weale A, Lee A, MacEachern A (2001) High tibial osteotomy using a dynamic axial external fixator. Clin Orthop Relat Res Jan(382):154-67
9. Magyar G, Toksvig-Larsen S, Lindstrand A (1999) Hemicallotasis open-wedge osteotomy for osteoarthritis of the knee. Complications in 308 operations. J Bone Joint Surg Br 81(3):449-51
10. Cameron H, Park Y (1997) Total knee replacement after supracondylar femoral osteotomy. Am J Knee Surg 10(2): 70-1 discussion 1-2
11. Nelson C, Saleh K, Kassim R et al (2003) Total knee arthroplasty after varus osteotomy of the distal part of the femur. J Bone Joint Surg Am 85(A-6):1062-5
12. Paley D (2002) Principles of Deformity Correction. Springer, Berlin
13. Specogna A, Birmingham T, Hunt M et al (2007) Radiographic measures of knee alignment in patients with varus gonarthrosis: effect of weightbearing status and associations with dynamic joint load. Am J Sports Med 35(1):65-70
14. Dugdale T, Noyes F, Styer D (1992) Preoperative planning for high tibial osteotomy. The effect of lateral tibiofemoral separation and tibiofemoral length. Clin Orthop Relat Res Jan(274):248-64
15. Phisitkul P, Wolf B, Amendola A (2006) Role of high tibial and distal femoral osteotomies in the treatment of lateral-posterolateral and medial instabilities of the knee. Sports Med Arthrosc 14(2):96-104
16. Hunt M, Fowler P, Birmingham T et al (2006) Foot rotational effects on radiographic measures of lower limb alignment. Can J Surg 49(6):401-6
17. Sabharwal S, Zhao C (2008) Assessment of lower limb alignment: supine fluoroscopy compared with a standing full-length radiograph. J Bone Joint Surg Am 90(1):43-51
18. McDermott A, Finklestein J, Farine I et al (1988) Distal femoral varus osteotomy for valgus deformity of the knee. J Bone Joint Surg Am 70(1):110-6
19. Wang J, Hsu C (2006) Distal femoral varus osteotomy for osteoarthritis of the knee. Surgical technique. J Bone Joint Surg Am 88(Suppl 1 Pt 1):100-8
20. Scuderi G, Windsor R, Insall J (1989) Observations on patellar height after proximal tibial osteotomy. J Bone Joint Surg Am 71(2):245-8
21. Billings A, Scott D, Camargo M et al (2000) High tibial osteotomy with a calibrated osteotomy guide, rigid internal fixation, and early motion. Long-term follow-up. J Bone Joint Surg Am 82(1):70-9
22. Westrich G, Peters L, Haas S et al (1998) Patella height after high tibial osteotomy with internal fixation and early motion. Clin Orthop Relat Res Sep(354):169-74
23. Wright J, Heavrin B, Begg M et al (2001) Observations on patellar height following opening wedge proximal tibial osteotomy. Am J Knee Surg 14(3):163-73
24. Noyes F, Mayfield W, Barber-Westin S et al (2006) Opening wedge high tibial osteotomy: an operative technique and rehabilitation program to decrease complications and promote early union and function. Am J Sports Med 34(8):1262-73
25. Puddu G, Cipolla M, Cerullo G et al (2007) Osteotomies: the surgical treatment of the valgus knee. Sports Med Arthrosc 15(1):15-22
26. Noyes F, Goebel S, West J (2005) Opening wedge tibial osteotomy: the 3-triangle method to correct axial alignment and tibial slope. Am J Sports Med 33(3):378-87
27. Amendola A, Panarella L (2005) High tibial osteotomy for the treatment of unicompartimental arthritis of the knee. Orthop Clin North Am 36(4):497-504
28. Giffin J, Shannon F (2007) The role of the high tibial osteotomy in the unstable knee. Sports Med Arthrosc 15(1):23-31
29. Zaidi S, Cobb A, Bentley G (1995) Danger to the popliteal artery in high tibial osteotomy. J Bone Joint Surg Br 77(3):384-6
30. Smith P, Gelinas J, Kennedy K et al (1999) Popliteal vessels in knee surgery. A magnetic resonance imaging study. Clin Orthop Relat Res Oct(367):158-64
31. McLaren C, Wootton J, Heath P et al (1989) Pes planus after tibial osteotomy. Foot Ankle 9(6):300-3
32. Flierl S, Sabo D, Hornig K et al (1996) Open wedge high tibial osteotomy using fractioned drill osteotomy: a surgical modification that lowers the complication rate. Knee Surg Sports Traumatol Arthrosc 4(3):149-53
33. Kirgis A, Albrecht S (1992) Palsy of the deep peroneal nerve after proximal tibial osteotomy. An anatomical study. J Bone Joint Surg Am 74(8):1180-5
34. Coventry M (1987) Proximal tibial varus osteotomy for osteoarthritis of the lateral compartment of the knee. J Bone Joint Surg Am 69(1):32-8
35. Clatworthy M, Amendola A (1999) The anterior cruciate ligament and arthritis. Clin Sports Med 18(1):173-98

36. Latterman C, Jakob R (1996) High tibial osteotomy alone or combined with ligament reconstruction in anterior cruciate ligament deficient knees. Knee Surg Sports Traumatol Arthrosc 4(1):32-8
37. Noyes F, Barber-Westin S, Hewett T (2000) High tibial osteotomy and ligament reconstruction for varus angulated anterior cruciate ligament-deficient knees. Am J Sports Med 28(3):282-96
38. Amendola A (2008) What Technical pearls do you have when performing a single-stage ACL reconstruction and high tibial osteotomy? In: Bach BR Jr, Verma NN (eds) Curbside Consultation of the ACL: 49 Clinical Questions. Slack Incorporated, Thorofare, NJ, pp 159-62
39. Aggarwal A, Panarella L, Amendola A (2005) Considerations for osteotomy in the ACL deficient knee. Sports Med Arthrosc Rev 13(2):109-15

Editors' Comments (Osteotomies of the knee)

Take your time when assessing the sagittal angle of the HTO. As the authors note when performing an HTO for genu varum and an associated PCL insufficiency, perform the HTO with an increased flexion angle in the sagittal plane; for an associated ACL insufficiency perform the HTO in a neutral to an extended angle. Navigation may prove helpful for this procedure.

Chapter 8
Avoiding and Managing Complications in Patella Surgery

Michael V. Elman, Scott Zimmer, and Anthony A. Schepsis

Top 10 Pearls

- Understand the "tissue homeostasis theory" when trying to explain the pathophysiology of patellofemoral pain.
- "Think soft tissues first" when examining patients with anterior knee pain.
- Do not use isolated lateral retinacular release for patellar instability.
- Do not perform a lateral release out of frustration in a patient with refractory anterior knee pain, unless you have a sound clinical basis to do so.
- When addressing recurrent lateral patellar instability, it should not be proximal vs. distal realignment, it should be proximal when indicated, distal when indicated, and both when indicated.
- In patients without a clear-cut diagnosis, get to know your patient well.
- Develop a consistent method for imaging of the patellofemoral joint.
- A dedicated CT patellar tracking study is invaluable in evaluating patellar instability and malalignment.
- Avoid medial instability of the patella.
- After patellofemoral realignment surgery of any sort, get the knee moving early and avoid early weight-bearing after anteromedialization of the tibial tubercle.

M.V. Elman (✉)
Department of Orthopedic Surgery, Boston University Medical Center, 720 Harrison Avenue, Boston, MA, 02118, USA
e-mail: Michael.elman@gmail.com

S. Zimmer
Sports Medicine, Boston University School of Medicine, Boston, MAssachusetts, USA

A.A. Schepsis
Orthopedic Surgery, Boston University Medical Center, Boston, MAssachusetts, USA

Introduction and Background

Afflictions of the patellofemoral joint are one of the most common conditions that the Sports Medicine Orthopedist will encounter in his practice. Anterior knee pain has many causalities, is often poorly understood, misdiagnosed, and, as a consequence, is often mistreated. Many consider anterior knee pain to be the "back pain" of the Sports Medicine Specialist. The etiology of the pain is often poorly understood, frequently leading to multiple operations that culminate in an unhappy patient as well as a frustrated physician. Although this chapter is focused on avoiding, managing, and treating complications in patellar surgery, the vast majority of patients with patellofemoral conditions should be managed with nonoperative measures. Rehabilitation is just about always at the top of the list in the vast majority of patellofemoral injuries and disorders. The patellofemoral joint is one of the most common areas where surgery can often make the patients worse rather than better and should be approached very carefully. In this chapter, we will focus on patellofemoral realignment and instability surgery. Over 100 operations have been described for the management of recurrent lateral patellar instability and, although there are many surgical methods to treat the same condition, performing the wrong operation can lead to a disastrous result. Select the operation wisely. This often requires multiple office visits to become acquainted with your patient physically as well as psychologically.

Remember that the etiology of anterior knee pain is very complex and poorly understood. As proposed and advocated by Dr. Scott Dye,[1] there is a myriad of possible pathophysiological processes that can account for the etiology of patellofemoral pain, including pain from the soft tissues, increased osseous metabolic activity, increased intraosseous pressure, and neural sources. These can lead to symptomatic loss of tissue homeostasis that may persist indefinitely. Probably the best clinical example of this is having a patient with recalcitrant anterior knee pain that has failed what would be considered adequate conservative measures, leaving a frustrated surgeon and patient. Thus, a lateral release is performed with little knowledge of what is actually causing the pain and little basis on which to perform the lateral release. This is probably where lateral release gets its bad name. Usually if these patients are outside their "envelope of function," surgery will not help them. Without getting into detailed discussion, the pearl here is to read the article!

It is not a good idea to automatically assume that articular cartilage changes seen at the time of arthroscopy are the cause of the patient's patellofemoral pain. Oftentimes the soft tissues are the culprit. Fulkerson[2] proposed that adaptive shortening of the lateral retinaculum occurs with patellofemoral malalignment and that recurrent stretching of this shortened lateral retinaculum causes nerve changes to occur. These nerve changes include demyelination and fibrosis resembling the histopathology of Morton's neuroma.

The relationship between anterior knee pain and neural damage and neurotransmitters has been elaborated by the work of Sanchis-Alfonso,[3] who demonstrated neural changes supporting the work of Fulkerson. Interestingly he found increased amounts of nerve fibers in patients with moderate knee pain as compared to those with severe pain. In addition the neurotransmitter substance P was also found in greater concentration in those with moderate pain. This suggests that patients with more severe symptoms experience a "burn out" of their nerve fibers, which may also explain a proprioceptive decompensation in cases with more severe instability. In comparing anterior knee pain patients to those with osteoarthritis or with ACL or meniscal pathology, Witonski[4] demonstrated increased amounts of substance P in the fat pad and medial retinaculum, rather than the lateral retinaculum. If nothing else, this demonstrates that our understanding of the neural contribution to anterior knee is rudimentary with more work needed to be done. Nonetheless, no evaluation of patellofemoral pain would be complete without consideration of the soft tissues. Try to use a careful clinical examination to differentiate articular from synovial or retinacular pain.

Reexamine your patients many times, and understand them physically and emotionally, particularly in patients with longstanding pain. Furthermore, if surgery is necessary, "start small, and start smart." Often times "staging or diagnostic arthroscopies" can be helpful, not only in maximizing an understanding of the patient's pathology, but also in understanding the patient's response to a simple procedure. Remember that there is no problem that surgery cannot make worse.

The authors are constantly surprised in terms of how poorly diagnostic imaging of the patellofemoral joint is utilized without proper AP, lateral, and axial views of the patellofemoral joint. A full-length weight-bearing lower extremity AP film allows for evaluation of the limb alignment. We prefer to obtain a 30° flexed true lateral film of the knee to evaluate patellar height and trochlear depth. The measurement techniques of Blackburn–Peel or Caton–Deschamps (Fig. 8.1) provide a more accurate assessment of patella height than that of Insall–Salvati as they are based on the articulating length of the patella. A true lateral will allow for observation of the crossing-sign or trochlear bump found in trochlear dysplasia[5] (Fig. 8.2a, b). Plain film axial views can prove helpful, and we routinely obtain them at 30°, 60°, and 90° of flexion to evaluate patellofemoral conditions. Although an abundance of radiographic measures can be performed for axial films flexed at 30°, we prefer to make the measurements of lateral patellofemoral angle, congruence angle, and tilt angle from axial CT scans at incremental degrees of flexion. Most malalignment and instability problems

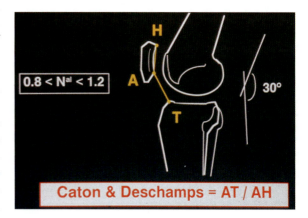

Fig. 8.1 Diagram representing the Caton–Deschamps ratio. Based upon an X-ray performed at 30° of flexion. A normal ratio is between 0.8 and 1.2

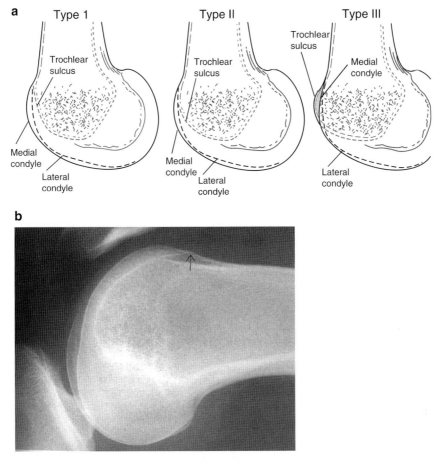

Fig. 8.2 (a) Diagram illustrating Dejour's classification of trochlear dysplasia demonstrating both the crossing sign and the trochlear bump seen with increasing severity. (b) X-ray with *arrow* pointing to crossing of trochlear and condylar lines with presence of trochlear bump

occur in early flexion and are not easily evaluated by plain X-ray. This also allows for more precise measurement of patellar subluxation, tilt, as well as the TT-TG or "radiographic Q-angle." (Fig. 8.3)

Regardless of the procedure or technique, patella contracture and patellar infera is a serious problem. Do not perform a procedure that is so tenuous that needs to be immobilized for a long period of time and allows the knee to get stiff. Several authors have reported proximal tibia fractures following anteromedialization of the tibial tubercle.[6–8] Stetson reported on six proximal tibial fractures that occurred on average at 7 weeks post-op when the rehab protocol was changed to immediate weight-bearing from nonweight-bearing to facilitate faster recovery. Bellemans reported on four proximal tibia fractures all occurring within 2 months after AMZ in patients who were performing unprotected full-weight-bearing activities. Eager reported on five fractures following AMZ occurring on average of 25 weeks post-op where transverse notching of the distal end of the osteotomy may have created a stress riser. In a cadaveric biomechanical model, Cosgarea[9] elegantly demonstrated the increased risk for tibial fracture and hardware pullout from the posterior cortex in an oblique osteotomy as compared to shingle fracture failure in a flat osteotomy. The mean load to failure was also significantly higher in the flat osteotomies. The authors recommend strict nonweight-bearing with protective bracing for 6 weeks followed by progressive protected weight-bearing.

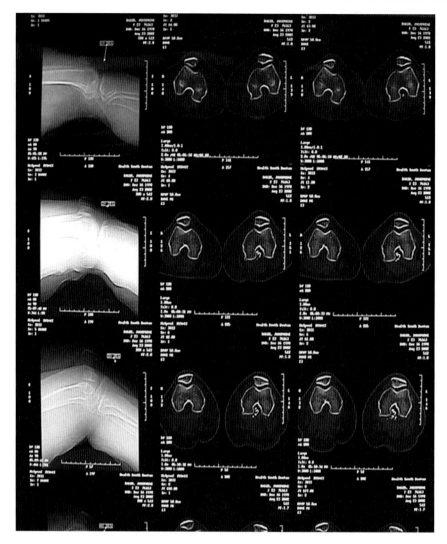

Fig. 8.3 CT scan at progressively increasing degrees of flexion. Diagram representing superimposed cuts of the trochlea and the tibial tubercle. This technique is commonly used to measure the TT–TG distance

Functional Anatomy at Risk

Fortunately, the anterior knee is blessed by not cohabitating with any of the major neurovascular structures. The principle structures to be aware of when addressing proximal soft tissue surgery are the location of the saphenous nerve and its branches and the branches of the lateral geniculate supplying the lateral retinaculum. When performing distal realignment surgery in the form of tibial tubercle osteotomies, the principle anatomy at risk includes the peroneal neurovasculature sitting right behind the lateral intramuscular septum, particularly when performing an anteromedialization, when subperiosteal dissection of the tibialis anterior off the lateral border of the proximal tibia is performed. Not violating the lateral intramuscular septum is paramount, either by dissection or with saw and osteotome. The septum should be carefully identified and protected.

The main anatomy at risk, however, is the posterior tibial artery and trifurcation as well as the posterior nerves when placing a bicortical screw or screws for fixation of tibial tubercle osteotomies. Kline[10] demonstrated the proximity of the vascular structures in cadaveric specimens to two drill holes used in tibial tubercle transfer, finding that the superior drill bit was a mean distance of 8.3 mm from the popliteal artery bifurcation while the inferior drill bit was a mean of 9 mm from the posterior tibial artery, with a range of approximately 0–20 mm for both drill holes. Drilling of the posterior cortex should be performed with the knee flexed to 90° to allow the neurovascular structures to fall back. However, we are unaware of any study indicating that this maneuver significantly increases the distance from the posterior cortex to the neurovascular bundles. Drilling through the posterior cortex should be performed very slowly and carefully to avoid "plunging" with the drill bit. Some authors recommend reverse drilling or drilling with a blunt drill bit to allow penetration of the posterior cortex in a slow, controlled fashion. Screw lengths should be carefully measured with the depth gauge at least twice, so that the appropriate length screw can be utilized to avoid a long screw protruding too far through the posterior cortex. If the surgeon is unsure, use of a C-arm is recommended.

Lateral Retinacular Release

Lateral retinacular release is the most commonly performed operation in patients with patellofemoral pain and instability. Unfortunately, it is probably one of the most overly used and misused procedures in orthopedic surgery. Lateral release has historically been used to treat patients with many types of patellofemoral disorders, including patellofemoral pain, malalignment, recurrent patellar dislocation, chondromalacia, and arthrosis.

The principle complication associated with lateral retinacular release is inappropriate use of this procedure. Oftentimes, surgeons and patients, particularly those with refractory patellofemoral pain, are frustrated by lack of response to treatment and often turn to lateral retinacular release as a potential solution. Without the proper indications, however, it usually follows the old adage "that nothing is so bad that you can't make it worse." The best way to avoid the complications of lateral retinacular release is not to perform it when it is not indicated.

In the authors' experience, which is well borne out in the literature, isolated lateral retinacular release should not be performed for treatment of recurrent lateral patellar instability. Statistically, the results of isolated lateral release for recurrent lateral patellar instability are unpredictable and likely deteriorate with time. Most of the evidence for lateral release in patellar instability is level III or IV. Ricchetti[11] performed a systematic review of the literature comparing lateral retinacular release to LRR with medial soft-tissue realignment in the treatment of recurrent patellar instability. The frequency-weighted mean success with respect to instability in the LRR studies was 77.3% vs. 93.6% in the LRR with MR studies. Of note, one or less than one failure was reported in three-eighth of the LRR alone studies that were reviewed.

Certainly surgeons and patients are tempted by the fact that this procedure can be done all-arthroscopically, thereby avoiding open surgery. Although this is tantalizing, it should be avoided.

The ideal indication for lateral retinacular release is excessive lateral pressure syndrome (ELPS) hallmarked by pain in the lateral part of the patellofemoral compartment, associated with negative passive patellar tilt (Kolowich sign), a negative Sage sign (medial glide of patella less than one quadrant, with the knee at 15–20° of flexion), and imaging evidence of lateral patellar tilt, either by radiographs, CT, or MRI (Fig. 8.4a, b). Lateral release may also be necessary in patellar realignment surgery for recurrent lateral patellar instability, with the above signs, when lateral release is necessary to re-center the patella. A survey of the International Patellofemoral Study Group performed by Fithian[12] indicates that, among experts in the field of patellofemoral surgery, surgeons who see a lot of patients with patellofemoral disorders, isolated lateral release only accounts for 1–5 surgical cases per year or about 2% of cases performed annually. Also, remember that lateral release requires specific informed consent.

The authors believe that even more important than understanding the indications of lateral retinacular release is to fully understand the *contraindications*. The most feared complication after lateral retinacular release is medial patellar instability, a very disabling condition, which is usually far worse than the condition that the patient started off with. By understanding the contraindications preoperatively, this usually can be avoided.

The main contraindication, in our experience, is *patellar hypermobility* or *generalized joint hyperlaxity*. These are hallmarked by the absence of negative passive patellar tilt and a positive Sage sign, as

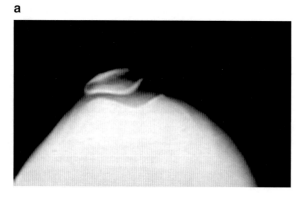

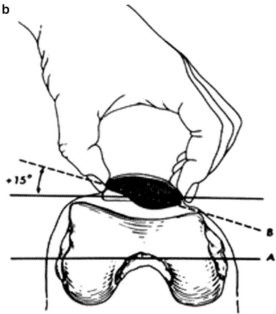

Fig. 8.4 (a) X-ray demonstrating lateral tilt on a sunrise view. (b) Diagram representing the Kolowich test. Performed by gripping the patella on either facet with the thumb and the index finger and internally rotating the patella on the long axis of the femur

the lateral retinaculum is extremely tight, associated with no passive patellar medial mobility or tilt and more severe degrees of tilt by imaging, lateral release that includes the area from the tubercle up to the superior pole of the patella is necessary for an adequate release. This has also been further substantiated in a biomechanics model by Marumoto.[13] Relative contraindications of lateral retinacular release include older-aged patients, patients with Grade IV disease of the lateral patellofemoral compartment, and patella alta.[14]

Avoiding and Managing Intraoperative Complications

Lateral retinacular release can be performed either in an arthroscopic or mini-open fashion. An underutilized technique is to perform a lateral retinacular lengthening rather than release, which is useful in the authors' experience in two scenarios. One is when the lateral retinaculum is only slightly tight and needs to be "fine tuned" with the fear that the situation will move from too tight to too loose, even with a limited release. The second is when performing a lateral approach to the patellofemoral joint for an intra-articular procedure, such as resurfacing, and the lateral retinaculum either is not tight or only slightly tight. This allows the surgeon to reapproximate the lateral retinaculum either anatomically or in a lengthened position.

The main intraoperative complication associated with lateral release is *hemarthrosis*. We routinely put a tourniquet on the thigh when contemplating a lateral retinacular release. We rarely inflate the tourniquet. However, it should always be applied for a stop-gap measure, in case of intraoperative arthroscopic bleeding that cannot be controlled by other measures. When placing the arthroscope in the standard anterolateral portal, we make the anterolateral portal in a longitudinal direction, which allows for enlargement, if necessary, and make the portal slightly lower than normal, so that more of the distal part of the retinaculum is included.

A spinal needle should be placed parallel with the superior pole of the patella to ensure that the vastus lateralis is not violated. The lateral retinacular release should never extend beyond the superior border of the

described above. Certainly, if the patella can be translated two quadrants or more medially, the possibility of ending up with medial patellar subluxation postoperatively becomes much higher. Remember also that a lateral retinacular release can be performed in what we call a "limited" fashion vs. an "extensive" fashion. The limited lateral retinacular release includes the lateral retinaculum from the superior pole of the patella below the vastus lateralis, down to the arthroscopic portal. An extensive lateral release includes this area, as well as the more distal portion of the retinaculum from the portal down to the tibial tubercle. In most cases where patella. Violation of the vastus lateralis significantly weakens the quadriceps mechanism and is associated with a higher incidence of medial patellar instability.

After other intra-articular procedures are performed, we routinely utilize a radiofrequency "saber" wand to perform the lateral retinacular release. Initially the saber wand is brought across from the anteromedial portal and placed in such a fashion to give the best direct access to the lateral retinaculum by localizing it with a spinal needle first (Fig. 8.5). The "bleeder" is usually encountered in the proximal third of the lateral release. Remember that there are two layers of lateral retinaculum, so careful sequential cutting of the fibers should be performed, taking the superficial fibers first and then the deeper fibers. We usually start off with a pump pressure of about 40–60, and utilization of a flow pump significantly decreases the chances of poor visualization from bleeding during a lateral retinacular release. Bleeders are cauterized as we go along. Arthroscopic electrocautery can also be utilized, but, some type of electrocautery or radiofrequency is paramount. After performing the proximal part of the lateral release from the medial portal, we then switch the arthroscope to the medial portal and perform the rest of the lateral release through the lateral portal. In cases where there is excessively tight retinaculum with excessive tilt, performing release distally from below the portal is important. This usually requires ablation and removal of the synovium and fat pad to allow visualization down to the tubercle. This should be performed carefully and slowly, cauterizing bleeders along the way. Frequently during the procedure, when we think we have done enough, we will remove the arthroscope and recheck the passive patellar tilt. We like to see the patella tilt 10–20° beyond neutral but no more. Some authors in the past have been able to evert the patella 90° after a lateral release. We believe this is excessive and know of no normal patella that can be everted 90°, so it does not make any sense to achieve this goal in these patients.

When the lateral release is completed, the most important step is to slowly lower the pump pressure, approximately 10 mm at a time, and cauterize bleeders along the way. We routinely do this until we get the pump pressure down to its minimum of 10–15 mm of mercury to cauterize all bleeders.

Postoperative hemarthrosis is not only associated with the immediate postoperative complications, but also associated with a poorer result for a long term.[14] Postoperatively we place a large compression pad over the site of the lateral release and use a constant ice application device. Cold therapy has been shown to decrease complications and improve results postoperatively.[15]

The other important point in the author's experience is to have the patient's first postoperative visit 3–4 days postoperatively, as opposed to the usual 7–14 days. Since swelling and hemarthrosis can still occur even with the above measures, it is important to pick it up early and aspirate the knee to avoid the negative effects of a prolonged hemarthrosis including stiffness and fibrosis. We usually tell the patients not to start range-of-motion exercises for about 48 h in order to control swelling, but then get the knee moving early.

Lastly, skin penetration has been reported with the arthroscopic technique. This can be easily avoided by having good visualization, releasing layer by layer, and keeping the outflow on slightly to cool the fluid.

Often patients with lateral patellofemoral pain may not have pain coming from the tilt, but rather, have a neural origin in the lateral retinaculum. The groundbreaking work of Sanchis-Alfonso and others provides a neuroanatomic basis for anterior knee pain in the active young patient. Furthermore, over 50% of those in the International Patellofemoral Study Group feel

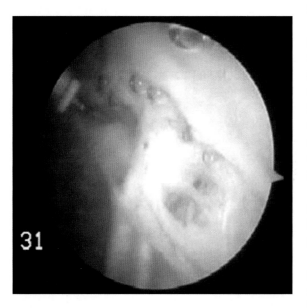

Fig. 8.5 Arthroscopic image of "saber" device in a lateral release procedure. We will routinely mark the superior pole of the patella with a spinal needle to limit the proximal extent of the release

that lateral release partially works by denervating the patella.[12]

Remember, there are seven surgically identifiable sensory nerves around the knee joint, with the medial and lateral retinacular nerves providing sensation to the joint, while the others do so to the skin. Neuromatous pain can occur also after lateral retinacular release. It is usually sharp and localized. Often patients have an isolated or multiple Tinel's sign. Careful one-finger palpation of the structures and the soft tissues is paramount, and diagnostically, a local trigger-point injection can be very helpful. In rare cases, the neuromatous tissue may need to be surgically excised.[16]

The most feared complication, however, after lateral retinacular release is medial patellar subluxation. This is an under-diagnosed condition in the authors' experience and is extremely disabling. It is frequently hallmarked by the fact that a patient being treated for instability in the first place feels a new onset instability that is distinct and much worse than the instability felt preoperatively. Although the senior author has seen a couple of cases of medial patellar instability in patients without previous surgery, just about all of this condition is iatrogenic after a lateral release that is either too excessive, inappropriate, or a lateral release with an overzealous medial tubercle tibial tubercle transfer. Most of the time by following the principles indicated above in the preoperative section, this can be avoided. It is associated with a paradoxical increase in pain after lateral release and disabling giving way and instability with activities of daily living. Physical findings include increased medial passive patellar mobility, a positive medial apprehension test, and a positive Fulkerson "jump" test (Fig. 8.6). The diagnosis usually must be suspected before it can be made, and then, if it is suspected and the signs are present, it is usually an easy diagnosis to make.

This complication usually cannot be managed nonoperatively. Wearing a patellar Buttress brace used for patellar instability "backwards," so that it provides a medial buttress with the patella lateral to it, can often serve as a diagnostic tool. Once a diagnosis is made, however, surgical intervention is just about always indicated.

Multiple procedures have been described in the literature, including medial retinacular release,[17] which is not recommended by the authors, repair and imbrication of the lateral retinaculum, which usually stretches out with medial subluxation usually reappearing within

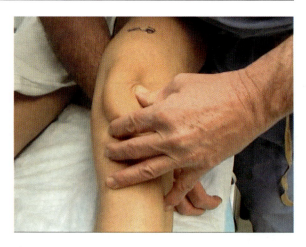

Fig. 8.6 Picture demonstrating the initial maneuver in Fulkerson's relocation or jump test. With a medial force on the patella the knee is then promptly flexed with simultaneous release of the medially directed force. The patient should express the feeling of instability as the patella engage the trochlea from medial to lateral

a year, or some type of reconstructive tether of the lateral patellofemoral ligament.

Procedures using a strip of the patellar tendon, iliotibial band, or a free anatomic tendon graft have been described. Utilizing a strip of the patellar tendon is recommended by Hughston. It is not recommended by the author, since it is not anywhere near anatomic. A free tendon graft with a piece of quadriceps tendon and bone block, an allograft, or a piece of patellar tendon with a bone block at one end has been described by Teitge.[18] This is an important article to read to understand the importance of isometry of lateral patellofemoral ligament reconstruction.

The authors' preference at the present time is a technique learned from Dr. Jack Andrish, utilizing a central strip of the iliotibial band leaving it attached distally and attaching it to the midpoint of the patella. The advantage of this technique, in the authors' experience, is that it allows "fine-tuning" of the tension by adding sutures laterally to further tighten the band and change the isometric position (Fig. 8.7a, b).The general trend at the present time, in the authors' experience, is utilizing a free tendon graft with careful testing of isometry to reconstruct the lateral patellofemoral ligament. We believe further basic science and clinical studies are necessary before we have the perfect technique.

The senior author has also encountered several cases, which he terms "multidirectional instability of

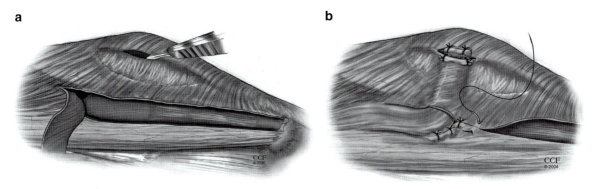

Fig. 8.7 (**a**) Illustration demonstrating Andrish's technique of lateral patellofemoral ligament reconstruction utilizing a strip of the ITB. (**b**) The completed lateral patellofemoral ligament reconstruction. An advantage of this technique is to precisely tension the reconstruction by adding sutures

the patella." This is usually seen in the scenario of a patient who preoperatively has had recurrent lateral patellar subluxation treated with an inappropriate and excessive lateral retinacular release. In these cases, the patella would be medially subluxed in extension, jump back into the groove in early flexion, and then laterally sublux at about 20–30° of flexion so the patella is going from too far medial to too far lateral. These cases have been treated with the above procedure, reconstructing the lateral patellofemoral ligament and also reefing and advancing of the medial patellofemoral ligament (MPFL) medially. Both of these can be "fine-tuned" to get the patella tracking correctly.

Lateral Patellar Instability: Deciding on the Right Operation

This chapter would not be complete without a separate discussion on choosing the correct operation when addressing patients with recurrent lateral patellar instability. With over a hundred operations described for treatment of patellar instability, it is not surprising that there is a lot of controversy in this area. The principle factor seems to be deciding on a proximal vs. a distal realignment. As mentioned at the beginning, it should not be proximal vs. distal, it should be proximal when indicated, distal when indicated, and both when indicated. It is not surprising, in the authors' experience, to see that many surgeons have a narrow-minded approach to recurrent patellar instability, always performing either a distal or proximal operation or both in their own practice. There is no question that both can work in many circumstances, but certainly there are some circumstances where the surgeon will definitely end up choosing the wrong operation and have a failure, requiring revision surgery. As we teach residents and fellows, there are many "right" operations to correct the problem, it is just important in certain circumstances to avoid the wrong ones. For example, a patient with recurrent lateral patellar dislocations with 4+ lateral glide of the patella (a completely "dislocatable patella") (Fig. 8.8), trochlear dysplasia, and a Q-angle and TT–TG within normal limits, will probably fail a distal realignment procedure. On the other hand, a patient with predominant pain, mild instability in the form of recurrent subluxations, fixed malalignment with tilt and subluxation through range of motion on imaging, a high Q-angle and TT-TG, and advanced arthrosis on the medial facet of the patella will not do

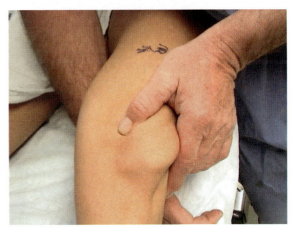

Fig. 8.8 Demonstration of 4+ lateral glide as the patella is completely dislocatable

well with a MPFL reconstruction alone. In general, a good axiom to remember is that proximal stabilizations are an operation for traumatic instability, whereas distal realignments are for pain and/or instability associated with tubercle malalignment as the primary inciting factor. Remember that fixed static malalignment with subluxation and a high congruence angle through a range of motion should not be corrected, and cannot be corrected, with a MPFL reefing or reconstruction. The MPFL reconstruction is meant to control excessive lateral movement of the patella, not "pull" the patella medially. This would only lead to increased loads on the medial facet of the patella.

After a careful history, a systematic physical examination is paramount. Remember to always look at the hip and the foot. Malalignment really comes from the hip and most of the time it is the femur that is internally rotated under the patella, rather than the patella being externally rotated over the femur. Although theoretically, osteotomies should be performed on the femoral side, for this reason, tubercle malalignment is best addressed through a much simpler operation of moving the tubercle over. The authors do agree that there are severe cases of femoral anteversion in patients with patellar instability that may require a derotational osteotomy of the femur as advocated by Teitge (Fig. 8.9a, b).

Evaluate patellar tracking, not only in the standing position, but in the sitting position as well. Medial and lateral patellar glide at 0 and 30° should be carefully recorded in both knees. The painful arc of motion in which the patient gets crepitus, if present, is important to note to help determine the symptomatic location of the disease. Early arc discomfort usually indicates distal patellar proximal trochlear disease and deep flexion arc crepitus and pain indicates the opposite. This may be helpful in determining whether or not an unloading and realignment procedure, such as an anteromedialization, may be helpful. As mentioned previously, passive patellar tilt and Sage sign will help determine clinically whether or not the lateral retinaculum is tight and needs to be addressed.

We performed a study looking at the interobserver reliability of the Q-angle as well as the correlation of the Q-angle with imaging measurement of tubercle malalignment (the TT–TG distance measured on CT scan). We found that the Q-angle should be carefully measured with the knee at 30° of flexion in the sitting or supine position with a long goniometer. We found, in these circumstances, the measurement is reliable and correlates the best with the TT–TG distance (Fig. 8.10).

We have a consistent method of performing patellofemoral radiographs. The authors recommend a true lateral at 30° of flexion to measure patellar height and also to determine whether or not trochlear dysplasia is present. In patients with recurrent lateral patellar instability, we routinely perform a CT patellar tracking study. This includes a set of images of mid-axial

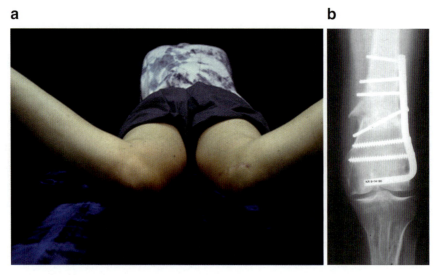

Fig. 8.9 (a) Demonstration of abnormally increased femoral anteversion. (b) X-ray of derotational distal femoral osteotomy for treatment of increased anteversion

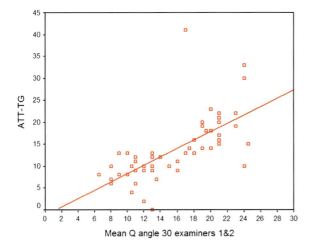

Fig. 8.10 Chart demonstrating high correlation of TT–TG with Q-angle measured at 30° of flexion

images from 0 to 60° in 10° increments (Fig. 8.3) to look at patellar tracking in this range. Since most patellar instability occurs in early flexion, we find the CT scan critical in looking at the patellar position from 0 to 30°, which is not possible by plain radiographs. A second set of images are what we call "fixed-frame images" from proximal to the trochlea distally through the tibial tubercle (Fig. 8.11). On this we can measure the TT–TG or the trochlear groove–tibial tubercle distance. This is really the "radiographic Q-angle." The classic study by Jones[19] indicates a TT–TG of greater than 20 mm is highly abnormal, 12–20 mm is borderline, and less than 12 mm is considered normal. In our study, we found that a TT–TG of more than 15 mm is considered abnormal and correlates with a Q-angle of more than 20°. Certainly when the TT–TG becomes more than 20 mm, one must seriously consider a distal realignment procedure as part of the operative regimen, either isolated or in combination with a proximal procedure. Furthermore, a patient with MPFL insufficiency who also has a high Q-angle and TT–TG distance may require a distal osteotomy as

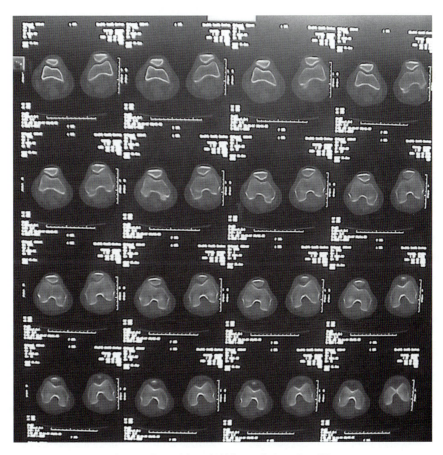

Fig. 8.11 CT tracking study demonstrating patella position at 10° intervals from 0 to 60°

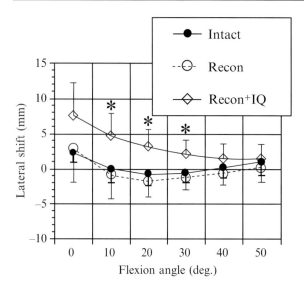

Fig. 8.12 Graph by Kuroda demonstrating nearly normal patella tracking after MPFL reconstruction in knees with normal Q-angles, while tracking remained abnormal with MPFL reconstruction in those with increased Q-angles

well as attention to the MPFL. Kuroda[20] has shown that MPFL reconstruction restores nearly normal tracking in aligned knees. However, when an increased Q-angle is present, there is still a lateral shift with MPFL reconstruction (Fig. 8.12).

Further discussion addressing proximal and distal realignments will be in the subsequent sections when talking about each separately. We like to think of Dr. Merchant's "Big Six" in assessing patellar instability. This includes increased Q-angle and TT–TG, patella alta, lax MPFL, deficient VMO, trochlear dysplasia or depth, and tight lateral retinaculum. Finally, remember that MPFL reefing or reconstruction is an operation for instability, not an operation for pain or arthrosis. Distal realignment can be an operation for instability but also can be an operation for pain and malalignment.

Proximal Patellar Realignment

Proximal patellar realignments are generally done for patients with lateral patellar instability. These include all-arthroscopic, arthroscopically assisted, mini-open or open reefing procedures, and reconstruction of the MPFL. The main complication to avoid is to pick the right operation for the particular patient. In general, we use all-arthroscopic techniques for patients with mild lateral patellar instability (an increased glide of 1–2 quadrants, with no trochlear dysplasia) and a mini-open "reefing" or advancement of the MPFL when there have only been a few episodes of dislocation, the integrity of the ligament is excellent, and the femoral attachment is intact. For more severe cases of 3 to 4+ lateral patellar instability, particularly when trochlear dysplasia is present, we prefer MPFL reconstruction since the tissue has already proven that it has failed. Remember that lateral retinacular release or lengthening is only necessary if there is negative passive patellar tilt, negative Sage sign, and the necessity to release the lateral retinaculum in order to re-center the patella in its groove.[21]

Arthroscopic Medial Reefing

Arthroscopic reefing of the MPFL and the medial retinacular restraints are generally performed by an arthroscopically assisted technique of imbricating the medial tissue. There are many techniques described. We prefer the technique described by Halbrecht,[22] since it is relatively simple and free of complications, although various techniques have been described. Other complications of all-arthroscopic technique include inadequate tissue advancement or excessive tissue advancement, with the former being more common. One of the shortcomings of arthroscopic imbrication is the surgeon has no idea of the quality of the tissue or any good quantitative idea of how much advancement or tightening of the ligament is being performed. Nor, is there any sense of the integrity of the femoral or patellar attachments. Nevertheless, good results have been reported with this technique, and this technique has worked in my hands in patients with mild increased lateral glide of the patella and in patients with subluxations without trochlear dysplasia.

Technically, the ability to tie knots arthroscopically is imperative, particularly using the Halbrecht technique. As far as surgical preparation, a tourniquet should be applied to the proximal thigh but not inflated, unless it is necessary. A controlled arthroscopic pump makes the procedure much easier to perform. If a lateral retinacular release is necessary, this should be performed after the sutures are passed but before they are tied. As the sutures are passed, the higher the degree of

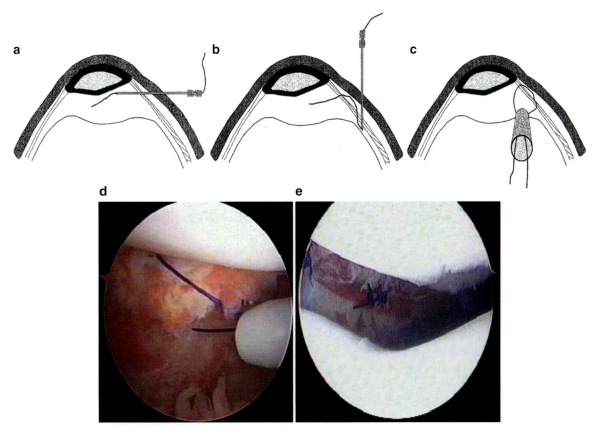

Fig. 8.13 (**a–e**) Illustrations of Halbrecht's arthroscopic imbrication using a cannulated needle to pass suture (**a**), withdrawing just outside of the capsule (**b**), and lastly tying an arthroscopic knot through a cannula

laxity, the more imbrication should be performed. Please refer to the excellent article by Halbrecht (Fig. 8.13a-e).

After the first suture is tied, usually from proximal to distal, the repair can be tested, and if there is adequate tissue tension, the suture can be removed and replaced. At the end of the procedure we usually prefer to slowly lower the pump pressure and cauterize any bleeders, particularly if a lateral release has been performed. The other complication that can occur is injury to some of the branches of the saphenous nerve. This can be avoided by making sure that the suture is passed just outside the capsule and does not capture any of the subcutaneous tissue. If there is any question, a mini-incision can be made to free up the suture from the subcutaneous tissue, by hand, before they are tied. When the knots are being tied intra-articularly, we recommend, as Halbrecht advocates, using absorbable suture. One of the problems with absorbable sutures is they tend to be weaker, and thus suture breakage could be a problem. This can occur if a sharp spinal needle is utilized to pass the sutures. This complication can be avoided by careful handling of the sutures and utilizing a Tuohey needle, usually 17–20 gauge, which has a beveled edge to avoid damage to the suture. These needles are often utilized by anesthesiologists and are readily available.

Postoperatively the patient should be seen within a few days, in case a hemarthrosis develops, which should be aspirated. In general, all-arthroscopic techniques are not associated with stiffness or loss of motion, like the open reefing or repairs. However, it still can occur. If the surgeon feels he has a good strong repair, we recommend early range of motion.

In general, the all-arthroscopic technique has relatively few complications if these rules are followed. It does not burn any bridges so that if this fails, the surgeon still has ability to perform a more extensive open reefing or, more likely, formal medial patellofemoral reconstruction. The authors have also found this technique very useful. In fact, the time we use it most frequently is in conjunction with distal realignments when both the distal and the proximal realignment are necessary if the proximal instability is only mild and used as a "fine-tuning" procedure.

Open Reefing

We utilize open reefing or advancement of the MPFL in cases where there is mild-to-moderate patellar instability and the integrity of the MPFL is still good with an intact femoral attachment. Often in cases where we are trying to decide whether reefing or advancement is adequate vs. a formal MPFL reconstruction, we will make the patellar incision that we would normally use either for a reefing or for the patellar side of the MPFL reconstruction, dissect down between layers 2 and 3, and palpate the MPFL. If there is a good femoral attachment and the ligament has good integrity, it just needs to be advanced; particularly if the degree of instability is only mild to moderate and there is no trochlear dysplasia or patella alta (Fig. 8.14). This can be performed in lieu of a formal MPFL reconstruction. In general, we no longer perform VMO advancements since the VMO advancement has not only a medial-to-lateral vector, but also a proximal-to-distal vector, which tends to tighten flexion. This only weakens the VMO and the contribution of the VMO to patellar instability is very unpredictable and is not the major stabilizer.

The main complication of reefing procedures is causing overtightening and excessive contact pressures in flexion. In the past, the literature described reefing or advancement going from not only medial to lateral but also slightly proximal to distal. We perform reefing not only medial to lateral, but also slightly distal to proximal to avoid tightening in flexion. This also follows the normal course of the more proximal aspect of the MPFL (Fig. 8.15). The main complication of reefing procedures is placing sutures such that they tighten in flexion. If and when the patient regains their range of motion, either the reefing will fail, will become lax in earlier degrees of flexion where it is most important, or the patient will lose range of motion. As each suture is placed, the repair should be tested and should allow a full range of motion. The authors' experience can be avoided by placing the sutures in a slight distal to proximal

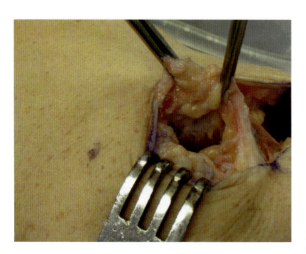

Fig. 8.14 Picture of a "tug test" assessing the integrity of the native MPFL. The ligament is more easily palpated when tension is pulled laterally from the femoral origin

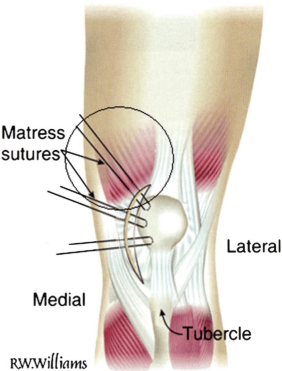

Fig. 8.15 A circle demonstrating a commonly used direction for medial reefing or VMO advancement. We warn against this direction as it can lead to excessive tightening in flexion and prefer to tighten from distal on the femoral side to proximal on the patella

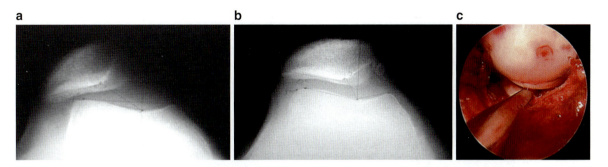

Fig. 8.16 (**a–c**) X-rays and arthroscopic image of the indications for acute operative intervention for patella instability (**a**) irreducible patella (**b, c**) osteochondral avulsion or fracture requiring repair

vector when advancing the tissues from medial to lateral. This is particularly important when there is diseased medial facet, as there oftentimes is, in patellar instability patients. It is also important after an acute dislocation with an osteochondral fracture that requires fixation or static asymmetrical alignment of the patella (Fig. 8.16a-c). In general, we advocate nonoperative treatment of acute patellar dislocations, unless one of these two factors is present. This is similar to operating on a "hot knee" after a multiple ligament injury and arthrofibrosis and potentially a patella infera complication. In general, ending up with a patella that is "too loose" is much easier to deal with than one that is "too tight."

Postoperatively, early full range of motion should be achieved. In general, if full range of motion has not been achieved or is not steadily improving by 12 weeks postoperatively, we recommend early lysis of adhesions to avoid patellar capture and a more serious arthrofibrosis. The other complication we see after reefing procedures is recurrence of instability. This is particularly true when there have been multiple dislocations and tissue has failed many times. This is also particularly true in the presence of trochlear dysplasia, where the other major static restraint, other than the MPFL is inadequate and thus the medial restraints, particularly the MPFL, are "doing all the work." If this procedure fails, a formal MPFL reconstruction should be performed.

In evaluating patients with failed patellofemoral surgery, I will always get a true lateral X-ray of the knee at 30° of flexion and compare both knees. This will always not only help diagnose patella alta or infera but also show the presence of severe trochlear dysplasia. Trochlear dysplasia can also be seen on MRI as well as CT scan. In Europe, surgical correction of trochlear dysplasia is much more common than in the United States, even though it is a common source of patellofemoral instability. The most common forms are a short lateral trochlea, a hypoplastic or flat lateral trochlea, or a flat groove (Fig. 8.17a, b). In our experience, although trochleoplasty addresses the anatomic abnormality causing the instability, it is fraught with complications and may lead to chondral or subchondral damage. We have experienced a couple of patients who would potentially benefit from an opening wedge osteotomy of the lateral trochlea for a flat lateral trochlea (Fig. 8.18a, b), which has, in our experience, a much lower complication rate than a "groove deepening" procedure (Fig. 8.19a, b). In our experience, trochleoplasty is rarely needed, in that careful medial/lateral balancing will generally manage these patients well. In particular, as mentioned previously, patients with recurrent lateral patellar instability and lax medial restraints with trochlear dysplasia are best managed by a formal MPFL reconstruction since they need a much stronger restraint to prevent recurrent lateral instability than simple reefing procedures. In fact, the work of Steiner[23] has shown that MPFL reconstruction performs well over the long term in patients with trochlear dysplasia.

The lateral X-ray is also helpful in delineating patients with severe patella alta (Fig. 8.20). Since the patella does not engage the groove until somewhere between 20 and 30° of flexion, recurrent instability, even in the face of careful reconstruction of the proximal restraints, is not an uncommon problem. We are often fearful of moving the tibial tubercle distally for fear of increasing patellofemoral contact pressures. In particular, our historical experience procedure with the

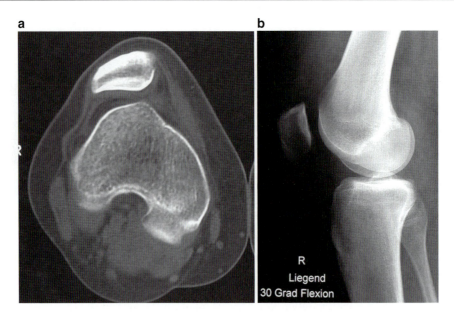

Fig. 8.17 (**a**, **b**) CT scan and X-ray demonstrating trochlear bump found in trochlear dysplasia

Hauser procedure where the tubercle was moved not only distally, but also posteriorly, had a clear association with a precocious patellofemoral arthrosis occurring. Again, we prefer to utilize a measurement based on the tibial plateau (the Caton-Deschamps or the Blackburn-Peel ratio, rather than the Insall-Salvati ratio, in defining patella alta. Although some authors recommend distalization for patients with a ratio of 1.2 or greater, I would reserve distalization for those patients with a ratio of 1.5 or greater. I would rarely move the tubercle more than 1 cm distally, and usually this is in association with a medial transfer. In particular, patients with chondrosis or arthrosis should be approached carefully in terms of distalization of the tubercle.

Another cause of medial instability, besides the more common excessive or inappropriate lateral retinacular release, is, as mentioned previously, medial or anteromedial tubercle transfer that has either been excessive or inappropriate. In these rare cases, an anterolateral (reverse) osteotomy of the tibial tubercle may be necessary to correct the instability pattern, if the lateral retinaculum is not or only partially responsible. Anterolateral transfer can also be utilized as a salvage procedure for a failed previous Hauser procedure with patellofemoral arthrosis. Another frustrating problem can be patients with patellar malalignment and arthrosis who have been treated with an anteromedialization of the tibial tubercle that has failed. First of all, patients should be

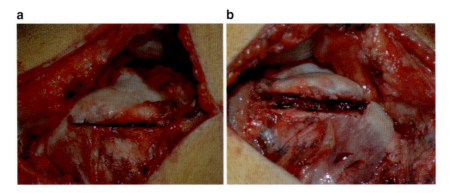

Fig. 8.18 (**a**, **b**) Pictures demonstrating an opening wedge osteotomy of the trochlea for a flat trochlea

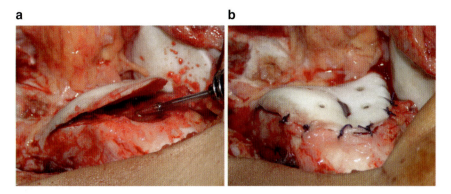

Fig. 8.19 (**a**, **b**) Photos of groove deepening procedure for a flat trochlea

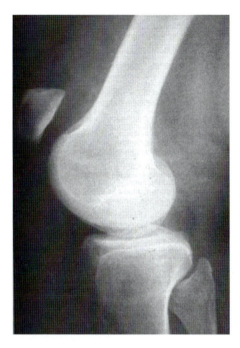

Fig. 8.20 Radiograph of severe patella alta

instructed that the results of the procedure, even in the best circumstance or pattern of arthrosis, are unpredictable This has been substantiated by the work of Henry,[24] showing that there is a variable effect in patient to patient, in terms of unloading effects of anteriorization and medialization of the tibial tubercle. Often, however, the arthrosis may be too advanced or extensive for the osteotomy to work. In younger patients, however, I still think this is a very reasonable option as a first-line procedure. In some cases, particularly when patients have a Grade IV trochlea or Grade IV disease extending proximally, either focal resurfacing, biological, or prosthetic, or patellofemoral replacement, if they are age and activity appropriate, may be helpful. We have treated several cases of patients with advanced disease combining an anterior medialization and tibial tubercle with focal resurfacing of the patellofemoral joint (Fig. 8.21a, b). In patients 60 years old or older and sedentary patients, total knee arthroplasty may be a better option than the less predictable patellofemoral arthroplasty.

Finally, in rare cases, straight anteriorization of the tibial tubercle may be helpful. The recent work of Beck[25] has shown that anteriorization of the tibial tubercle will unload or decompress the trochlea, and it can be particularly helpful in patients with advanced trochlear disease, either performed in association with a chondroplasty, microfracture, or performed in association with formal resurfacing, whether it be autologous, chondrocyte implantation or fresh osteochondral allograft implantation. Anteriorization can also be helpful in patients with distal patellar disease that is advanced with good articular cartilage on the proximal trochlea, if there is no malalignment or poor lateral restraints and medialization is not desired. This can be performed utilizing either a flat elevating osteotomy with bone graft or an oblique osteotomy with an off-set bone graft[26] (Fig. 8.22a–c).

We have also had experience with straight anteriorization in treating patients for postpatellectomy with postpatellectomy pain secondary to "trochleomalacia," where the extensive mechanism has increased contact pressures in the trochlear groove. Anteriorization of the tibial tubercle also improves the lever arm of the

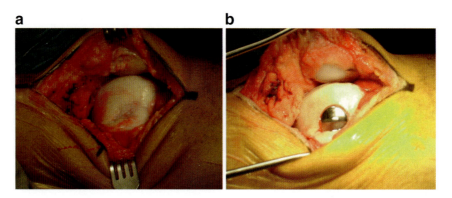

Fig. 8.21 (**a**, **b**) Pictures of severe trochlear disease treated by a focal resurfacing of both the trochlea and patella

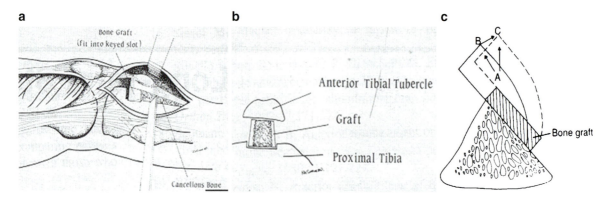

Fig. 8.22 (**a–c**) (**a** and **b**) Diagram represent the bone graft technique for elevation of the tubercle without translation, while (**c**) demonstrates the off-set bone used in oblique osteotomy for anteriorization

extensor mechanism and partially negates the negative effects of the patellectomy. Straight anteriorization can also be helpful in patients who had previous Hauser procedures where any medialization is not desired.

A last important point in patients who have had previous failed patellofemoral surgery is to utilize diagnostic or "staging" arthroscopy before making a definitive treatment plan for more major patellofemoral surgery. This can be further helpful not only in the diagnosis and discussion with patients in terms of surgical options and potential outcomes, but also in delineating what I call "the patient profile," in terms of the patient's response to minor surgery, pain, and rehabilitation before undertaking a more major procedure. Lastly, one should not be afraid to tell a patient that surgery is not the solution to their problem. In these cases, an honest approach to the patient in terms of recommendations and outcomes may be to their best benefit in the long term.

MPFL Reconstruction

MPFL reconstruction has received increased popularity and attention over recent years, primarily because of studies showing that the MPFL is a primary static soft tissue restrain against lateral patellar loads and that reconstruction of the MPFL restores tracking to near normal when medial restraints are deficient.[27–29] If done properly, reconstruction of the MPFL closely reproduces the normal anatomy and biomechanics more than imbricating or nonanatomic restraining procedures. Furthermore, it does not depend on the quality of the soft tissues. Finally and most importantly, the surgeon has better control over proper tensioning and tracking of the patella with this procedure. As mentioned in the previous section, reefing or advancements are acceptable with good soft tissue quality and attachments. However, they tend to create varying and nonisometric vectors of tension and often times tend to tighten flexion. Furthermore, when the degree of laxity is severe, the quality of the tissue is poor, and particularly when there is the presence of trochlear dysplasia, MPFL reconstruction is a more reliable and more reproducible technique to treat lateral patellar instability in my hands than reefing procedures. Our present indications for MPFL reconstruction are lateral patellar instability secondary to *moderate-to-severe* deficiencies of the medial restraints, lax medial restraints when trochlear dysplasia is present, failed reefing or imbrication procedures, poor tissue quality, and failed distal realignments. The most important point to remember is this is not an operation for pain or arthrosis, but an operation for instability. If the patient does not have instability, in general, this procedure should not be performed. Relative contraindications or warnings are the presence of severe medial facet arthrosis that would lead to increased contact pressures on the medial patella because of the posterior vector involved with MPFL reconstruction, patients with no symptoms of instability, and patients with permanent tilt, subluxation, or arthrosis with tubercle malalignment that are better dealt with a distal procedure, as will be discussed subsequently.

It is important to remember that the MPFL functions primarily in the first 30° of flexion and should become progressively lax (shortened) in higher degrees of flexion. It is meant to act as a restraint or checkrein to prevent abnormal lateral displacement not meant to "pull" the patella medially. Therefore, one of the most common mistakes is overtensioning the reconstruction (Fig. 8.23). The goal should be to restore the normal physiological lateral patellar glide of the patella and still allow the patella to enter the trochlea slightly from the lateral side. As mentioned before, severe medial facet arthrosis is a relative, but not an absolute, contraindication. A common scenario is to have a patient with recurrent dislocations, where the most common chondral damage pattern is in the distal medial portion of the patella. If there is 4+ lateral glide of the patella, indicating poor medial restraints, particularly in the presence of trochlear dysplasia, MPFL reconstruction can still be performed, but often in these cases I will make sure that the reconstruction is "underconstrained;" in other words "loose or sloppy" to prevent abnormal lateral displacement, but to just act as a checkrein. More importantly, it should become progressively lax beyond 30° of flexion where the medial

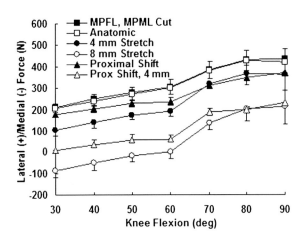

Fig. 8.23 Graph by Elias demonstrating the relationship between shifting the femoral attachment and increasing tension and associated increase medial forces with flexion

facet will see its most contact pressures. Furthermore, in cases of patients with any type of typical malalignment indicated by a high Q-angle or an increased TT–TG or a lateral tilt and subluxation, as documented by the CT scan, I will combine it with a medialization or an anteromedialization of the tibial tubercle. In this situation, the reconstruction is only constraining the patella in early flexion, becoming lax in 30° of flexion, with the anterior medial tubercle transfer not only unloading the damaged area but also adding further restraint. By adding a tubercle transfer, the amount of tensioning performed during the MPFL reconstruction is much less.

In terms of graft choice, the most commonly used graft is an autograft semitendinosis or gracilis. The procedure can also be performed with a strip of quadriceps tendon or a strip of adductor tendon. The most important point to remember is that these grafts, in general, are many magnitudes stiffer/stronger, with a higher load to failure, than the native MPFL.[28] This has its advantages and disadvantages. The advantages are that it will not stretch out over time and will be able to perform in long-term and "high-demand" situations (e.g., trochlear dysplasia). The disadvantage is that it can place high compressive loads on the patella, if placed improperly or overtensioned. This point emphasizes again the fact that the MPFL should not be overconstrained.

We have switched from utilizing a semitendinosis autograft to a semitendinosis allograft, avoiding the morbidity of harvesting the semitendinosis tendon.

We have not noticed any difference in results utilizing a soft tissue allograft in a rich extra-articular environment. In selected cases, particularly in young, petite females with a very small patella, a gracilis graft is also sufficient, whether it be autograft or allograft.

In terms of technique, as in most procedures, an accurate knowledge of the anatomy and biomechanics of the MPFL is paramount. Remember that the MPFL insertion on the femur is really in the "saddle" between the adductor tubercle and the medial epicondyle, not up at the adductor tubercle. Also, remember that the MPFL is not an isometric structure, and we like to use the term described by Dr. Jack Farr of "anatomometric" when delineating the proper points in length characteristics of the graft.[30] Remember that the length/tension characteristics of the graft are much more sensitive to the femoral attachment to the graft more than the patellar attachment to the graft, which is wider and spans the proximal half of the patella. There are many procedures described for MPFL reconstruction.[31-33] We presently utilize a technique that we have published,[34] utilizing a free semitendinosus graft with a closed socket fixation on the femur utilizing a Biotenodesis screw (Arthrex, Naples, Florida) and bio-suturetaks ("reverse loaded") on the patella in a trough on the proximal half of the patella, utilizing a double-limb graft. Although we have utilized sockets or tunnels in the patella in the past, we have switched to use of suture anchors in a trough. We found that the utilization of "reverse-loaded" anchors, a technique taught by Dr. Jack Farr, allows excellent fine tuning of the tensioning of the graft. It is a little easier and more user-friendly, it is easy to "bail out," if inadequate or there is failure of fixation, it is easier for a double-strand fixation, and, most importantly, there is less risk of patellar tunnel fracture. We have seen a couple of cases of patellar fracture (fortunately, not ours) from large tunnels in the patella, particularly smaller patellae in young, petite females. The biomechanical studies by Amis[31] show that this technique should have more than adequate fixation strength. Obviously, the major disadvantage is that you have less tendon/bone contact area, but this is offset by using a trough and the reverse loaded technique, as described in our paper.

We utilize a two-incision technique, with the first incision being over the proximal medial border of the patella and a second small incision over the femoral insertion. It is important to place the reconstruction extra-articularly, and we place it between layers 2 and 3 of the medial structures. Intra-articular placement could cause "snapping" of the tendon with range of motion over the medial femoral condyle or epicondyle and should be avoided. Careful dissection over the medial border of the patella to identify the interval between layers 2 and 3 is paramount. After placing a trough over the medial border of the patella, we then place a Biotenodesis pin over the proposed femoral insertion point. This is usually over the proximal slope of the medial epicondyle, which is usually more in the central to distal portion of the insertion of the MPFL. Placing the femoral fixation point too proximally is probably the most common technical error in our experience. This would cause the graft to tighten in flexion, which either would cause both increased forces on the medial facet of the patella or also may cause loss of flexion of the knee.

After placing the pin at the proposed femoral attachment, we run a suture around the pin up to the two points of fixation on the patella and secure and tension it at 30° in flexion to eliminate the abnormal patholaxity. What we like to see is, with extension from 30 to 0, that the length stays the same or possibly lengthens just slightly. However, more importantly, from 30° to full flexion, the distance shortens and the sutures become "lax." The most critical step is to get this point exactly right, and it is not infrequent to have to adjust this several times before getting the point right. Even a couple of millimeters of change in fixation point can make a difference. In very obese patients, where their landmarks are less distinct, fluoroscopy can be helpful with the use of *Schottle's point*[35] (Fig. 8.24). Radiographically, a reproducible center of attachment lies 1.3 mm

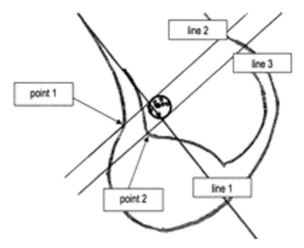

Fig. 8.24 Illustration representing Schottle's point, or a radiographic landmark for the femoral origin of the MPFL

anterior to the posterior cortical extension and 2.5 mm distal to the posterior origin of the medial femoral condyle, just proximal to the posterior extension of Blumensaat's line on a lateral X-ray with condylar overlap. Once the appropriate femoral point is found, the graft is taken and the doubled end sutured together for a distance of 25 mm and sized. A table is available in our publication for the correct socket size to make, depending on the doubled graft size. This usually provides very strong fixation, and the screw should be placed posterior to the doubled end of the graft on the femur. We have never had a failure of fixation here. However, if this did occur, the best "bail out" would be to drill a Beath pin from the floor of the socket through to the lateral side and utilize a screw fixation with backup of suture fixation over an endobutton or a bone bridge on the lateral side. Alternatively, a couple of suture anchors could be added for fixation. Washers or plates over the medial epicondyle should be avoided, as prominent hardware here is poorly tolerated.

The two limbs of the graft are then brought back to the patella and two reverse-loaded biosuturetak anchors are placed in the trough, one at the proximal medial extent of the patella and the other at 2 cm distal to this. Each separate limb is brought through a loop that is coming through the suture anchor and is then tensioned at 30° of flexion. Again, this technique allows for "fine-tuning" of the graft length and tension. This should eliminate the abnormal lateral patellar glide and restore the normal physiological glide (Fig. 8.25a–i).

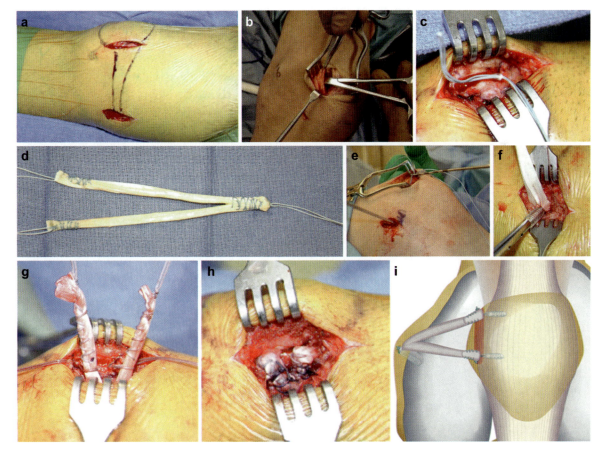

Fig. 8.25 (a) Photo demonstrating the two incisions used in our preferred MPFL reconstruction technique. (b) Careful dissection between layers 2 and 3 of the medial side of the knee avoiding synovial penetration for creation of the plane across which to pass the graft. (c) Photo showing a 3.0 reverse-loaded biosuturetak (arthrex) placed within a trough for patellar attachment. (d) A semitendinosus allograft doubled over into a Y-configuration with two limbs for the patella and one for the femur. (e) Anatomometric tensioning at 30° of flexion with suture looped around a biotenodesis pin. A probe is helpful in determining if the suture tightens or slackens with flexion and extension from 30° and the pin is then moved accordingly. (f) Biotenodesis pin securing the graft to the femoral socket. (g) Reverse loops holding the two limbs of the graft allowing for further fine-tuning of the tension with anatometry already being achieved. (h) Limbs are then doubled back toward the femoral side and sutured. (i) Representation of the final MPFL reconstruction

This can be thoroughly fixed, and patellar tracking can be assessed to make sure it is appropriate and, furthermore, that there is no medial tracking of the patella, particularly if a lateral release was necessary. We have found that, in general, if it seems that the MPFL reconstruction requires quite a bit of tension to get the patella to track properly, this is usually in association with tubercle malalignment, and I would prefer, at this point, to move the tubercle medially to decrease the tension on the MPFL reconstruction.

Usually the bone on the patella is quite strong, and usually these are young patients, so the use of standard glenoid-based anchors is sufficient. The 3.0 biosuturetak (Arthrex, Florida) has a loop that allows it to be reverse loaded loop-to-loop to perform this technique. We know of no other anchor at the present time that can be utilized. If the bone is slightly softer, we will use a 3.7-mm biosuturetak. If there is inadequate fixation with the use of this anchor, a larger metal anchor can be utilized or U-shaped tunnels can be utilized, as in Dr. Fithian's technique (Fig. 8.26). Another bail out would be to place a socket and then dock the sutures on the lateral side of the patella or to utilize an endobutton. Another thing to avoid is when making the small incision over the femoral attachment, sometimes one can encounter branches of the saphenous nerve. These must be carefully sought out and isolated to avoid painful neuromas. If a painful saphenous neuroma is recognized postoperatively, this can be treated with physical therapy modalities, tincture of time, local injections, and, in rare cases, excision of the neuroma.

If utilizing a bone tunnel technique and one gets an intraoperative fracture affecting the integrity of the bone tunnel, probably the best bail out is to utilize a reverse suture anchor, as described above. If utilizing the U-shaped tunnel described by Dr. Fithian and the bone bridge fractures, one can easily utilize suture anchors or drill a hole through the bottom of the socket to the lateral side of the patella and utilize a "docking technique" on the lateral side of the patella or utilize an endobutton.

The most common postoperative complication is loss of motion or stiffness of the knee. The best way to prevent this is to aggressively start early range of motion. We utilize a home CPM for the first 2–3 weeks postoperatively and have the patient start on this immediately upon discharge. I cannot think of any patellar realignment surgery that I do where I do not initiate immediate passive range of motion to the knee. Remember that your fixation should always be strong enough to withstand early range of motion and make the easy adjustments intraoperatively, so that early range of motion can be performed. If the femoral fixation point has been placed just proximally, this is another technical reason for loss of flexion to the knee and should be avoided and recognized by carefully testing length change characteristics intraoperatively before placement of the graft.

If the patient has sufficient loss of flexion that is not making any gains in PT after 3 months post-op, we would probably not wait any longer to bring the patient to the operating room and do a gentle arthroscopic lysis of adhesions and manipulation to regain motion of the knee.

Tibial Tubercle Osteotomy

Translation of the tibial tubercle, either medially, anteromedially, or even distally, is a frequently used procedure in patellofemoral realignment surgery. The main indications for distal realignment include patellar

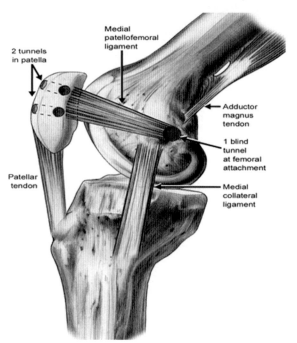

Fig. 8.26 A representation of Dr. Fithian's technique for MPFL reconstruction using a U-shaped tunnel in the patella for passage of graft

instability and/or pain from malalignment associated with tubercle or rotatory malalignment. In the study by Ramappa[36] on the effects of medialization and anteromedialization of patellofemoral mechanics, they showed that increased Q-angle increases the patellofemoral contact pressures, transfers forces to the lateral facet of the patella, and tilts and subluxes the patella laterally. Medialization corrects maltracking and partially corrects the increased contact pressures. In general, the most frequently used operations are medial tubercle transfer (a variation of the Elmslie-Trillat procedure) (Fig. 8.27a, b) for patients with patellar instability and malalignment with little or no pain or arthrosis, or anteromedialization of the tibial tubercle as popularized by Fulkerson (Fig. 8.28a, b), which not only corrects malalignment, but also is useful in patients with pain from arthrosis. Remember that the location of the arthrosis is more important than the extent, since anteromedialization transfers forces from the distal lateral to the proximal medial patella. In Fulkerson's study it was shown that patients who faired best with this procedure were patients with either lateral or distal arthrosis. Furthermore, in patients with severe forms of patella alta associated with pain and/or instability, distalization of the tibial tubercle can be performed as well.

Obviously the goal of this discussion is to discuss complications of tibial tubercle osteotomy rather than an extensive review of indications. Lastly, straight anteriorization of the tibial tubercle can be performed. This is a rare procedure but can be useful in patients with no malalignment, poor lateral restraints, where the idea is to unload either the distal patella or the trochlea. Other indications include patients with postpatellectomy pain and/or weakness or patients with post-Hauser procedure.[26] When deciding which operations to do for patellar instability, it should not be proximal vs. distal; it should be proximal when indicated, distal when

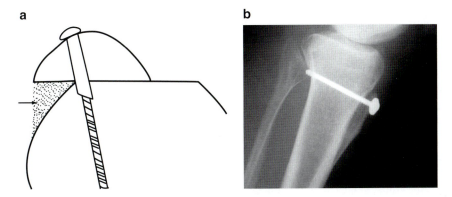

Fig. 8.27 (**a**, **b**) A diagram and X-ray demonstrating a medial tibial tubercle transfer

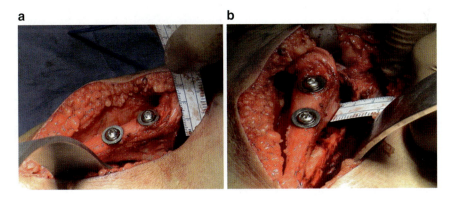

Fig. 8.28 (**a**, **b**) Pictures demonstrating the anteriorization and medialization achieved by the oblique osteotomy popularized by Fulkerson

indicated, and both when indicated. In general, proximal stabilizations are operations for traumatic instability, whereas distal realignments are for pain and/or instability associated with tubercle malalignment as the primary inciting factor. Furthermore, the presence of painful arthrosis associated with malalignment puts a distal procedure in more favor.

When deciding whether or not a patient has tubercle malalignment, obviously the most clinically useful parameter is the Q-angle. In our study, we found that the Q-angle is best measured at 30° of flexion since this is the point where the patella becomes centered (or as well centered as it will be) in the trochlear groove. As mentioned previously, we always utilize a CT scan, which includes fixed-frame images so we can measure the TT–TG, which is really the radiographic Q-angle or the CT measurement of the distance between the center of the trochlear groove and the center attachment of the patellar tendon on the tibial tubercle. According to our study, in general, the parameters that we use to delineate patients with tubercle malalignment are a Q-angle of greater than 20° and a TT–TG of greater than 15 mm.

The principle contraindication to a tibial tubercle osteotomy is a patient who is skeletally immature. Also, caution must be taken when performing a medial tubercle transfer in patients with a normal Q-angle, a low TT–TG, or a varus knee.

As mentioned previously, the two most common tibial tubercle osteotomy directions are either straight medial or anteromedial. The straight medialization is a flat osteotomy, which usually involves less cross-sectional area of the tibia, whereas the anteromedialization is an oblique osteotomy has an increasingly higher cross-sectional area, depending on the obliquity of the cut. It has been well shown in the literature as well as biomechanical studies[6,8,9,16,37] that the risk of postoperative fracture is much higher with an oblique osteotomy.

Intra-operatively, the first thing to remember, regardless of the exact incision used, is to respect the soft tissues. In general, we avoid incisions directly over the top of the tibial tubercle, where the subcutaneous tissues are most scant. In general, we prefer lateral approach to the tibial tubercle. A full-thickness dissection is important down to the deep fascia before undermining. We usually utilize a tourniquet during the critical portion of the procedure, but always release the tourniquet before closure to identify bleeders. In general, for large anteromedialization osteotomies, we always utilize a drain postoperatively because of the large surface area of the bone exposed, and with smaller, flat osteotomies, we do not utilize a drain, unless there is an indication to do so at the end of the procedure. Also, releasing the tourniquet before closure will allow inspection of the blood supply to the skin and subcutaneous tissues upon closure and particularly with highly oblique osteotomy with anteromedialization, this will increase pressures on the soft tissues. This is paramount in avoiding the occurrence of skin necrosis.

When performing a flat osteotomy, we usually perform a small shingle osteotomy approximately 5 cm long, tapering distally. It is important to have a complete transverse cut under the patellar tendon to avoid propagation of fracture toward the tibial plateau. (Fig. 8.29) When performing an anteromedialization, which is a much larger osteotomy, we feel it is *critical* to utilize a cutting guide. One would not perform a total knee arthroplasty cut without a guide, and, furthermore, there is no reason to perform this osteotomy without a guide. This ensures a nice flat cut, and we usually utilize the AMZ tracker guide (Depuy-Mitek, Warsaw, IN) (Fig. 8.30). The tracker guide will also tell you exactly where the cut is going to come out laterally, since the obliquity cut is limited to 60° by the intramuscular septum and neurovascular structures behind this. When performing an anteromedialization, it is critical to expose subperiostally the lateral cortex of the tibia down to the intramusclar septum and protect this with a large retractor). The tracker guide also

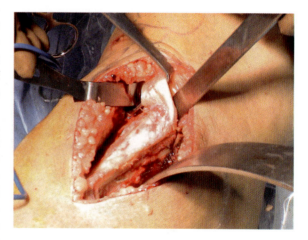

Fig. 8.29 Picture demonstrating an osteotome passing transversely just proximal to the patella tendon insertion completing the osteotomy

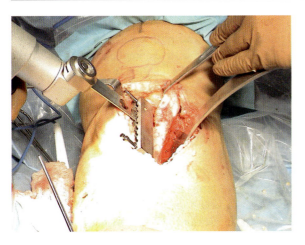

Fig. 8.30 Picture demonstrating the AMZ tracker guide (Depuy-Mitek). A slotted cutting guided is secured by pins ensuring a smooth cut and a large retractor protects the lateral musculature and neurovascular structures

allows the cut to be made exactly in the obliquity that is indicated (Fig. 8.31a, b). In general, a highly oblique cut is useful for patients with more arthrosis than malalignment and instability and a less oblique cut for vice versa. When performing anteromedialization after making the initial oblique cut, it is important to have a transverse cut on the patellar tendon and then a connecting cut between the lateral edge of the attachment of the patellar tendon and the proximal extent of the oblique osteotomy to prevent propagation into the tibial plateau. Furthermore, the osteotomy should be tapered distally for a distance of 8 cm, and notching should be avoided (Fig. 8.32). Also, utilizing a guide will take the osteotomy completely flat, whereas when performing this free-hand when transferring the tubercle anteromedially, one will end up with less bone-to-bone contact and a higher instance of delayed or nonunion. The next tip is, if utilizing a slot guide, one should avoid using drill holes. One technique that has been popular is just to put a series of drill holes along the planned osteotomy direction and then to connect the "dots" between the drill holes. We feel this should be avoided, as the drill holes provide a stress riser to the shingle of the tibial tubercle.

Multiple studies have shown that bicortical screw fixation is probably the best way to fix these osteotomies and that the use of wires or cerclage is not quite as strong.[38,39] Utilizing a bicortical screw, however, has the risk of injury to the posterior neurovascular structures since they are very close to the posterior tibial cortex.

After we perform the osteotomy, either medially or anteromedially, we usually provisionally fix this with a 3.2 drill bit to, but not through, the posterior cortex (Fig. 8.33). We then check the tracking of the patella, and once we are sure that the extent of displacement of the osteotomy is correct, we will flex the knee past 90° and carefully and slowly drill through the posterior cortex of the tibia to prevent "plunging" and perform a careful measurement of the length. We routinely use a metal washer with a screw for fixation of the tibial

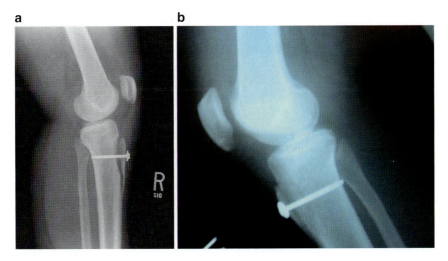

Fig. 8.31 (a) A lateral X-ray demonstrates the irregularity of a free-hand osteotomy for medial tibial tubercle transfer. (b) A lateral X-ray showing a smooth medial osteotomy achieved with a cutting guide

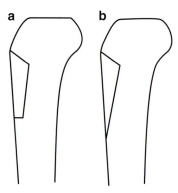

Fig. 8.32 Illustrations of two osteotomies for anteromedialization. The notched osteotomy is associated with increased fracture complications compared to the tapered one

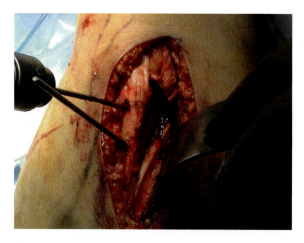

Fig. 8.33 Demonstration of the 2 drill bit technique of securing the tibial tubercle. First the distal 3.2 drill bit is drilled to but not through the posterior tibial cortex and tracking is assessed. The knee is then flexed to 90° and the proximal drill hole is made followed by placing the appropriate proximal screw and washer. The distal hole is then completed and screw and washer placed. The tubercle is palpated at all times when passing screws to ensure no lift-off is occurring due to missing the posterior drill holes with screw passage

tubercle osteotomy. In general, for a medial tubercle transfer, we will either use one or two screws, but with the anteromedialization always use two bicortical screws. Although some authors have advised "countersinking" to make the screws on the anterior tibia less prominent, we found this to not be very helpful in decreasing the incidence of hardware removal, and, furthermore, with the large countersink hole anteriorly, this weakens the shingle further, so we avoid this. We tell all patients that there is a high likelihood that the screws will be bothersome and that they will have to be removed about 1 year postoperatively.

The next intraoperative complication that should be looked for is medial instability of the patella, particularly in patients for whom you are performing a lateral retinacular release in conjunction with the osteotomy or who have had a lateral retinacular release previously. Transferring the tibial tubercle medially too far or inappropriately can cause medial instability of the patella. That is why it is important to provisionally fix the osteotomy temporarily and check patellar tracking. If one gets a large "clunk" or jump of the patella from extension to flexion, this usually indicates medial instability. In patients where I feel that either the lateral retinaculum is tight, but not excessively so, I would prefer to perform a lateral retinacular lengthening rather than a release so that I have the option of controlling the tension on the lateral retinaculum. In some cases, when performing anteromedialization primarily for arthrosis, the patient may not have a high degree of malalignment and then when transferring anteromedially, the medialization causes a medial tracking pattern. In this case, one has the option after temporarily fixing the osteotomy, if it is felt that the medialization effect is excessive but the anteriorization effect is desirable, an offset bone graft could be used to decrease the amount of medialization but preserve the anteriorization (Fig. 8.22c). Therefore, it is always important to provisionally fix the osteotomy and check the tracking carefully before definitive fixation to prevent this complication from occurring.

The next important point is to have the patient always consented for local bone grafting, either allograft or autograft, if there are areas of gapping or deficiency that need to be filled in. Again, make sure upon closure that the tourniquet is released so that hemostasis can be achieved and careful observation of the blood supply to the anterior tibial skin can be observed upon closure.

Postoperatively we feel all patients with a tibial tubercle osteotomy should be admitted for overnight observation. Radiographs should be obtained postoperatively and then at 2 weeks, 6 weeks, 12 weeks, and 24 weeks. Postoperatively, the amount of bleeding should be monitored as well as the devastating complication of compartment syndrome. Remember that upon closure no attempt should be made to close the fascia that was opened for the osteotomy. We do not usually routinely do a complete fasciotomy down the leg. With careful respect to the soft tissues, obtaining hemostasis after taking the tourniquet down, and the use of a drain for anteromedialization, we have not had any problems with compartment syndrome. Obviously, with any signs of compartment syndrome it is imperative to immediately return to the operating room in order to perform a decompressive fasciotomy.

The principle postoperative complication is fracture, nonunion, and delayed union. There are many case reports and literature of fracture after tibial tubercle osteotomy. The chief risk factor, particularly after anteriorization, is to allow early weight-bearing. For patients with anteromedialization, we routinely keep patients nonweight-bearing for 6 weeks and then partial, protected weight-bearing for another 4 weeks afterward. Furthermore, strenuous activities should be avoided for at least 4 months, and we do not encourage contact or collision sports until approximately 6 months postoperatively. A careful series of postoperative radiographs will ensure radiographic union to utilize as a guide for returning to activity. For a flat osteotomy, we allow protected weight-bearing in a brace for 6 weeks. However, we use the same guidelines for return to strenuous activities or sports.

In a study by Eager,[7] delayed fracture of the tibia following anteromedialization osteotomy was described in five patients. They felt that the primary factor was a distal notching technique used to create the osteotomies and that they subsequently started performing a tapering osteotomy and felt this avoided fracture (Fig. 8.32).

In Cosgarea's[9] study, they showed that the failure mechanisms for a flat osteotomy was usually a tubercle "shingle" fracture and for an oblique osteotomy, a proximal tibial fracture, or posterior cortical pull out. Interestingly, in clinical situations for the oblique osteotomy, proximal tibial fractures can be seen; however, posterior cortical pull-outs are not really reported. In Stetson's[8] article in 1997, he had a 2.6% fracture rate and felt that immediate weight-bearing was responsible.

The other complication that can occur is if the transverse cut of the osteotomy is not made directly at the proximal extent of the attachment of the patellar tendon on the tibial tubercle, there is a shingle of bone above the attachment of the tibial tubercle that is attached to the osteotomy that can provide a stress riser. This small fragment can fracture off, and, although it does not have any biomechanical effect since it is above the patellar tendon attachment, it can cause a painful loose ossicle. Therefore, the osteotomy should be transverse cut right flush with the patellar tendon attachment. If this complication does occur, usually excision of this painful fragment of bone is indicated.

If a fracture does occur despite these precautions, and if the fracture is nondisplaced, it usually can be treated nonoperatively, either with casting or bracing. At this point, emphasis should be made on bony healing rather than rehabilitation and that rehabilitation of the patellofemoral realignment surgery should be suspended until the fracture is well healed, even at the expense of atrophy, weakness, and stiffness, which may need to be addressed later on. If there is displacement of the fracture, open reduction and internal fixation may be necessary.

The other thing that can occur is loss of fixation. We have seen this most commonly when bicortical screws are not utilized and the osteotomy "lifts off." We would recommend treating this by the placement of a compressive bicortical screw with the possible addition of bone grafting. Delayed union or nonunion may require bone grafting as well as further compressive screw fixation or plate fixation if it does occur.

Painful hardware in our practice is really not considered a complication. We warn all patients with tibial tubercle osteotomies that the screws will be quite prominent and that there is a good chance that they will have to be removed. We usually wait a full year before removing the hardware, unless there is a reason to wait longer. The other complication that can occur is chronic medial instability of the patella, particularly in patients who have had overzealous medialization in association with a lateral retinacular release. Usually this can be recognized intraoperatively, if one follows the rules of provisionally fixing the shingle and carefully assessing the tracking of the patella. However, sometimes it may not occur statically under anesthesia but becomes a dynamic problem postoperatively. If this does occur in a subacute or chronic situation, this needs to be addressed surgically, since it usually will not improve with rehabilitation and will be quite disabling, as mentioned previously. If the medialization has not been excessive, this can be treated by the methods mentioned in the previous section, by lateral retinacular repair, or reconstruction. If the amount of medialization has been excessive or inappropriate, in rare chronic cases an anterolateral tubercle osteotomy can be performed, keeping the anteriorization in the tibial tubercle and even increasing it at the same time, lateralizing the tibial tubercle (as described by Fulkerson).

Revision Surgery

Failed patellofemoral surgery, unfortunately, is not an uncommon occurrence in the orthopedic knee specialist's practice. The first thing we teach residents and fellows is that, if a patient has already had eight surgeries for patellofemoral pain, malalignment, or instability, it is unlikely the ninth is going to cure them, so a careful approach is paramount. Each patient is different and it is important to use a careful history, examination, and use of imaging to guide you to the appropriate diagnosis. By following the principles outlined previously to avoid inappropriate or wrong surgical procedures, a lot of these complications certainly can be avoided. In particular, avoid surgery in the patients with chronic patellofemoral pain that include poorly responsive worker's compensation patients, diffuse ill-defined pain, patients with hyperesthesia, RSD, or regional pain syndromes, patients who are inadequately rehabilitated, and what we call the Type A "can't deal with this" patients. Remember that weight loss and rehabilitation are particularly effective methods to deal with patients with chronic patellofemoral pain.

The first salient point is to realize that the source of pain may not always be intra-articular, particularly in patients with chondral or osteochondral lesions. As taught by Dr. John Fulkerson, always "think soft tissues first." In patients who had previous surgery, often retinacular neuromas may be a source of pain. Carefully palpate all the soft tissues around the knee to see if you can find any "trigger points." As described by Fulkerson[2], these parapatellar neuromas often can be very painful and easy to treat. Carefully palpate everything, particularly all the incisions, and ask if the palpation "reproduces pain." Diagnostically, a local trigger-point injection can be helpful to delineate sources of pain. In some cases, if this is successful, local excision of the neuroma can be helpful. Likewise, tendinosis, either in the quadriceps tendon, particularly the vastus lateralis, or the patellar tendon, may be a source of pain. Again, local injection with an anesthetic may be helpful in differentiating referred pain to the patellar tendon from a chondral lesion vs. actual patellar tendinosis or tendinitis. Another frequently used tool in our practice, with patients with undiagnosed patellofemoral pain, is to give an intra-articular injection of a local anesthetic to help differentiate intra-articular vs. extra-articular pain.

As described in the beginning of the chapter, again, remember Scott Dye's "tissue homeostasis" theory. Often times a bone scan may be helpful in these patients who have had multiple surgeries, as patients with a very hot bone scans in the patellofemoral joint are generally not good candidates for surgical intervention.

Medial subluxation is a common reason for revision surgery and has been well described in previous sections. On a further note, we have encountered, not infrequently, patients with what we term "multidirectional instability." The most common scenario is a patient who suffers from recurrent lateral patellar instability who undergoes an isolated, inappropriate, lateral retinacular release. In this setting, the lateral retinacular release not only increases medial glide to an inappropriate level but also increases lateral glide by approximately 20%. We have seen several cases of patients who have a medial instability pattern in terminal extension and then a lateral instability pattern in slight flexion, so the patella is going from too-far-medial to too-far-lateral. In these cases, repair or reconstruction of the lateral retinaculum, in association with medial reefing, similar to capsular shifts in the shoulder can be quite helpful.

Fulkerson has described two forms of multidirectional instability. The first type is grossly unstable or Type A, as described in the previous case example. The second is a patient with chronic pain or Type B, which are more difficult to discern. These patients are similar to those with multidirectional shoulder instability and often present with hyperelasticity and hypermobility of the joints. Often times they do not have any evidence of malalignment. Similar to multidirectional instability of the shoulder, extensive rehabilitation should be exhausted before surgical intervention is entertained. In these cases, a careful capsular shift in the patellofemoral joint, either arthroscopically or with a mini-open approach of the medial retinaculum, may eliminate the problem. Often in these patients we will use a lateral buttress as well as medial Buttress bracing diagnostically to help diagnose the problem. One word of caution, however, is that in patients who have some chondrosis, imbricating both medial and lateral sides may lead to increased contact pressures and may trade an instability problem for a pain problem.

Three other common sources of recurrent instability in patients who have had previous patellar instability surgery are severe femoral anteversion, severe trochlear dysplasia, and patella alta, all of which are rarely managed with standard proximal and distal realignments. Careful examination of hip rotation is an essential step in evaluating any patient with patellar pain and instability. We encourage all surgeons who commonly manage patellar malalignment and instability to read Dr. Robert Teitge's[40] work on the role of femoral derotation osteotomy and the treatment of patellofemoral instability. In our practice, we would only recommend femoral derotation osteotomy in patients with an excess of 30-35° of femoral anteversion.

No chapter on patellofemoral complications would be complete without discussing chondral injury. However, it is beyond the scope of this chapter to address diffuse arthrosis of the patellofemoral joint. Treatment options for focal lesions of the patella or trochlear mirror the options available for femoral condyle lesions, varying from reparative to restorative, and lastly arthroplasty. Consequently the controversies, complications, and pitfalls of various techniques correspond to those applications in other compartments of the knee. There are several studies in the literature that investigate various chondral treatments, specifically in the patellofemoral joint, and we recommend taking a look at them.[41–43] One should keep in mind that the patella and trochlea present a challenge in the complexity of their contours. In addition, we believe that the thickness of patellar cartilage renders the patella less amenable to reparative techniques, thus we prefer osteochondral allografts for the treatment of focal lesions. We do, however, feel that reparative techniques are very useful in the treatment of trochlear lesions.

It cannot be understated that any surgical management of articular cartilage in the patellofemoral joint must take into account factors of malalignment or instability that may have cause the injury originally. Just as a meniscal transplant, a high tibial osteotomy, or an ACL reconstruction may be necessary in the survival of any technique aimed at treating a femoral condyle lesion, a lateral release, tibial tubercle transfer, or an MPFL reconstruction may be crucial concomitant procedures in the treatment of patellofemoral lesions. We commonly combine an unloading tibial tubercle osteotomy with resurfacing procedures, whether biologic or focal prosthetic.

References

1. Dye S (2005) The pathophysiology of patellofemoral pain: a tissue homeostasis perspective. Clin Orthop Relat Res Jul(436):100-10
2. Fulkerson J, Tennant R, Jaivin J et al (1985) Histologic evidence of retinacular nerve injury associated with patellofemoral malalignment. Clin Orthop Relat Res Jul-Aug(197): 196-205
3. Sanchis-Alfonso V, Roselló-Sastre E, Monteagudo-Castro C et al (1998) Quantitative analysis of nerve changes in the lateral retinaculum in patients with isolated symptomatic patellofemoral malalignment. A preliminary study. Am J Sports Med 26(5):703-9
4. Witoński D, Wagrowska-Danielewicz M (1999) Distribution of substance-P nerve fibers in the knee joint in patients with anterior knee pain syndrome. A preliminary report. Knee Surg Sports Traumatol Arthrosc 7(3):177-83
5. Dejour H et al (1994) Factors of patellar instability: an anatomic radiographic study. Knee Surg Sports Traumatol Arthrosc 2:19-26
6. Bellemans J, Cauwenberghs F, Brys P et al (1998) Fracture of the proximal tibia after Fulkerson anteromedial tibial tubercle transfer. A report of four cases. Am J Sports Med 26(2):300-2
7. Eager M, Bader D, Kelly JIV et al (2004) Delayed fracture of the tibia following anteromedialization osteotomy of the tibial tubercle: a report of 5 cases. Am J Sports Med 32(4):1041-8
8. Stetson W, Friedman M, Fulkerson JP et al (1997) Fracture of the proximal tibia with immediate weightbearing after a Fulkerson osteotomy. Am J Sports Med 25(4):570-4
9. Cosgarea A, Schatzke M, Seth A et al (1999) Biomechanical analysis of flat and oblique tibial tubercle osteotomy for recurrent patellar instability. Am J Sports Med 27(4):507-12
10. Kline A, Gonzales J, Beach W et al (2006) Vascular risk associated with bicortical tibial drilling during anteromedial tibial tubercle transfer. Am J Orthop 35(1):30-2
11. Ricchetti E, Mehta S, Sennett B et al (2007) Comparison of lateral release versus lateral release with medial soft-tissue realignment for the treatment of recurrent patellar instability: a systematic review. Arthroscopy 23(5):463-8
12. Fifthian D, Paxton E, Post W, International Patellofemoral Study Group et al (2004) Lateral retinacular release: a survey of the International Patellofemoral Study Group. Arthroscopy 20(5):463-8
13. Marumoto J, Jordan C, Akins R (1995) A biomechanical comparison of lateral retinacular releases. Am J Sports Med 23(2):151-5
14. Simpson L, Barrett J Jr (1984) Factors associated with poor results following arthroscopic subcutaneous lateral retinacular release. Clin Orthop Relat Res Jun(186):165-71

15. Bert J, Stark J, Maschka K et al (1991) The effect of cold therapy on morbidity subsequent to arthroscopic lateral retinacular release. Orthop Rev 20(9):755-8
16. Fulkerson J (1999) Fracture of the proximal tibia after Fulkerson anteromedial tibial tubercle transfer. A report of four cases. Am J Sports Med 27(2):265
17. Shannon B, Keene J (2007) Results of arthroscopic medial retinacular release for treatment of medial subluxation of the patella. Am J Sports Med 35(7):1180-7
18. Teitge R, Torga Spak R (2004) Lateral patellofemoral ligament reconstruction. Arthroscopy 20(9):998-1002
19. Jones R, Barlett E, Vainright J et al (1995) CT determination of tibial tubercle lateralization in patients presenting with anterior knee pain. Skeletal Radiol 24(7):505-9
20. Kuroda R, Kambic H, Valdevit A et al (2001) Articular cartilage contact pressure after tibial tuberosity transfer. A cadaveric study. Am J Sports Med 29(4):403-9
21. Miller J, Adamson G, Pink M et al (2007) Arthroscopically assisted medial reefing without routine lateral release for patellar instability. Am J Sports Med 35(4):622-9
22. Halbrecht J (2001) Arthroscopic patella realignment: An all-inside technique. Arthroscopy 17(9):940-5
23. Steiner T, Torga-Spak R, Teitge R (2006) Medial patellofemoral ligament reconstruction in patients with lateral patellar instability and trochlear dysplasia. Am J Sports Med 34:1254-61
24. Cohen Z, Henry J, McCarthy D et al (2003) Computer simulations of patellofemoral joint surgery: patient-specific models for tuberosity transfer. Am J Sports Med 31:87-98
25. Beck P, Thomas A, Farr J et al (2005) Trochlear contact pressures after anteromedialization of the tibial tubercle. Am J Sports Med 33(11):1710-5
26. Schepsis A, DeSimone A, Leach R (1994) Anterior tibial tubercle transposition for patellofemoral arthrosis. Am J Knee Surg 7(1):13-20
27. Burks R, Desio S, Bachus K et al (1998) Biomechanical evaluation of lateral patellar dislocations. Am J Knee Surg 11:24-31
28. Conlan T, Farth W Jr, Lemons J (1993) Evaluation of the medial soft tissue restraints of the extensor mechanism of the knee. J Bone Joint Surg Am 75:682-93
29. Hautama P, Fithian D, Kaufman K et al (1998) Medial soft tissue restraints in lateral patellar instability and repair. Clin Orthop Relat Res Apr(349):174-82
30. Farr J, Schepsis A (2006) Reconstruction of the medial patellofemoral ligament for recurrent patellar instability. J Knee Surg 19(4):1-10
31. Amis AA, Firer P, Mountney J et al (2003) Anatomy and biomechanics of the medial patellofemoral ligament. Knee 10:215-20
32. Muneta T, Sekiya I et al (1999) A technique for reconstruction of the medial patellofemoral ligament. Clin Orthop Relat Res Feb(359):151-5
33. Schock E, Burks RT (2001) Medial patellofemoral reconstruction using a hamstring graft operative techniques. Sports Med 9:169-75
34. Farr J, Schepsis A, Cole B et al (2007) Anteromedialization: review and technique. J Knee Surg 20(2):120-8
35. Schöttle PB, Schmeling A, Rosenstiel N et al (2007) Radiographic landmarks for femoral tunnel placement in medial patellofemoral ligament reconstruction. Am J Sports Med 35(5):801-4
36. Ramappa A, Apreleva M, Harrold F et al (2006) The effects of medialization and anteromedialization of the tibial tubercle on patellofemoral mechanics and kinematics. Am J Sports Med 34(5):749-56
37. Gödde S, Rupp S, Dienst M et al (2001) Fracture of the proximal tibia six months after Fulkerson osteotomy. A report of two cases. J Bone Joint Surg Br 83(6):832-3
38. Caldwell P, Bohlen B, Owen J et al (2004) Dynamic confirmation of fixation techniques of the tibial tubercle osteotomy. Clin Orthop Relat Res Jul(424):173-9
39. Davis K, Caldwell P, Wayne J et al (2000) Mechanical comparison of fixation techniques for the tibial tubercle osteotomy. Clin Orthop Relat Res Nov(380):241-9
40. Teitge R (2006) Osteotomy in the treatment of patellofemoral instability. Tech Knee Surg 5(1):2-18
41. Kreuz P, Steinwachs M, Erggelet C et al (2006) Results after microfracture of full-thickness chondral defects in different compartments in the knee. Osteoarthritis Cartilage 14(11):1119-25
42. Minas T, Bryant T (2005) The role of autologous chondrocyte implantation in the patellofemoral joint. Clin Orthop Relat Res Jul(436):30-9
43. Owens B, Stickles B, Balikian P et al (2002) Prospective analysis of radiofrequency versus mechanical debridement of isolated patellar chondral lesions. Arthroscopy 18(2):151-5

Editors' Comments (Patella)

On use of MRI vs. CT

Although CT scanning can be very useful to assess the TT–TG distance, MRI scanning provides the same measurement, avoids radiation, and is often obtained in any event.

Treatment of OA

It is the editors' experience that patients with early degenerative disease of the lateral patellofemoral joint can benefit from patella surgery if the correct surgery is performed. If the arthrosis is indeed localized to the lateral PF joint, unloading this area can be very effective. A lateral release and anteromedialization osteotomy of the tubercle should be performed if the disease is distal on the patella. If the disease is more proximal, we would perform a release along with an arthroscopic medial reefing to tilt the patella away from the degenerative lateral facet, without overloading the proximal patella as would occur with an osteotomy. We also carefully evaluate a preoperative Merchant view looking for lateral facet osteophytes, and resect these as necessary. A partial facetectomy is also considered if there is significant lateral overhang of the patella or if the Grade IV disease is isolated to the lateral most portion of the facet.

Synovectomy

Dye has demonstrated that much of the pain associated with patellofemoral disease emanates from synovial irritation. Certainly one should remove impinging or inflamed synovium identified at the time of surgery. However, it is the editors' opinion that excessive fat pad debridement should be avoided so as to prevent postoperative scarring and iatrogenic Hoffa's syndrome.

Chapter 9
Avoiding and Managing Complications Associated with Arthroscopic Knee Surgery: Miscellaneous Knee Conditions

Eric J. Strauss and Robert J. Meislin

Introduction and Background

Secondary to improvements in instrumentation, operative techniques and surgeon experience, knee arthroscopy has gained significant popularity amongst orthopedists for the management of a variety of pathologic conditions affecting the knee. In the United States, knee arthroscopy is the most commonly performed operative orthopedic procedure, with more than 2 million cases occurring annually.[1–5] As the indications for operative knee arthroscopy have increased, so have complications associated with the surgery. Although the vast majority of knee arthroscopic procedures occur without incident, recent reports have cited complication rates ranging from <1% to 8% of cases.[1,4,6–9]

Arthrofibrosis, infection, osteonecrosis/bone marrow edema syndrome, broken/retained hardware, and issues with portal healing are among the possible complications associated with arthroscopic knee procedures. The following chapter reviews each of these potential problems associated with operative knee arthroscopy and provides suggestions for appropriate management.

E.J. Strauss
Department of Orthopaedic Surgery, NYU Hospital for Joint Diseases, 301 East 17th Street, New York, NY
e-mail: straued1@med.nyu.edu

R.J. Meislin
Orthopedic Surgery, NYU Hospital for Joint Diseases, New York, New York, USA

Arthrofibrosis Following Arthroscopic Knee Procedures

The development of arthrofibrosis following arthroscopic assisted ligamentous reconstructions of the knee is a significant source of postoperative morbidity.[10–16] Patients who do not regain full range of motion following ligament surgery commonly report persistent anterior knee pain, weakness, alterations in their gait pattern, difficulty regaining their preinjury level of function, and overall dissatisfaction with their outcome.[10,12,15] Recently, there has been increased recognition and interest in identifying the risk factors and pathophysiology associated with the development of postoperative arthrofibrosis. Advances in the understanding of this potential complication has led to better prevention strategies in addition to improved management techniques once the diagnosis has been made.

Typically defined as postoperative loss of range of motion secondary to the development of abnormal intra-articular scarring, the diagnosis of arthrofibrosis includes a wide spectrum of disease involving both intra-articular and extra-articular pathology. Its reported incidence in the orthopedic literature varies, ranging from 4 to 57% after ligament reconstruction procedures.[10,13,17] Studies have demonstrated that patients with multi-ligamentous injuries are most prone to the development of postoperative arthrofibrosis. Noyes et al., in their retrospective review of 207 arthroscopic assisted anterior cruciate ligament reconstructions, found that cases in which an additional medial collateral ligament repair was performed had a 23% incidence of postoperative loss of motion.[13] In a review of seven patients who underwent anterior and posterior cruciate ligament reconstruction after traumatic knee dislocation,

Shapiro and Freedman reported that four patients (57%) developed significant arthrofibrosis requiring additional treatment.[14]

Postoperative loss of extension after ligament surgery is often more disabling than a corresponding loss of flexion. Patients who develop flexion contractures as little as 5–10° may experience changes in their gait pattern, quadriceps strain, early fatigue, and patellofemoral pain.[10,12] Those who develop severe postoperative loss of flexion (<90°) often report difficulty with stair climbing. In athletes, loss of more than 10° of knee flexion when compared with the normal contralateral knee may impact stride length and running speed.[12] Various classification schemes based on the extent of postoperative motion loss have been developed. Del Pizzo et al. described mild loss of motion as less than 5° of extension with maintenance of flexion past 110°.[12] Moderate loss was defined as a 5–10° flexion contracture coupled with 90–110° of knee flexion. Greater than 10° of extension loss and lack of flexion past 90° represents severe postoperative motion loss. Shelbourne et al. reported their system, which classified motion loss into four types.[15] Type 1 represents patients who maintain normal flexion and have a loss of less than 10° of extension. Those with normal flexion and a flexion contracture greater than 10° have type 2 loss, while patients with loss of flexion greater than 25° and loss of extension greater than 10° are classified as type 3. Type 4 motion loss is defined as flexion loss greater than 30° coupled with extension loss greater than 10° and associated patella infera.

Recently, investigators have identified a number of risk factors associated with the development of arthrofibrosis.[10,12] One commonly discussed risk factor is the acute reconstruction of a torn anterior cruciate ligament (ACL). In a retrospective review of 244 patients treated with arthroscopic ACL reconstruction, Harner et al. found that those operated on within one month of injury had a significant, nearly sevenfold increased incidence of arthrofibrosis compared with those managed with delayed reconstruction.[18] Similar findings were reported by Shelbourne et al. in their review of 213 consecutive ACL reconstructions.[19] The authors reported that compared with reconstructions performed at least 21 days after injury, those operated on within 1 week had a significantly higher incidence of symptomatic postoperative loss of motion requiring intervention. Technical issues during ligament reconstruction including errors in tunnel placement, failure to completely excise remnants of the torn ligament leading to the development of a cyclops lesion anteriorly, failure to remove drilling debris and possibly choice of graft type (allograft versus autograft) have all been identified as potential sources for postoperative loss of motion.[10,12,15,18] Whether it is associated with a greater extent of initial soft tissue or additional trauma from a more extensive surgical procedure, the addition of a concomitant posterior cruciate ligament (PCL) or medial collateral ligament (MCL) repair/reconstruction to an isolated ACL reconstruction has been shown to correlate with an increased incidence of arthrofibrosis.[17,18] Additional risk factors include prolonged postoperative knee immobilization, delayed or impaired rehabilitation secondary to complex regional pain syndrome and postoperative infection.[10,12] Recent studies have proposed the theory that certain patients may have a genetic predisposition to the development of postoperative arthrofibrosis. In a retrospective cohort study comparing blood samples from 17 patients with arthrofibrosis after ACL reconstruction to samples from the general population, Skutek et al. found that patients who developed arthrofibrosis had differences in certain HLA alleles.[16]

Three varieties of postoperative arthrofibrosis have been described based on the extent of pathology.[10,12] Loss of extension secondary to the development of an ACL nodule, also known as a cyclops lesion, has been termed localized anterior intra-articular arthrofibrosis.[12,20] The nodule, which is typically a fibroproliferative scarred mass located anterolateral to the tibial tunnel, is believed to occur with anterior placement of the graft, failure to completely excise remnants of the torn native ligament or from bony debris left in the joint following drilling of the tibial tunnel. In cases of anterior graft placement, repetitive trauma to the graft in the notch during extension is thought to cause graft tissue hypertrophy and proliferation of fibrous tissue. When present, the fibrous cyclops lesion acts as a mechanical block to extension. A second type of arthrofibrosis is localized intra-articular disease with extra-articular extension. First described by Paulos et al., this variant of arthrofibrosis is also called infrapatellar contraction syndrome or patellar entrapment syndrome.[21] Deficits of both flexion and extension coupled with decreased patellar mobility and patella infera occur secondary to pathologic hypertrophic fibrous tissue developing anteriorly. The normally mobile and pliable infrapatellar fat pad becomes increasingly adherent to the proximal tibia limiting knee motion. In a review of 75 patients with infrapatellar contraction syndrome, Paulos et al. found that acute ACL surgery, use of patellar tendon autograft, and prolonged immobilization were predisposing fractors.[21] Diffuse intra-articular and extra-articular disease or global arthrofibrosis is the third type of motion loss following arthroscopic ligament procedures. This subtype is believed to occur secondary to an exaggerated inflammatory response leading to extensive periarticular fibrous scar formation.[10,12,22] The development of extensive scar tissue throughout the joint and associated capsular fibrosis with their subsequent contraction acts to decrease the volume of the suprapatellar pouch and gutters severely limits knee range of motion and patellar mobility.

Despite the development of various treatment protocols to manage postoperative arthrofibrosis, prevention remains the most effective management strategy.[10,12,15,18,19] Currently, most authors recommend avoiding acute ligament reconstruction, delaying the surgical procedure until the inflammation and swelling associated with the injury have completely resolved. Most often this requires a delay of at least 3–6 weeks postinjury, during which time preoperative physical therapy can be instituted. Formal preop therapy employing quadriceps strengthening and restoration of knee range of motion with active-assist and passive protocols can be helpful in avoiding postoperative loss of motion. Once the patient has achieved/regained full extension and flexion to at least 125°, the elective arthroscopically assisted ligament reconstruction can be undertaken. Exception to these rules would be an extension block due to a displaced bucket handle meniscal tear. Avoidance of intraoperative technical errors including anteriorly placed femoral and tibial tunnels can help prevent the development of impingement and associated cyclops lesions. Postoperative factors including adequate control of pain and swelling in addition to improved rehabilitation protocols which promote immediate knee range of motion, patellar mobilization, and quadriceps strengthening have also been shown to help prevent the development of arthrofibrosis. In a prospective review of 443 ACL reconstructions, Noyes et al. reported that the institution of immediate knee motion postoperatively led to 93% of patients regaining full 0–135° range of motion.[13] Many published post-ACL reconstruction protocols include extension or hyperextension bracing for the first 2–3 weeks. Mikkelsen et al., in a prospective randomized study comparing postoperative bracing in full extension versus hyperextension (−5°), found that 3 weeks of hyperextension bracing led to a significant reduction in extension loss at 3 months of follow up.[23]

We have found that use of a locked extension brace at night helps avoid postoperative loss of extension, intercondylar notch scarring, or cyclops formation. The brace is set in the OR to equal the extension or even hyperextension of the opposite normal knee. The brace is utilized at all times during the first 2–3 weeks when the patient is not otherwise doing range of motion exercises and physical therapy. If a patient still has difficulty maintaining postoperative extension, we have had success utilizing a knee extension board (Instrument Maker), which is provided to the patient for home use.

Once identified, the management of arthrofibrosis depends on the extent of motion loss, the extent of inflammation, and the duration of the symptoms. In the early postoperative period, it is recommended that patients are seen weekly to objectively evaluate the progress of range of motion therapy. Adequate control of pain and swelling can be achieved using nonsteroidal antiinflammatory medications, judiciously prescribed narcotics, cryotherapy, and oral steroids in cases of persistent inflammation. The physician should review the rehabilitation program to ensure that overly aggressive therapy is avoided in the perioperative period. Patients who fail to reach flexion past 90° and develop flexion contractures greater than 10° between the four and eight week follow up time points are candidates for manipulation under anesthesia with or without an associated arthroscopic lysis of adhesions.[10,12] Manipulation under anesthesia alone has been shown to be effective in regaining some of the motion deficits associated with early arthrofibrosis. It is imperative to ensure that the physical therapist mobilizes the patella. Dodds et al., in their review of manipulations performed in 42 knees with motion loss after ACL reconstruction, reported a mean increase of 41° of flexion and 8° of extension after the procedure.[11] Interestingly, the authors found that patients with more significant preprocedure motion loss (flexion contractures > 15°) benefited less from manipulation than those with less severe arthrofibrosis.

Published surgical indications in cases of arthrofibrosis include knee flexion of less than 125°, flexion contractures greater than 10°, and failure to progress with nonoperative management by the 8-week follow up timepoint.[10,12] Operative arthroscopy provides the surgeon with the opportunity to debride a focal cyclops lesion, an adherent/contracted infrapatellar fat pad, and lyse adhesions associated with more global arthrofibrosis. A systematic arthroscopic approach to managing cases of arthrofibrosis has been proposed by Kim et al.[24] The authors start by reestablishing the suprapatellar pouch followed by reconstituting both the medial and lateral gutters. Next the pretibial recess is recreated followed by a medial or lateral retinacular release in cases of patellar entrapment. Next, the surgeon evaluates the intercondylar notch looking for graft impingement in extension. When present a notchplasty is performed. The graft is then examined for evidence of hypertrophy or scarring, which can then be debrided. The knee is then taken through a range of motion, with or without a gentle manipulation. Persistent flexion loss can be further addressed by releasing the superior or proximal suparapatellar capsule with a heat thermal device. Cases of persistent extension loss following arthroscopic debridement and manipulation will often require either an arthroscopic or open posterior capsular release. Utilizing a 70° scope for visualization through the intercondylar, the posteromedial and posterolateral portals can be utilized to incise the surrounding posterior capsule with a heat thermal device. The posteromedial compartment is visualized by passing the arthroscopic from the anterolateral portal at the interval between the PCL and the medial femoral condyle and gently joysticking one's hand upwards several degrees. Be careful not to forcefully plunge as the neurovascular bundle remains close to the posterior capsule. The posterolateral compartment is best seen by passing the arthroscope from the anteromedial portal at the interval between the lateral femoral condyle and the ACL. Under direct visualization with either a 30 or 70° scope the posteromedial or posterolateral portal can be established. The knee should be flexed to 90° to allow for the neurovascular structures on either the medial or lateral side to fall further away. The posteromedial portal is bounded by the medial head of the gastrocnemius, semimembranosis, and MCL. The posterolateral portal is bounded by the lateral head of gastrocnemius, LCL, and posterolateral tibial plateau.

If a patient loses motion after surgery and surgical treatment is undertaken, the approach needs to be comprehensive and needs to address both flexion and extension deficits. To regain flexion, release of the supra patella pouch, medial and lateral gutters, and possibly retinacular releases are often necessary. If the graft itself is poorly placed, in rare cases the graft will need to be released or removed. To regain extension, the surgeon will need to clear out the intercondylar notch to ensure that there is no mechanical block anteriorly preventing extension. If this is still not effective, the posterior capsule is often the culprit, particularly if a meniscus repair was done, which may capture the capsule. In this instance, the surgeon needs to be prepared to perform a posterior capsular release. This is performed arthroscopically in our hands, utilizing a posterior medial portal. Through this portal, the posterior medial and posterior lateral capsule can be released by penetrating through the septa behind the PCL, while viewing with the arthroscope through the notch.

Open treatment is usually reserved for recalcitrant cases as a salvage procedure, often those with associated extra-articular sources of motion loss such as heterotopic ossification and myositis ossificans.[10,12] Open treatment typically involves large exposures with a parapatellar arthrotomy. A similar systematic approach is utilized with the addition of a subperiosteal posterior capsular release at both the femoral and tibial insertion sites. An alternative approach is the use of a mini-open posterior approach following arthroscopic lysis of adhesions utilizing the interval between the medial head of the gastrocnemius and semimembranosus. A capsular incision is made along the trailing edge of the medial collateral ligament opening up the meniscofemoral interval.[10] From this position, the fibrotic capsule can be elevated off of the distal femur and proximal tibia along with removal of remnant posterior scar tissue. Other salvage procedures have been described for severe cases of arthrofibrosis unresponsive to other treatments.[10,12,25,26] Quadricepsplasty in which the vastus intermedius is released while the quadriceps tendon is z-lengthened has been reported to significantly improve postprocedure flexion.[26] For cases of recalcitrant patella infera, tibial tubercle osteotomies have been described.[12]

Postoperative rehabilitation protocols following treatment of vary depending on the type of arthrofibrosis present and the procedure performed. After manipulation under anesthesia, some authors recommend casting the patient in full extension or hyperextension for a brief period (1–2 days) prior to resumption of range of motion therapy. Following an arthroscopic debridement of a cyclops lesion, patients are typically restarted on their prescribed physical therapy regimen.

For more severe cases requiring extensive surgical releases, Dehaven et al. recommend placing the patient in an extension cast, which is bivalved on postoperative day number one.[10] The patients are taken out of the cast 4–5 times per day for range of motion therapy (with a continuous passive motion machine if available) over a 2-week period. Next, physical therapy for additional range of motion and strengthening is performed, with the patients using the extension cast or a spring-loaded extension brace at night. The use of postoperative NSAIDs and short courses of oral steroids have been recommended to minimize postoperative inflammation and scar tissue reformation. In refractory cases, the patients may have to be admitted for pain control that may also include an indwelling epidural catheter. Although outcome studies following treatment of arthrofibrosis are limited in the orthopedic literature, many authors report continued gains in post-treatment range of motion for up to six months.

Postoperative Infection

Infection following knee arthroscopy is a relatively rare complication. The reported incidence in the orthopedic literature ranges from 0.007 to 3.4%.[7,27–32] Judd et al., in a recent retrospective evaluation of 1,615 arthroscopically assisted anterior cruciate ligament reconstructions, identified 11 cases of postoperative infection (incidence of 0.007%).[32] Skin flora such as *Staphylococcus* and *Streptococcus* species account for the vast majority of infecting organisms. Rarely, other organisms such as *Pseudomonas aeruginosa*, *Clostridium perfringens*, *Neisseria meningitidis*, and *Candida albicans* have been cultured from infections postarthroscopy.

Careful attention to sterile technique coupled with the use of prophylactic antibiotics (typically a first-generation cephalosporin) has helped keep the risk of infection associated with operative knee arthroscopy low. The results of recent studies have questioned the utility of antibiotic prophylaxis for arthroscopic knee cases. Bert et al., in a retrospective review of 2,780 cases, compared the infection rate between patients who received antibiotic prophylaxis within 1 h before the procedure and those who were not prophylaxed.[29] The authors found that the infection rate was 0.15% among the patients receiving antibiotics compared with an incidence of 0.16% in those who did not. Additionally, as the complexity of the cases being treated arthroscopically increases, the ability of an experienced arthroscopist to reduce the overall operative time becomes important in preventing contamination and the development of subsequent infection.[7,31]

Classic signs of joint infection include the presence of a knee effusion or an acute increase in its extent, knee pain, erythema, warmth, and drainage from the portal sites. The management of a suspected postoperative septic arthritis following knee arthroscopy includes a full set of infection labs, including a complete blood count with differential, erythrocyte sedimentation rate, and C-reactive protein level. A knee aspiration provides fluid for culture and gram stain, and an intra-articular cell count. Once an infection has been identified, treatment options include arthroscopic irrigation and debridement or open irrigation and debridement coupled with an organism-specific intravenous antibiotic regimen. The decision to retain or remove an implanted graft remains controversial in the literature, with most authors choosing on a case by case basis.[32] In the acute (<6 weeks) and subacute (<3 months) infected setting of an ACL reconstruction an arthroscopic I & D of the knee can be performed as in initial intervention with retention of the graft. Proper cultures must be obtained and the infectious disease specialist must be alerted to properly design the type and duration of antibiotics. Often time the patient will have to receive a PIC line to receive home antibiotics. Signs of persistent infection after an initial arthroscopic or open I&D should prompt graft and hardware removal. Expeditious identification and treatment of an infectious complication enables the surgeon to decompress the associated knee effusion, remove the destructive proteolytic bacterial enzymes, and eradicate the infection.[31]

Osteonecrosis of the Knee Following Knee Arthroscopy/Bone Marrow Edema Syndrome

First described in 1968 by Ahlback et al., spontaneous osteonecrosis of the knee has been recognized as a distinct clinical entity and a rare potential complication of arthroscopic knee surgery.[33–37] An association between arthroscopic meniscectomy and subsequent development of osteonecrosis of the distal femur has been described.

Brahme et al. reported on seven cases of postmeniscectomy distal femoral osteonecrosis.[38] In each case, initial MRI evaluation demonstrated complete meniscal tears with normal bone marrow signal intensity. Within 2–14 months following arthroscopic partial meniscectomy, all seven patients returned with recurrent knee pain and associated effusions limiting ambulatory ability. Repeat MRI demonstrated lesions in the subchondral area of the distal femoral condyle consistent with osteonecrosis. Similar presentations have been reported by Prues-Latour et al., Muscolo et al., and Santori et al.[36,37,39] In each of these series, the patients who developed osteonecrosis tended to be older (>50 years) with degenerative meniscal pathology and associated chondromalacia in the compartment where the lesion subsequently developed. Although an association between the meniscal injury itself and the development of osteonecrosis cannot be ruled-out, the authors of these reports theorize that the alteration in the distribution of forces following arthroscopic partial meniscectomy in cases with baseline degenerative changes is the likely etiology. Repetitive microtrauma from increased bone-to-bone contact following meniscectomy in patients with compromised or deficient articular cartilage may lead to the subchondral microfractures believed to be the pathologic precursor to osteonecrosis lesions.

Various staging systems have been developed for osteonecrosis affecting the knee. Koshino et al. define stage 1 disease as incipient, with patients reporting pain with activity. Plain X-rays in this stage are negative for pathology; however, bone scan is positive in the affected region. Stage 2 osteonecrosis, or the avascular stage, is demonstrated by subchondral lucency in the weight-bearing area with associated surrounding sclerosis. Arthroscopic evaluation during this stage typically finds minimal articular changes. During the collapse stage of disease (stage 3), X-rays demonstrate a calcified plate with radiolucency surrounded by a sclerotic halo. Subchondral collapse heralds stage 3 osteonecrosis. Further collapse with associated development of arthritic changes in the affected compartment defines stage 4 disease. Similar classification systems published by Aglietti et al. and Mont et al. describe the spectrum of disease running from normal imaging and arthroscopic findings to full collapse and joint degeneration.[40,41]

Bone marrow edema syndrome, thought to represent an early, reversible stage of osteonecrosis has also been noted to occur following arthroscopic knee surgery.[34] The pattern of bone marrow edema syndrome tends to be more diffuse than isolated osteonecrosis, with progression to full blown AVN possibly inhibited by abundant new bone formation.[34,42] It is likely that a similar etiology of altered force distribution following meniscectomy results in changes within the subchondral region of the distal femoral condyles. In an MRI evaluation of normal volunteers, Schweitzer and White were able to produce diffuse bone marrow edema by changing gait mechanics with a shoe insert that caused foot overpronation.[34,43]

Bone marrow edema syndrome involves three stages.[34] Stage one is described as pain usually following an usual or atypical activity, which is worsened by weight-bearing and relieved by rest. Plain X-rays in stage one are negative for any detectable pathology. Persistent symptoms and X-rays in which osteopenia is evident defines stage two disease. This stage can last up to two months in duration. Stage three bone marrow edema syndrome follows, and is defined as resolution of symptoms with corresponding restoration of normal bone density. The overall course of disease ranges from 6 months to 2 years.

In patients who return following arthroscopic meniscal surgery with recurrent knee pain and swelling, the spectrum of bone marrow edema syndrome and post-arthroscopy osteonecrosis must remain in the differential diagnosis. Repeat MRI helps identify the presence of these potential post-arthroscopy complications, allowing for early diagnosis and appropriate management. For cases of early disease, nonoperative treatment is appropriate, with protected weight-bearing, nonsteroidal antiinflammatory medications and physical therapy for quadriceps and hamstring strengthening. Smaller lesions caught early, appear to respond well to nonoperative management. In a review of 79 patients with medial femoral condyle osteonecrosis, Lotke et al. reported that of 31 of 33 knees with stage 1 disease managed with protected weight bearing and symptomatic treatment had good to excellent results.[44] Persistent symptoms not responding to nonoperative treatment may be indicated for repeat surgical intervention. Available options include repeat arthroscopy with debridement/chondroplasty of unstable cartilage lesions, core decompression with or without bone grafting, high tibial osteotomy if there is weight-bearing malalignment and prosthetic replacement (unicompartmental arthroplasty vs. total knee arthroplasty).

The choice of procedure must be tailored to the individual patient with the extent of their symptoms, their functional status, the severity of their disease, and expectations taken into consideration.

Broken Instrumentation/Retained Hardware

Although rare, failure of arthroscopic instrumentation within the knee joint has been described. In Small's large series of cases, he reported an incidence of intra-articular hardware failure of 0.05%.[8,9] Case reports in the orthopedic literature describe the potential for breakage of scalpel blades during the creation of portals,[45] arthroscopic knives used in meniscectomy, and even detachment of the tip of a motorized shaver.[46] Unless the broken instrumentation can safely be grabbed and removed from the joint using an arthroscopic grasper, arthrotomy is often required. A magnetic wand is a "must have" instrument to have in one's toolkit as this may obviate the need for an open arthrotomy to attract a broken hook or tool. Beware that nitinol is titanium based and does not display magnetic properties.

Portal Issues

In addition to the risks of nerve injury and infection associated with arthroscopy portals, healing complications of these sites may also occur, postoperatively. The small size of most arthroscopy portals limits the morbidity associated with portal opening secondary to suture breakage or portal scarring. Rare cases of synovial cyst formation related to an arthroscopic portal have been reported.[47] When present, a portal site synovial cyst can cause anterior knee pain with activity. Shaikh et al., in their case report describe successful treatment of a portal site synovial cyst with repeat arthroscopy. Intraoperatively, the authors identified a capsular defect laterally as a remnant of their previous anterolateral portal, which contributed to cyst development. Cyst excision coupled with capsule repair led to a successful clinical outcome.

Conclusion

Arthroscopy of the knee is a safe and effective treatment for a number of soft tissue and intra-articular pathologies. The overall reported incidence of complications associated with operative knee arthroscopy is <2% in most large case series. Although rare, arthrofibrosis, infection, osteonecrosis/bone marrow edema syndrome, broken hardware, and issues with portal healing may occur in association with arthroscopic knee procedures. Knowledge of the potential complications seen with this commonly utilized procedure can aid the arthroscopist in avoiding their development, identifying them when they present, and applying appropriate treatment protocols.

References

1. Kim T, Savino R, McFarland E et al (2002) Neurovascular complications of knee arthroscopy. Am J Sports Med 30(4):619-29
2. McGinty J, Johnson L, Jackson R et al (1992) Uses and abuses of arthroscopy: A symposium. J Bone Joint Surg Am 74(10):1563-77
3. Rodeo S, Forster R, Weiland A (1993) Neurological complications due to arthroscopy. J Bone Joint Surg Am 75(6):917-26
4. Small N (1988) Complications in arthroscopic surgery performed by experienced arthroscopists. Arthroscopy 4(3):215-21
5. Booth R Jr (2004) Arthroscopy before arthroplasty: A con or a comfort? J Arthroplasty 19(4 Suppl 1):2-4
6. Collins J (1989) Knee-joint arthroscopy--early complications. Med J Aust 150(12):702-706
7. Sherman O, Fox J, Snyder S et al (1986) Arthroscopy--"no-problem surgery". An analysis of complications in two thousand six hundred and forty cases. J Bone Joint Surg Am 68(2):256-65
8. Small N (1990) Complications in arthroscopic meniscal surgery. Clin Sports Med 9(3):609-17
9. Small N (1993) Complications in arthroscopic surgery of the knee and shoulder. Orthopedics 16(9):985-8
10. DeHaven K, Cosgarea A, Sebastianelli W (2003) Arthrofibrosis of the knee following ligament surgery. Instr Course Lect 52:369-81
11. Dodds J, Keene J, Graf B et al (1991) Results of knee manipulations after anterior cruciate ligament reconstructions. Am J Sports Med 19(3):283-7
12. Magit D, Wolff A, Sutton K et al (2007) Arthrofibrosis of the knee. J Am Acad Orthop Surg 15(11):682-94
13. Noyes F, Berrios-Torres S, Barber-Westin S et al (2000) Prevention of permanent arthrofibrosis after anterior cruciate

ligament reconstruction alone or combined with associated procedures: a prospective study in 443 knees. Knee Surg Sports Traumatol Arthrosc 8(4):196-206
14. Shapiro M, Freedman E (1995) Allograft reconstruction of the anterior and posterior cruciate ligaments after traumatic knee dislocation. Am J Sports Med 23(5):580-7
15. Shelbourne K, Patel D, Martini D (1996) Classification and management of arthrofibrosis of the knee after anterior cruciate ligament reconstruction. Am J Sports Med 24(6):857-62
16. Skutek M, Elsner H, Slateva K et al (2004) Screening for arthrofibrosis after anterior cruciate ligament reconstruction: analysis of association with human leukocyte antigen. Arthroscopy 20(5):469-73
17. Cosgarea A, Sebastianelli W, DeHaven K (1995) Prevention of arthrofibrosis after anterior cruciate ligament reconstruction using the central third patellar tendon autograft. Am J Sports Med 23(1):87-92
18. Harner C, Irrgang J, Paul J et al (1992) Loss of motion after anterior cruciate ligament reconstruction. Am J Sports Med 20(5):499-506
19. Shelbourne K, Wilckens J, Mollabashy A et al (1991) Arthrofibrosis in acute anterior cruciate ligament reconstruction. The effect of timing of reconstruction and rehabilitation. Am J Sports Med 19(4):332-6
20. Fullerton L Jr, Andrews J (1984) Mechanical block to extension following augmentation of the anterior cruciate ligament. A case report. Am J Sports Med 12(2):166-8
21. Paulos L, Wnorowski D, Greenwald A (1994) Infrapatellar contracture syndrome. Diagnosis, treatment, and long-term followup. Am J Sports Med 22(4):440-9
22. Zeichen J, van Griensven M, Albers I et al (1999) Immunohistochemical localization of collagen VI in arthrofibrosis. Arch Orthop Trauma Surg 119(5-6):315-8
23. Mikkelsen C, Cerulli G, Lorenzini M et al (2003) Can a post-operative brace in slight hyperextension prevent extension deficit after anterior cruciate ligament reconstruction? A prospective randomised study. Knee Surg Sports Traumatol Arthrosc 11(5):318-21
24. Kim D, Gill T, Millett P (2004) Arthroscopic treatment of the arthrofibrotic knee. Arthroscopy 20(Suppl 2):187-94
25. Millett P, Williams RIII, Wickiewicz T (1999) Open debridement and soft tissue release as a salvage procedure for the severely arthrofibrotic knee. Am J Sports Med 27(5):552-61
26. Wang J, Zhao J, He Y (2006) A new treatment strategy for severe arthrofibrosis of the knee. A review of twenty-two cases. J Bone Joint Surg Am 88(6):1245-50
27. Armstrong R, Bolding F (1994) Septic arthritis after arthroscopy: The contributing roles of intraarticular steroids and environmental factors. Am J Infect Control 22(1):16-8
28. Armstrong R, Bolding F, Joseph R (1992) Septic arthritis following arthroscopy: Clinical syndromes and analysis of risk factors. Arthroscopy 8(2):213-23
29. Bert J, Giannini D, Nace L (2007) Antibiotic prophylaxis for arthroscopy of the knee: Is it necessary? Arthroscopy 23(1):4-6
30. McAllister D, Parker R, Cooper A et al (1999) Outcomes of postoperative septic arthritis after anterior cruciate ligament reconstruction. Am J Sports Med 27(5):562-70
31. Wind W, McGrath B, Mindell E (2001) Infection following knee arthroscopy. Arthroscopy 17(8):878-83
32. Judd D, Bottoni C, Kim D et al (2006) Infections following arthroscopic anterior cruciate ligament reconstruction. Arthroscopy 22(4):375-84
33. DeFalco R, Ricci A, Balduini F (2003) Osteonecrosis of the knee after arthroscopic meniscectomy and chondroplasty: A case report and literature review. Am J Sports Med 31(6):1013-6
34. Gorczynski C, Meislin R (2006) Osteonecrosis of the distal femur. Bull Hosp Jt Dis 63(3-4):145-52
35. Muscolo D, Costa-Paz M, Ayerza M et al (2006) Medial meniscal tears and spontaneous osteonecrosis of the knee. Arthroscopy 22(4):457-60
36. Muscolo D, Costa-Paz M, Makino A et al (1996) Osteonecrosis of the knee following arthroscopic meniscectomy in patients over 50-years old. Arthroscopy 12(3):2737-9
37. Santori N, Condello V, Adriani E et al (1995) Osteonecrosis after arthroscopic medial meniscectomy. Arthroscopy 11-2:220-24
38. Brahme S, Fox J, Ferkel R et al (1991) Osteonecrosis of the knee after arthroscopic surgery: diagnosis with MR imaging. Radiology 178(3):851-3
39. Prues-Latour V, Bonvin JC, Fritschy D (1998) Nine cases of osteonecrosis in elderly patients following arthroscopic meniscectomy. Knee Surg Sports Traumatol Arthrosc 6(3):142-47
40. Aglietti P, Insall J, Buzzi R et al (1983) Idiopathic osteonecrosis of the knee. Aetiology, prognosis and treatment. J Bone Joint Surg Br 65(5):588-97
41. Mont M, Tomek I, Hungerford D (1997) Core decompression for avascular necrosis of the distal femur: long term followup. Clin Orthop Relat Res 334:124-30
42. Plenk H Jr, Hofmann S, Eschberger J et al (1997) Histomorphology and bone morphometry of the bone marrow edema syndrome of the hip. Clin Orthop Relat Res 334:73-84
43. Schweitzer M, White L (1996) Does altered biomechanics cause marrow edema? Radiology 198(3):851-3
44. Lotke P, Abend J, Ecker M (1982) The treatment of osteonecrosis of the medial femoral condyle. Clin Orthop Relat Res 171:109-16
45. Gambardella R, Tibone J (1983) Knife blade in the knee joint: a complication of arthroscopic surgery. A case report. Am J Sports Med 11(40):267-8
46. In Y, Bahk W, Park J (2003) Detachment of the tip of a motorized shaver within the knee joint: A complication of arthroscopic surgery. Arthroscopy 19(6):E25-7
47. Shaikh N, Abdel-Galil K, Compson J (2004) An unusual complication of knee arthroscopy: Portal site synovial cyst. Knee 11(6):501-2

Editors' Comments (Misc.)

Arthrofibrosis

Prevention: We have found that use of a locked extension brace at night helps avoid postoperative loss of extension, intercondylar notch scarring, or cyclops formation. The brace is set in the OR to equal the extension or even hyperextension of the opposite normal knee. The brace is utilized at all times during the first 2–3 weeks when the patient is not otherwise doing range of motion exercises and physical therapy. If a patient still has difficulty maintaining postoperative extension, we have had success utilizing a knee extension board (Instrument Maker), which is provided to the patient for home use.

Treatment of Arthrofibrosis

If a patient loses motion after surgery and surgical treatment is undertaken, the approach needs to be comprehensive and needs to address both flexion and extension deficits. To regain flexion, release of the supra patella pouch, medial, and lateral gutters and possibly retinacular releases are often necessary. If the graft itself is poorly placed, in rare cases the graft will need to be released or removed. To regain extension, the surgeon will need to clear out the intercondylar notch to ensure that there is no mechanical block anteriorly preventing extension. If this is still not effective, the posterior capsule is often the culprit, particularly if a meniscus repair was done, which may capture the capsule. In this instance, the surgeon needs to be prepared to perform a posterior capsular release. This is performed arthroscopically in our hands, utilizing a posterior medial portal. Through this portal, the posterior medial and posterior lateral capsule can be released by penetrating through the septa behind the PCL, while viewing with the arthroscope through the notch.

Chapter 10
Avoiding and Managing Complications in Shoulder Labral Repair

Jeffrey S. Abrams

Top 10 Pearls

- Surgical repair prior to multiple instability events has greater potential for success due to less structural damage.
- The number of fixation anchors and sutures is determined by the amount of labral detachment and desired capsular correction.
- Intraoperative evaluation of the degree of soft tissue deformity, glenoid bone loss, and Hill-Sachs engagement positions is critical to proper surgical procedure selection.
- Soft tissue mobilization and releases from the rotator cuff and glenoid neck is critical to repositioning the inferior glenohumeral ligament along the glenoid articular margin.
- Any suture anchor can be problematic and catastrophic to the articular surface. Early recognition and treatment of exposed hardware is critical to limit this injury.
- Suture anchor and plication repairs need to reduce a capsular pouch deformity with proper spacing between fixation points and to create a "balanced repair."
- Intraoperative evaluation with the arm out of traction and placed through a range of motion is important to evaluate the humeral head position relative to the glenoid, security of the repair, and anticipated range of motion. A Hill-Sachs deformity should have rotated posteriorly to the glenoid after proper retensioning of the glenohumeral ligaments.

- Postoperative healing of the detached soft tissue structures on an abraded glenoid neck is a biologic process that cannot be accelerated by our current techniques.
- Recovery and return-to-activities is a combination of static restraint healing, dynamic scapular and cuff rehabilitation, and activity-specific preparation.
- Athletes successfully treated are at risk for additional injuries and possibly recurrence. Multiple procedures may be necessary to complete a career. Surgical techniques should be able to be revised with minimum trauma to the shoulder complex.

Introduction and Background

As participation in overhead and collision athletics increases, so does the risk of shoulder instability. Many young and middle-age individuals are interested in activities that place their shoulders at risk. Since age is a factor, there is a limited window of opportunity to return to playing a sport. Sports medicine physicians need to apply the best possible techniques to allow the athlete to continue his or her participation while minimizing the risk of developing premature degenerative arthritis.[1] The athletes' expectations are high and many feel that most can be returned to full participation. The obstacle that stands in the way of a full recovery is recurrence of instability and avoiding complications. This chapter will address commonly seen complications that can limit successful surgical repair of an unstable shoulder. The complications included are recurrence of instability, shoulder stiffness, implant complications, articular destruction due to inflammation or chondrolysis, and degenerative arthritis.

J.S. Abrams (✉)
Princeton Orthopaedic and Rehabilitation Associates,
Princeton, New Jersey
e-mail: rxbonz@aol.com

The literature does not supply sufficient data on the incidence of these complications. Most of the peer review literature and textbook chapters refer to individual case reports and potential catastrophes. However, there is longitudinal data on patients with instability recurrence. Long-term studies show an increase in the number of patients who sustain recurrence of instability, which would have escaped a short-term study. Recurrence of instability with the most current techniques is in the single-digit incidence including arthroscopic and open reconstructive techniques.[2-6] An operation that was successful in returning an athlete back to the offending sport is at risk for sustaining additional injuries.

New technical advances have been helpful in understanding the potential pitfalls in treatment. The solutions include a number of newer modified procedures applied to both open and arthroscopic procedures. Often accompanying new advances are risks of additional complications. Capsular ablation from thermal devices, absorbable implant synovitis, and chondrolysis associated with postoperative pain pumps are examples of catastrophic events that may occur in the youthful shoulder. Nevertheless, the search for the perfect mousetrap continues to emphasize precise evaluation, patient selection, and optimal technique to repair and rehabilitate the unstable shoulder.

Sports medicine physicians need to have a menu of surgical procedures to address the unstable shoulder including open and arthroscopic techniques. The most popular surgical procedures include arthroscopic anterior stabilization, open Bankart repair with capsular shift, and surgeries that address bone loss from the articular surfaces. Proficiency in all of these techniques will provide sports medicine surgeons the opportunity to select the best procedure for the individual patient. Understanding the patient's situation should include the anatomical deficit, anticipated activities following treatment, and the potential for additional treatment in the athlete's future.

Functional Anatomy at Risk

The shoulder is often thought of as a difficult structure to repair because of its great degree of mobility and proximity to important neurologic and vascular structures. Shoulder stabilization may place certain structures at risk, including the axillary nerve, musculocutaneous nerve and brachial plexus, rotator cuff tendons, and vascular structures.

Open surgical repair is most commonly approached through the deltopectoral interval. The axillary nerve drapes the subscapularis medially and travels along the inferior glenoid neck prior to exiting through the quadrilateral space. The nerve arborizes to branches to the capsule, posterior structures, and the deltoid. Proper identification of the nerve and careful placement of retractors may avoid an unexpected injury during tissue mobilization and repair.

The axillary nerve to the arthroscopist is adjacent to the midportion of the inferior capsular pouch.[7,8] As the inferior pouch enlarges due to multiple recurrences or an inherited syndrome creating an enlarged pouch, the nerve may be in proximity to the inferior capsule. Special care is needed to work parallel to the capsule rather than perpendicular to minimize the risk of plunging through.

The musculocutaneous nerve passes the short head of the biceps approximately 5 cm inferior to the coracoid incision.[9] Instruments used to retract the short arm flexors (short head of the biceps and coracobrachialis) need to be placed superior to this structure after finger palpation confirms the safe placement. There is additional risk to this nerve during the procedures that require a coracoid transfer with the attached tendons. Careful mobilization of the pedicle prior to augmenting the glenoid rim will reduce risk of injury to the attached structures. Revision surgery following a coracoid transfer can be hazardous to the musculocutaneous nerve. There is often scar tissue making the nerve particularly difficult to identify and mobilize.

Although little is mentioned about injury to the brachial plexus, there are some data to suggest that this can be injured following an open repair.[10] This is likely due to medial retraction for improving the exposure of the anterior structures. These are often stretching injuries resulting in temporary neuropraxia. Since many surgeries today are being performed with interscalene regional anesthesia, there may be some "shared" risks if nerve injuries are detected postoperatively. There have also been reported cases of trauma creating a plexus injury. Surgery should be delayed, when possible, until after resolution of these injuries.

Vascular problems and complications are uncommon. The cephalic vein is a large structure that is a common landmark during the open deltopectoral approach. This is most often mobilized and retracted laterally with the anterior portion of the deltoid. Circumflexed arterial vessels are located along the humeral neck and ascend along the bicipital groove. These can be encountered if the surgical procedure extends distal to the subscapularis tendinous insertion.

The subscapularis is a common doorway leading to the entrance of the anterior glenoid. Open procedures often divide, mobilize, and split this tendon to gain access to the anterior glenoid rim and lateral attachment of the capsule to the humeral head. Injury to the subscapularis can occur including tendon insertion detachment and muscle weakness without dehiscence.[11,12] Certain arthroscopic techniques have penetrated the subscapularis without detachment, and it is uncertain whether this may place the subscapularis at risk as well. Careful reattachment or repair of the subscapularis approaches will minimize the risk of injury.

Techniques to Avoid Complications

Proper preparation is important to reduce the risk of intraoperative complication and be in the best position possible to have the maximum number of options if problems are detected. Preparation would include patient positioning and setup, available equipment, and patient selection.

Patient positioning is determined by the anticipated procedure and potential for changing the approach intraoperatively (i.e., converting arthroscopic surgery to an open procedure). Surgeons choosing arthroscopy can perform this procedure in the lateral decubitus or beachchair position. Both of these setups will allow diagnostic arthroscopy, reconstructive surgery, and the conversion to open stabilization. A popular position for performing arthroscopic stabilization is the lateral decubitus position, placing the glenoid parallel to the floor. The torso is supported with a beanbag and tape, approximately 20° backwards from the vertical. The arm is supported at 45° of abduction and flexed 20°. The ability to rotate the humerus throughout the procedure may be beneficial. A second lateral traction device can be added to distract the humerus from the glenoid and assist reduction of the Hill-Sachs lesion if engaged with the glenoid rim defect. Other options include using a surgical assistant to provide this lateral traction intermittently or use a rolled-up blanket in the axillary region to provide leverage. The cervical area should be supported to maintain the neck in a neutral position to minimize any potential traction. At times, the surgeon may elect to perform diagnostic arthroscopy and convert to an open procedure. Even if this is not expected, this position can be modified intraoperatively by applying a sterile stockinette around the hand and forearm and releasing of the tape supporting the torso with deflation of the beanbag via a circulating nurse. A gentle posterior pressure on the proximal humerus will allow the torso to roll posteriorly. It is important to properly prep and drape the patient to avoid potential crowding if this mid-operative conversion is applied.

Surgeons who prefer the beach chair position for arthroscopy need to have a proper table setup, allowing the patient to be seated and with adequate exposure to the anterior, lateral, and posterior quadrants of the shoulder. Proper cervical support is important, as well as padding and protection to the other extremities. Conversion to open surgery is performed by reducing the inclination of the table Although lateral decubitus and beach chair each have certain benefits, surgeons should utilize the best position to gain access to the damaged regions and be able to create a surgical result with proper correction to multiple regions of the glenohumeral articulation.

Open techniques are most commonly being performed in the supine or modified beach chair position. The chest wall is either flat on the table or mildly elevated to allow the humerus posterior translation during the anterior repair. The inclination of the back of the table is determined by the best approach to the anterior glenoid rim and potentially the coracoid if transfer is being considered. Table inclination can be changed during the procedure, allowing surgeons the best possible position for individual steps of the procedure. When positioning the patient, the surgeon should be able to alter the position of the shoulder during the surgical procedure. This would include abduction and rotation. Traction devices may make this inconvenient, and assessment should be performed preoperatively and intraoperatively by a mobility examination rather than a static "snapshot."

Equipment used for shoulder stabilization is based on the anticipated procedure and the potential additional techniques based on intraoperative findings. Many of these surgeries begin arthroscopically. The basic instruments include a motorized shaving system, articular soft tissue elevators, cautery and a cutting instrument, suture anchors with their particular insertion equipment, a drill, suture, and shuttling device systems, and knot-tying devices. Saline pump, axillary and torso padding, and Venodyne support may be helpful. Open equipment would include proper instruments to create arthrotomy and soft tissue restraint. Special retractors have been designed for the glenohumeral joint, allowing for improved exposure and less subscapularis detachment. The additional oscillating saw with half-inch blade should be available if coracoid transfer is being considered. Cannulated screws, drills, and taps should also be available if bone grafting is undertaken.

Selection of implants and sutures are important to reduce risk of complications. Suture anchors have become a popular way of repairing a detached capsular labral complex from the glenoid as well as humeral attachments of the capsule and rotator cuff. The anchors can be made of metal, plastic, or PEEK (polyetheretherketone), or absorbable polymers. The metal anchors were the first implants and were quite successful, although problems with anchor insertion, anchors backing out, magnetic resonance imaging difficulties due to hardware artifact, and degenerative arthritis led to other alternative designs.[13] The radiographic invisible anchors have had problems as well. Joint destruction as a result of implant debris can occur.[14] This was first recognized with the tack, which had an exposed portion of the implant, which could loosen or break during the absorption process. Later suture anchors were being reported as having similar problems with microscopic debris being released into the joint and creating synovitis that may clinically resemble an infection.[15] Anchor absorption has a combination of factors, which include a host response. Giant cells attempt to clean up the anchor debris since this is recognized as foreign to the body. This lytic response may produce a weakness in the bone. Multiple anchors that are in proximity to each other may create a potential weakness of the glenoid rim.

The search for the ideal material for suture anchor continues. This material will provide sufficient strength for easy insertion strong enough to maintain the repair until healing occurs and then reincorporate into the native glenoid. The inert implants have allowed revision surgery, ease of application, avoidance of bony reaction, but do not display the ability to assimilate into the bone.

Suture material has also evolved. Braided multifilament sutures and monofilament sutures are commonly used. Selection of sutures that are strong in combination with anchor eyelet and soft enough to be adjacent to articular surface is important. The newer reinforced multifilament sutures provide improved strength and are less abrasive when inserted through an absorbable anchor.[16] Ideally, an absorbable suture that is present long enough for tissue remodeling will become available.

There is an ongoing discussion on the ideal procedure of arthroscopy vs. open repair to the unstable shoulder. Rather than lumping all shoulders into a single category, it may be beneficial to recognize the individualized treatment based on preoperative factors, and intraoperative findings may be the athlete's best option.[17] Indications and contraindications to various techniques have changed, based on modification of the original procedure descriptions. They are likely to continue to change in the future as techniques continue to improve. Sports medicine surgeons should become adept at multiple techniques to repair the unstable shoulder, allowing them more options to individualize treatment.

Patient selection begins with the history of the initial event, treatment rendered, and history of recurrences. If there was a prior surgery, an operative report can identify intraoperative findings and the technique used to repair or reconstruct the shoulder. The anticipated activities and sports may persuade selection to emphasize or maintain maximal range of motion or stabilization strength. Patients with numerous instability events and failed surgical procedures may need additional alternatives in the operating room. Physical examination can be helpful to identify potential problems that may arise. Translation testing is performed by multiple techniques including the load-and-shift maneuver.[18] In a relaxed patient, the humeral head can be centered and translated in various directions of abduction and rotation to identify looseness and structural deficiency. The contralateral extremity is used to compare. This procedure is repeated as an examination under anesthesia. Placing the arm at 45° abduction and 45° externally rotated can reproduce anterior subluxation when applying this maneuver (Fig. 10.1). Shoulders that dislocate with more abduction may have additional static restraint deficiency including bone loss. Although most procedures are determined preoperatively, the anticipated findings are often

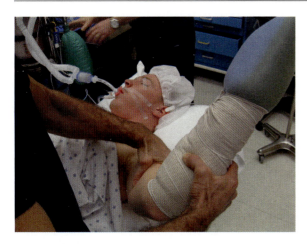

Fig. 10.1 The load-and-shift exam can be done with the arm abducted 45° and externally rotated 45° to examine the integrity of the anterior static restraints

confirmed following examination under anesthesia. Changing a surgical approach due to an unexpected event is less common as greater experience is gained with the preoperative evaluation.

Intraoperative Complications

Diagnostic Arthroscopy

One of the benefits of arthroscopy is to be able to utilize multiple portals to visualize and quantitate articular injury. It is not uncommon to have multiple lesions in multiple quadrants. Soft tissue assessment will include capsular labral avulsions, humeral capsular avulsions, mid-capsular tears, superior or posterior labral lesions, and rotator cuff lesions including subscapularis and articular partial tears of the supraspinatus. Bone loss can be further assessed with measurements of the articular surface of the glenoid, positions of engagement of the Hill-Sachs lesion, and visualize location of displaced glenoid rim fracture. In patients who present with failed stabilization, reasons for failure can be visualized prior to embarking on revision surgery. If a problem is discovered that may suggest a change in approach, then conversion to an open procedure may follow. The most common problems that may lead to this decision include large bone losses limiting the potential for stability with a soft tissue repair and soft tissue deficiency (i.e., following prior thermal capsular necrosis).

Capsular Mobilization

There are several injury patterns that can create an incompetent inferior glenohumeral ligament. Potential findings include a Bankart lesion, an extensive lesion that is either contiguous with a posterior labral tear or superiorly to the biceps, mid-capsular tears, lateral capsular tears or avulsions, medially-fixed capsules, or thin atrophic capsules.

The typical Bankart avulsion is a labral detachment that occurs anteriorly and inferiorly. A shaver blade can be used to assess mobilization and release adhesions. A grasping instrument or traction stitch can help reposition the capsular ligaments prior to repair. A group of patients will appear to have a thin atrophic capsule that appears insufficient. This can be due to scar tissue following an L-shaped tear in the anterior capsule. Visualizing the posterior inferior capsule and rotating the scope anteriorly, the inferior extent of the capsular tear can be appreciated. As the capsule deviates from the normal contour with the glenoid, the free edge of the capsule can be identified. As this tissue is carefully separated from the subscapularis, proper tissue transfer and repair can take place.

A group of patients will have either a very small Bankart lesion or a small crack between the labrum and the glenoid. Patients with confirmed dislocation either by preoperative X-ray or by the presence of a Hill-Sachs lesion may need repair that extends beyond the obvious small lesion. This small lesion may be partially healed and look innocuous, but in reality allows for excessive humeral head translation. Surgeons should place an elevator into the defect and accentuate the lesion. This is followed by capsular plication combined with labral repair.

The discovery of a mid or lateral capsule tear may be repaired arthroscopically or require conversion to open surgery. This is in proximity of the axillary nerve, and portals attempting to place suture anchors in the humeral head may be difficult (Fig. 10.2). A localization suture placed arthroscopically may be helpful to locate during an open approach. The conversion to open surgery is performed with a deltopectoral approach. Rather than dividing and elevating the majority of the subscapularis, the superior subscapularis tendon can be left intact, and the inferior half of the subscapularis can be elevated to complete the capsular repair and reattachment. Other approaches

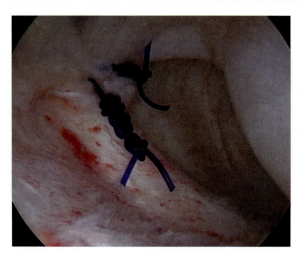

Fig. 10.2 Inferior capsular repair. An additional posteroinferior cannula allows side-to-side suture placement to close this tear

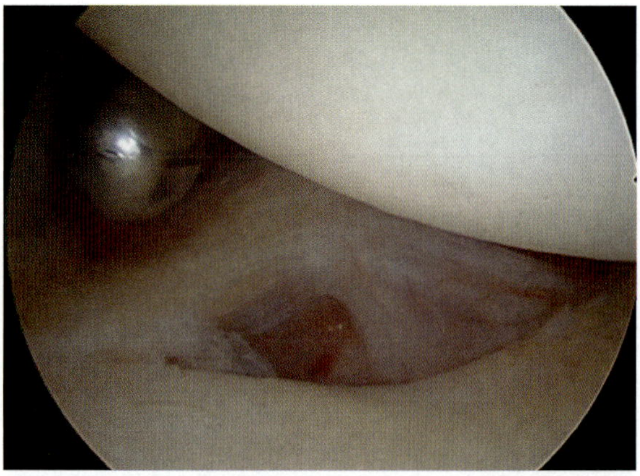

Fig. 10.3 A large anterior fovea between the labrum and the glenoid. If instability is encountered, capsular plication inferiorly and laterally is preferred over anchor reattachment, to prevent loss of external rotation

include a subscapularis tendon split or a side-to-side arthroscopic approach.

Surgeons need to avoid closing anatomic variants of the labrum. Here, there is a large fovea naturally occurring in the anterior quadrant, and closure would create a significant restricted range of motion. Capsular plication inferiorly to superiorly can restore proper tensioning and can avoid the risk of sacrificing external rotation if this variant is encountered (Fig. 10.3).

Capsules that are scarred medially along the glenoid neck are often attached to rim fractures that have healed inferiorly and medially. The soft tissue may need to be elevated and mobilized to allow for proper tensioning and positioning. The capsule may be traumatized during the attempts at releasing adhesions. The best visualization will occur with the scope anterosuperiorly and the working portal anteroinferiorly (Fig. 10.4). Placing a traction suture through the superior edge of the inferior glenohumeral ligament and retrieving through a percutaneous stick will allow full use of your cannulas for further instrumentation.

At the completion of a repair, the shoulder should be tested to confirm humeral head centralization and the absence of a Hill-Sachs contact with the glenoid articular surface. If the head does not remain centered or if the humeral head defect contacts the articular surface, additional capsular tension is suggested. This can be accomplished with inferior sutures placed through the posterior cannula and rotator interval closure anteriorly.

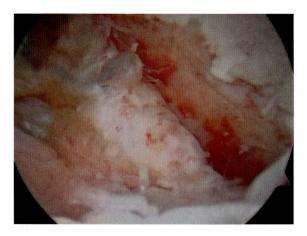

Fig. 10.4 A glenoid rim fracture with capsular tissue healed medially to the scapular neck

Suture Anchors

One of the great advances in arthroscopic and open stabilization is the common practice of placing suture anchors. Hardware problems become a concern as the ideal anchor position is felt to be on top of the glenoid articular margin. A dilemma is a partially-inserted metallic anchor that cannot be advanced or retrieved (Fig. 10.5). This is often due to stripping of the anchor during the insertion with the driver. The removal of a partially-inserted anchor can be achieved with a number of techniques. Some instrument trays supply an additional device that has a small-diameter retriever to assist easy placement below the level of the articular cartilage,

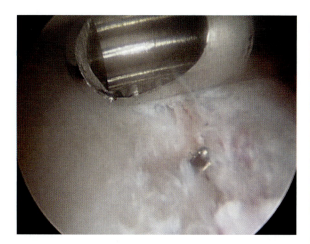

Fig. 10.5 A metallic glenoid anchor that became detached from the driver during insertion. This will need to be treated by removal and not covering with transferred labrum

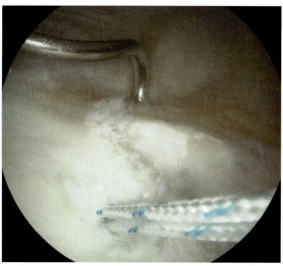

Fig. 10.6 A low posterior portal can allow suture hook placement to grasp the capsule distal to the anchor

permitting a better grip on the screw. Another option is to use a circular bone-cutting device similar to that used in the OATS procedure. A bone plug is obtained that includes the anchor. The anchor is then removed and the plug is replaced. Last, if the anchor is adjacent to the edge of the articular margin, a microfracture punch can be used to weaken the bone wall medially and then to loosen the anchor sideways through the defect.

Glenoid Rim Fractures

Labral detachment can occur in combination with a glenoid rim fracture. This fracture can heal inferiorly at the level of the glenoid or medially. Tissue mobilization is difficult, and specific releases should be considered. If the rim fracture has healed adjacent to the inferior glenoid rim, separate the labrum with an elevator and leave the fragment in its current location. Place anchor drill holes at the fragment glenoid seam and transfer the labrum over the fragment, fixing the soft tissue to the native glenoid. If the bone fragment has medially located, elevation of the fragment with the labrum and anatomically repairing them is a good option. There are certain shoulders that are difficult to assess the inferior quadrant when applying an arthroscopic technique. The options include reducing the distal arm traction, internally rotating the upper extremity and posterior translating the humerus. If there is continued difficulty, consider using a posterior portal approach. Leave the arthroscope in the anterior portal, place a spinal needle from the posterolateral position, and identify a favorable angle to the inferior glenoid. Place the anchor through the percutaneous puncture. The hooks can be used through the posterior portal to reduce the pouch and advance the inferior ligament in an anterior direction (Fig. 10.6). The distance between this anchor and the anteroinferior anchor is usually less than 1 cm.

Chondral Injuries

Anchor placement on the articular face of the glenoid may be altered when certain situations arise. Chondral injuries may occur anteriorly or posteriorly following traumatic dislocation or recurrent subluxations. If these lesions are adjacent to the labral attachment, the capsular labral complex can be transferred over the defect. In this case, an anchor hole is placed medially to the defect. The tissue is mobilized and transferred over the defect. Prior to the transfer, one may consider to microfracture the surface to increase healing potential. This is similar to the labral transfers over healed glenoid rim fractures.

Suture Problems

A relatively new problem being discovered is knot impingement, as the newer reinforced sutures are creating larger bulkier knots when used in conjunction

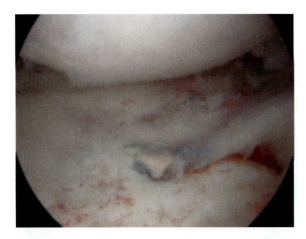

Fig. 10.7 Suture impingement. Sutures were placed down the anchor arm or migrated from lateral to medial creating friction with the humeral head. Mattress sutures may be a preferred alternative

with suture anchors (Fig. 10.7). It is always important to slide the knot down the post suture that has passed through the inferior glenohumeral ligament and under the labrum. Another choice may be to use mattress sutures. This can maximize the distance of the knot from the articular surface and reduce the risk of suture-loop rotating, permitting the knot to be adjacent to the articular surface.

During the process of suture passage or anchor placement, the suture can break, pull out of the eyelet, or anchor eyelet breakage. Many of the anchors today are nonmetallic. Rather than creating a new hole, we use the drill through the previously drilled hole and retap it if a screw-in anchor is selected, and replace with a new anchor and test pullout strength. This may be similar to revision cases. Prior holes and anchors can be ignored; recreate new holes adjacent or through prior tunnels. Suture management can be problematic if entanglements occur and surgeons are attempting a single cannula. Options include creating a second cannula anteriorly or posteriorly to separate the two arms of the suture.

Knot-Tying

Knot-tying can be challenging. Loop security can generally be visualized as sliding knots or push-in knotless anchors are used. On occasion, the knot cannot be cinched up as tight as desired. Surgeons have several choices. If possible, a suture grasping instrument is placed in the anterior portal to see if the knot can be potentially retrieved or potentially untied to allow additional half-hitches and progression of the knot. Prior to redoing the knot, slide the length of the suture to attempt creating the knot at a different location along the length of the suture. If the knot cannot be loosened, additional tension can be created by an additional plication with a separate stitch. Occasionally, the loop of the plication stitch can reach inside the anchor stitch and create additional tension. The other option is placing an additional anchor on the glenoid superior inferior to the loose stitch and place a mattress suture to avoid a large knot near the articular surface.

Open Repairs

Open surgical repairs have unique problems. When creating a deltopectoral approach, the subscapularis needs to be separated from the underlying capsule. On occasion during the subscapularis tenotomy, the capsule is inadvertently cut. If the two structures are separated from the lesser tuberosity as a unit, place a traction suture along the free edge, place an index finger medially inferior to the coracoid process while applying traction on the suture. There is a more natural interval between the subscapularis muscle and anterior capsule. This interval is easily developed with the digit, and dissection can be further developed from medial to lateral, preserving both structures. A horizontal arthrotomy can then be created to create a T-plasty repair.

When performing an open repair, the anchor sutures are tied externally to the capsule creating mattress sutures. If the humeral head retractor is removed to assess capsular mobility, the humeral head tends to glide anteriorly. This may compromise the security of these important fixation points. A posterior directed force on the proximal humerus will allow improved visualization and security of the capsule labral complex repair against the abraded glenoid neck. This may restrict security of these important fixation points. A posterior-directed force on the proximal humerus will allow improved security of the complex against the abraded glenoid neck.

Bone Graft

Bone graft transfers may be necessary in deficient shoulders with recurrent instability. During the process of harvesting a graft or during glenoid fixation, it is possible to discover a fracture in the graft. Surgeons have several options including substituting another graft (i.e., either iliac or allograft) or attempt to salvage the graft. The latter would be preferred due to the addition of augmentation that occurs with the tendon transfer and interposition through the subscapularis. One technique allows multiple sutures passes around the graft and at the junction of the coracoid tendon articulation; the sutures are placed through the glenoid in a transglenoid stabilization technique with the sutures being tied posteriorly. Another technique is to use larger rotator cuff anchors to secure the graft fragments to the anterior glenoid.

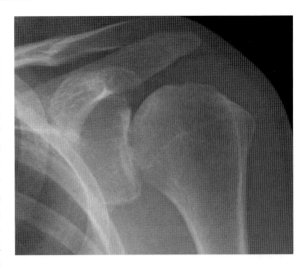

Fig. 10.8 Radiograph of chondrolysis of a 19-year-old athlete's shoulder (Photo of Dr. R. Burks)

Postoperative Complications

There have been unique complications to both arthroscopic and open repairs. Arthroscopic complications that develop in the postoperative period include chondrolysis, recurrent instability due to premature return to activities, and stiffness. Chondrolysis was originally discovered with certain articular thermal procedures.[19] Other patients were discovered in the postoperative period following continuous bupivacaine infusion with an articularly-placed pain pump (Fig. 10.8).[20] Both of these problems led to the recommendation of avoiding articular pain pumps and minimum use of thermal devices near the articular surfaces.

Patient compliance has been emphasized in the postoperative period, but particularly following arthroscopic stabilization. During the early developmental stages, fewer anchors were used and suture strength was not capable of significant strain, in addition to the common practice of using tacks. As the procedures became more refined and better anchors and sutures were introduced, there has been less concern with protected range of motion. Nevertheless, suture anchors placed on top of the articular rim are designed to position the ligament and periosteum against the abraded glenoid. There is no direct compression or fixation, and healing is a biological event with fixation placed along the articular perimeter. Sling use, delay in mobilization, and other restrictions have continued to be recommended.[1]

Open surgery has had reported problems with the subscapularis following arthrotomy and detachment. Dehiscence can occur if premature stretching exceeds the fixation strength of the repair.[11] Postoperative restrictions following a secure repair should minimize risk of detachment.

Articular problems may develop in the postoperative period. Placement of suture anchor includes proper depth into the bone and below the articular surface. Many devices contain a line illustrating the proper depth of anchor insertion. Additional depth during anchor insertion needs to be considered if acute angulation or increased thickness of articular cartilage to avoid potential humeral head contact. Flattening or detachment of articular cartilage can occur as activities are restored. Delayed anchor loosening has been discovered with metal anchors in rare instances. This is less likely to occur with nonmetallic anchors making them a popular alternative. However, nonmetallic anchors can also become dislodged and cause articular problems with difficult imaging identification. Any sense of grinding should be aggressively pursued unless anchor hardware position can be confirmed. If this is uncertain, early removal should be considered.

The squeaky shoulder can occur months after shoulder stabilization. This is felt to be related to suture material abrading against the humeral head with shoulder elevation and/or rotation. Since one can assume that the problem evolved during the postoperative course, it may relate to a suture loop rotating through the eyelet and around the labrum. The knots are no longer lateral to the labrum but become more medial and adjacent to articular surfaces (Fig. 10.7). Placement of mattress sutures rather than simple sutures makes articular suture impingement less likely. Preference for suture material that is softer and less abrasive will cause less friction, possibly creating lower profile knots.

A potential problem can be created with multiple absorbable anchors placed in proximity to each other along the glenoid rim. The host reaction will attempt to resorb the foreign polymer and may cause lysis around the anchors. Magnetic resonance imaging of the glenoid may demonstrate decreased bone uptake, and increased rehabilitation activity may predispose these structural changes. Other researchers felt that this may relate to disuse osteopenia. Continued search for safe polymers or inert materials and a gradual approach to return to physical activity may minimize this affect.

New techniques to repair an unstable shoulder have emphasized range of motion. Since most of the arthroscopic and open repairs address damaged structures anatomically, significant loss of rotation and elevation is uncommon. Marked stiffness in the early postoperative period may represent capsulitis. After the initial healing period, antiinflammatory medications, pendulum exercises, and self-stretches can be started after hardware position is confirmed. Stiffness that develops three months or later following surgery may be related to articular changes, either due to implant synovitis or chondrolysis (Fig. 10.9). Reduction of therapy and continued pendulums for a short period of time may be helpful prior to returning to therapy. Late stiffness that is not associated with a great deal of pain may be due to scar tissue, fovea closure, or asymmetric repair. Arthroscopic release of adhesions, physical therapy progression, and home therapy are alternatives that can be considered approximately six months postoperatively.

Revision Surgery

Reasons for revision surgery include instability recurrence, shoulder pain with a stable shoulder, stiffness, and implant complications including chondrolysis.

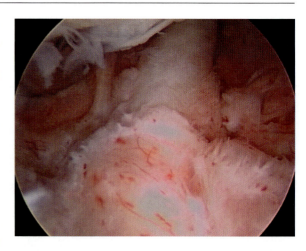

Fig. 10.9 Glenohumeral joint sterile synovitis after arthroscopic stabilization felt to be related to anchor debris

Although shoulder dislocation recurrence after surgical repair is not considered a complication, it has been included as the most common adverse event.

Evaluation of instability recurrence in an athlete begins with the patient's history. Important factors include previous operative findings and treatment during the postoperative interval, activities following the previous repair, the amount of trauma and shoulder position when dislocation or subluxation occurred, and the effort required to reduce the recent event. The patient's selection can be arthroscopic, open, bone grafting, or nonoperative treatment. Compelling factors are whether there is sufficient trauma to create a recurrence and whether the athlete wishes to pursue contact and collision sports. In patients with recurrent instability from collision sports following an arthroscopic repair, one may consider a reinforced repair including articular repair, capsular flap overlap, and possibly bone augmentation if indicated. Overhead athletes are more likely to pursue an arthroscopic revision, and those who are considering a less-aggressive lifestyle may choose a nonoperative approach. The operative evaluation includes examination under anesthesia and diagnostic arthroscopy. Further evaluation of bone loss and lesion engagements are important criteria to consider a bone-grafting procedure during revision (Fig. 10.10).[21] Other potential findings include a capsular tear either medially or laterally. Depending on its location, surgeons may choose an arthroscopic or open approach. Arthroscopic revision surgery requires tissue mobilization similar to an index operation. The capsule is often stiffer and needs traction to reposition along the glenoid. There is no great need for posterior plication unless labral detachment or capsular injury is discovered. There is, however, a need for tensioning the inferior glenohumeral ligament with additional sutures inferiorly (Fig. 10.11a). Tissue mobilization is a time-consuming and tedious procedure but critical to the outcome. The glenoid preparation can be done with the arthroscope posteriorly and anteriorly to visualize a proper surface for reattachment. Avoid aggressive burring and emphasize removal of devitalized tissue that may interfere with healing. If old anchors are not visible, they can be ignored. Remove any prominent hardware – metallic or absorbable. Suture anchor placement is based on soft tissue desired reattachment. There may be a need for additional anchors to complete a routine repair (average of four anchors).[22] Additional closure of the rotator interval should be performed in patients with persistent sulcus with the arm placed in external rotation (Fig. 10.11b).

Pain and stiffness may be a reason for revision surgery, even if stability has been established. The greatest concern is hardware and articular cartilage injury (Fig. 10.5). A diagnostic exam should confirm anchor security below the surface from multiple portals. Sutures causing abrasion to the humeral head and suture knots near the articular surface should be removed (Fig. 10.7). Visualize the glenohumeral joint with the arm out of traction and through a full range of motion. Translate the humeral head and see if cartilage defects become apparent. Microfracture may be helpful. More likely, a choice should be made to cover the defect with adjacent labrum or tighten adjacent ligaments to limit terminal rotation. Another choice is to cover the articular defect with a dermal allograft in combination with tissue retensioning. The postoperative instructions following revision surgery should be tailored to the problem. If instability recurrence was the problem, then consider a longer period of immobilization and restricted activities. If stiffness is being treated, then early mobilization should be considered. Rehabilitation is a combination of restoring static restraints and a gradual approach to recovery of the dynamic process. This will include bone density, cuff

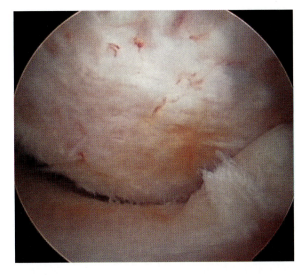

Fig. 10.10 Arthroscopic evaluation includes bone loss and engagement of a Hill-Sachs lesion, in addition to soft tissue disruption

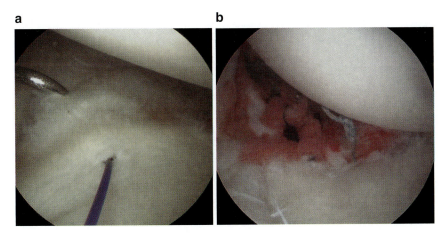

Fig. 10.11 Additional sutures are placed to increase capsular tension, reduce pouch deformities, and close tears. (**a**) inferior plication; (**b**) rotator interval tear closure

and scapular strength, proprioception qualities that are needed to return to demanding activities. The future is likely to add to the biological process of healing. Visualization and tissue mobilization have advanced to the level of predictably restoring the glenoid, labrum, and capsular restraints. Additional capsular treatment can thicken the capsule in selective areas. New technology has been very helpful in strengthening the repairs. Other technology, as in thermal or pain pump introduction of analgesics, have led to serious complications requiring salvage surgery. This is a young population and the likelihood of further injury from continued participation is present. The avoidance or delay of degenerative changes while permitting a desired active lifestyle should be the goal. We should not "burn bridges" with surgery but rather have a thoughtful plan that will include short-term and long-term goals of this active population.

References

1. Abrams J (2007) Role of arthroscopy in treating anterior instability of the athlete's shoulder. Sports Med Athrosc Rev 15:230-8
2. Bottoni C, Smith E, Berkowitz M et al (2006) Arthroscopic versus open stabilization for recurrent instability: A prospective randomized clinical trial. Am J Sports Med 34:1730-7
3. Karlsson J, Magnusson L, Ejerhed L et al (2001) Comparison of open and arthroscopic stabilization for recurrent shoulder dislocation in patients with a Bankart lesion. Am J Sports Med 29:538-42
4. Mohtadi N, Bitar I, Sasyniuk T et al (2005) Arthroscopic versus open repair for traumatic anterior shoulder instability: A meta-analysis. Arthroscopy 21:652-8
5. Pagnani M, Dome D (2002) Surgical treatment of traumatic anterior shoulder instability in American football players. J Bone Joint Surg Am 84:711-15
6. Mazzocca A, Brown F Jr, Carreira D et al (2005) Arthroscopic anterior shoulder stabilization of collision and contact athletes. Am J Sports Med 33:52-60
7. Yoo J, Kim J, Ahn J et al (2007) Arthroscopic perspective of the axillary nerve in relation to the glenoid and arm position: A cadaveric study. Arthroscopy 23(12):1271-7
8. Eakin C, Dvirnak P, Miller C et al (1998) The relationship of the axillary nerve to arthroscopically placed capsulolabral sutures: An anatomic study. Am J Sports Med 26:505-9
9. Flatow E, Bigliani L, April E (1989) An anatomic study of the musculocutaneous nerve and its relationship to the coracoid process. Clin Orthop Relat Res 244:166
10. Boardman NIII, Cofield R (1999) Neurologic complications of shoulder surgery. Clin Orthop Relat Res 368(1):44-53
11. Greis P, Dean M, Hawkins R (1996) Subscapularis tendon disruption after Bankart reconstruction for anterior instability. J Shoulder Elbow Surg 5(3):219-22
12. Sachs R, Williams B, Stone M et al (2005) Open Bankart repair: Correlation of results with postoperative subscapularis function. Am J Sports Med 33:1458-62
13. Rhee Y, Lee D, Chun I et al (2004) Glenohumeral arthropathy after arthroscopic anterior shoulder stabilization. Arthroscopy 20:402-6
14. Athwal G, Shridharani S, O'Driscoll S (2006) Osteolysis and arthropathy of the shoulder after use of bioabsorbable knotless suture anchors: A report of four cases. J Bone Joint Surg Am 88:1840-5
15. Freehill M, Harms D, Huber S et al (2003) Poly-L-lactic acid tack synovitis after arthroscopic stabilization of the shoulder. Am J Sports Med 31:643-7
16. Wüst D, Meyer D, Favre P et al (2006) Mechanical and handling properties of braided polyblend polyethylene sutures in comparison to braided polyester and monofilament polydioxanone sutures. Arthroscopy 22(11):1146-53
17. Cole B, L'Insalata J, Irrgang J et al (2000) Comparison of arthroscopic and open anterior shoulder stabilization: A two- to six-year follow-up study. J Bone Joint Surg 82A:1108-14
18. Abrams J (2007) Arthroscopic anterior instability repair. In: Levine W, Blaine T, Ahmad C (eds) Minimally-Invasive Shoulder and Elbow Surgery. Informa, New York, NY, pp 91-104
19. Levine W, Clark A Jr, D'Allesandro D et al (2005) Chondrolysis following arthroscopic thermal capsulorrhaphy to treat shoulder instability: A report of two cases. J Bone Joint Surg 87:616-21
20. Gomoll A, Kang R, Williams J et al (2006) Chondrolysis after continuous intra-articular bupivacaine infusion: An experimental model investigating chondrotoxicity in the rabbit shoulder. Arthroscopy 22:813-19
21. Burkhart S, DeBeer J (2000) Traumatic glenohumeral bone defects and their relationship to failure of arthroscopic Bankart repairs: Significance of the inverted-pear glenoid and the humeral engaging Hill-Sachs lesion. Arthroscopy 16:677-94
22. Kim S, Ha K, Kim Y (2002) Arthroscopic revision Bankart repair: A prospective outcome study. Arthroscopy 18:469-82

Editors' Comments (Labral)

The use of double loaded suture anchors for routine labral repairs is not necessary, save for SLAP repairs as suture management becomes an unnecessary issue. Arthroscopic rotator cuff interval closure may be considered for associated multidirectional instability (MDI) in the face of labral pathology. One, though, can address MDI with a secure and shifted labral repair concomitant with capsular plication using the 7 O'Clock portal.

Beware of the engaging Hill-Sachs lesion as this can be better served with an initial open stabilization that would include possible bone grafting. In certain instances, a preoperative CT scan with 3D reconstruction is helpful. The glenoid should also be assessed for possible bone grafting.

When labral tearing is associated with a rotator cuff tear, address the labral tear first followed by the rotator cuff repair. Watch the clock! View the glenohumeral space from both the posterosuperior and anterosuperior portals to avoid missing a HAGL lesion.

Occasionally, a bone defect will be identified intraoperatively that is more significant than anticipated. If after Bankart reconstruction, a Hill Sachs lesion still engages, one option we prefer is to perform an arthroscopic infraspinatous transfer. Viewing from an anterior superior portal, the Hill Sachs lesion is abraded, and two anchors are utilized. The anchor is inserted into the lesion, the cannula is withdrawn outside the capsule and infraspinatous tissue. A retriever device is used to withdraw suture and extracapsular/extra muscular knot tying is performed, advancing the tissue into the defect. This typically incorporates the infraspinatus. This acts as a posterior tether, reducing anterior translation, filling the defect, and eliminating the Hill Sachs from engaging on the anterior glenoid rim.

HAGL lesions are often missed on MRI and found only at surgery. We have had success utilizing one of two arthroscopic methods for this repair. Anchors can be utilized for repair of the lateral edge of the anterior capsule to bone, or sutures can be retrieved percutaneously and tied over the anterior deltoid fascia.

For best visualization of the anterior glenoid, we recommend that an anterior superior viewing portal be utilized, while working through an anterior inferior portal. The placement of the anterior inferior working portal is crucial to avoid an improper drilling angle for anchor insertion, which can lead to great frustration and skiving of the drill. Always place the cannula for anchor insertion just above the leading edge of the subscapularis, lateral enough to get a good drilling angle. Too medial a portal will cause the drilling approach to the glenoid to be too parallel to the articular surface. In tight shoulders, or when there has been extravasation limiting access from the originally placed cannula, it is occassionally useful to utilize a "trans subscapularis" portal directly through the subscapularis. This will give a direct shot to the inferior glenoid and has been shown to be both safe and effective.

Failure to adequately release the scarred down inferior GH ligament/labral complex off the anterior glenoid neck is a common cause of failure of repair (i.e., ALPSA lesion). Take time to release this tissue adequately. One must see the subscapularis muscle or the release has not been completely performed.

Make sure that the patient has at least 30° of external rotation while still on the table after your stabilzation procedure. If the patient is over tightened in the OR, there is little chance that acceptable motion will be achieved postop. Use of an abd/er sling and pillow will help avoid scarring of the anterior capsule and coracohumeral ligament and should be utilized postoperatively. We titrate the length of immobilization time based on the postoperative exam. We examine the patient at 3 weeks, and if the patient cannot easily be externally rotated to 30° with the arm at the side, we discontinue the sling. If the patient feels overly loose, we will continue the sling for 6 weeks.

Chapter 11
Avoiding and Managing Complications for Shoulder Superior Labrum (SLAP) Repair

Michael S. Bahk and Stephen J. Snyder

Top 10 Pearls

- The diagnosis of SLAP lesions can be challenging. There is no specific test or imaging study that is perfect. Arthroscopy is the key when the clinical situation requires a remedy.
- SLAP lesions often have additional pathology.
- There are numerous anatomic variants that can be confused for SLAP lesions, and they must be understood to avoid misdiagnosis and treatment.
- Creation of the anterosuperior portal is critical and allows proper anchor placement. The ideal location is superior to the biceps tendon at the posterior aspect of the rotator interval. Use a spinal needle for an outside-in technique.
- Avoid rotator cuff injury with the anterior superior portal.
- Place the punch or drill posterior to the biceps and angle it directly into the bone at the center of the biceps tubercle.
- The punch must ideally penetrate the superior glenoid exactly at the center of the biceps anchor just below the edge of the cartilage at an angle of 45° relative to the glenoid surface.
- One low profile double-loaded suture anchor with a suture anterior and one posterior to the biceps is typically sufficient and ideal.
- Do not leave any anchors proud.
- Use a 15° external rotation sling with no aggressive strengthening until 6 weeks.

S.J. Synder (✉)
Southern California Orthopedic Institute, Van Nuys, CA
e-mail: mbahk@scoi.com

Introduction and Background

Clinically significant injuries to the superior labrum are uncommon. Most arthroscopic shoulder series report an incidence around 6%.[1-3] In 1985, Andrews et al. described tears of the anterosuperior labrum in 73 overhead athletes.[4] They recommended debridement alone as an effective treatment but made no mention or need for fixation of the biceps anchor. Snyder et al. in 1990 first described superior labral and biceps anchor pathology as a Superior Labrum Anterior and Posterior (SLAP) lesions. They characterized and classified these lesions as injuries occurring posteriorly, extending anteriorly to *and including* the biceps anchor.[1] Subsequent laboratory studies have defined the biomechanical importance of the biceps anchor,[5-10] while clinical data report significant pain and prolonged disability in patients with untreated SLAP tears.[1,2,4] However, diagnosis of SLAP lesions is still challenging even when based on history, physical examination, and modern imaging modalities. Knowledge of the numerous normal anatomic variations diminishes the likelihood of over diagnosis of SLAP tears and unnecessary surgical treatment of normal anatomy. Proper surgical repair technique requires understanding and arthroscopic skill and is fraught with potential complications.

Functional Anatomy at Risk

The glenoid labrum is a fibrocartilaginous ring along the edge of the glenoid fossa.[11,12] The anatomy of the superior labrum is unique and different from that of the other three quadrants. The superior labrum is often meniscoid or triangular in shape with a sublabral recess in 73% of shoulders.[13–15] The sublabral recess is most common at the 12 o'clock position and decreases in incidence inferiorly.[15] The superior labrum is also more mobile with variable attachment in the anterosuperior quadrant. Conversely, the inferior labrum is rounded, firmly attached, and continuous with the glenoid.[14] Cooper et al. felt that the superior labrum may act as a mobile extension of the superior glenoid, while the inferior labrum may act as a stabilizing bumper.[14]

The long head of the biceps tendon originates from the superior labrum and supraglenoid tubercle in varying degrees.[11,16,17] However, the biceps arises predominantly from the labrum with little contribution from the supraglenoid tubercle in some shoulders.[11,16] The supraglenoid tubercle lies 5 mm medial to the superior glenoid rim.[11,17] The biceps origin may vary from the 11–1 o'clock position; however, in 55% of shoulders it arises posteriorly. It has an equal anterior and posterior origin in 37% of shoulders.[17]

The superior glenohumeral ligament predominantly arises from the supraglenoid tubercle with some fibers arising from the biceps-superior labral origin.[15] The middle glenohumeral ligament attachment is variable. It may arise from the superior labrum at the biceps anchor, the anterior superior glenoid, or the adjacent labrum, and is described as sheet-like typically and obliquely draped over the subscapularis tendon.[18]

There are three normal variations of the anterosuperior quadrant of the glenoid having an overall incidence of 13–14%.[19,20] The most common variation is a sublabral foramen (9%) with a cord-like middle glenohumeral ligament attaching directly to the anterosuperior labral tissue.[19,20] Three percent of shoulders have a sublabral foramen and 1.5% include a Buford complex. This important variation consists of complete absence of all anterosuperior labral tissue but possesses a robust *cord-like* middle glenohumeral ligament that attaches directly to the base of the biceps tendon/labral junction.[19,20] It is important to understand these normal variations to avoid over diagnosis of SLAP lesions or "repair" of normal anatomy, which may severely restrict motion.

The blood supply of the labrum is peripherally based and predominately radial in flow. It originates from the surrounding periosteum and capsule and not from the underlying bone.[14] The anterosuperior and superior labrum have less vascularity compared with the rest of the labrum.[14] The blood supply ultimately originates from the suprascapular, circumflex scapular, and posterior circumflex humeral arteries.[14] Vascularity decreases with increasing age.[11,12]

Biomechanics

The long head of the biceps and its glenoid-labral anchor contribute to the stability of the glenohumeral joint. Biomechanical studies have shown that a competent biceps labral complex provides translational and rotational stability. Proper repair of a SLAP tear should restore normal biomechanics.[21]

With biceps contraction, the short head causes proximal humeral migration. However, this is counterbalanced by the biceps long head contraction, which results in humeral head depression. With elbow flexion and supination, release of the long head of the biceps results in proximal humeral migration by 15.5%.[5]

In the abducted externally rotated position, the shoulder is vulnerable to anterior dislocation. At 90° abduction, increased biceps tension significantly reduces anterior displacement at 60° and 90° of external rotation.[6] With 120° external rotation, increased biceps tension reduces anterior displacement when a Bankart lesion is present.[6] In other words, biceps contraction helps to stabilize the unstable shoulder anteriorly. Similarly, EMG studies have reported peak biceps activity in the late cocking phase of throwing for pitchers and noted higher biceps activity in pitchers with known chronic anterior instability.[7,8] Rodosky et al. also reported that creation of a SLAP lesion in a cadaveric model decreases anterior shoulder stability by decreasing torsional rigidity in the overhead position. They also reported that a SLAP tear increases inferior glenohumeral strain.[9]

Pagnani et al. reported increased superoinferior and anteroposterior translation in the lower and middle ranges of abduction with a SLAP lesion.[10] Detachment of the superior labrum with its concomitant superior and middle glenohumeral ligaments may help explain the increase in translation. In addition, loss of an intact labral complex reduces concavity compression with loss of biceps contraction.[10]

Similarly, Panossian et al. reported SLAP tears increased anteroposterior and superoinferior translation along with increased external rotation in a cadaveric model. Arthroscopic repair was able to return range of motion to normal levels afterwards without the need for additional capsular plication.[21]

Classification

In 1990, Snyder et al. classified SLAP tears into four types (Fig. 11.1a-d).[1] There have been numerous additions to this classification system since then.[22–24]

Type I lesions have degenerative fraying but the labrum and biceps anchor are firmly attached to the glenoid. Snyder reported a 21% incidence in their study population.[2] This lesion is part of the degenerative process and more common in middle-aged to older patients. It is a possible but uncommon source of clinical symptoms.

Type II lesions are the most common lesion (55%) and represent a significant detachment of the biceps labral anchor from the glenoid.[2] The superior and middle glenohumeral ligaments may be detached as well, so evaluation for instability is important.

Type III lesions occurred in 9% of the study population.[2] This lesion includes a bucket-handle tear of a meniscoid superior labrum. The biceps is normal and firmly attached to the rest of the labrum and supraglenoid tubercle. Type IV lesions occur in 10% of patients and consists of a bucket-handle tear of the meniscoid superior labrum with extension of the tear into the biceps tendon.[2]

There may be complex SLAP tears or combinations of these lesions. Most commonly, type III and type IV tears may have detached biceps anchors or a type II component. They can be described as type II and III or type II and IV.[25]

Type II SLAP tears have also been subclassified into three groups by Morgan et al. as anterior, posterior, and combined anterior and posterior lesions.[22] Type II SLAP tears with posterior extension more commonly occurred in younger overhead or throwing

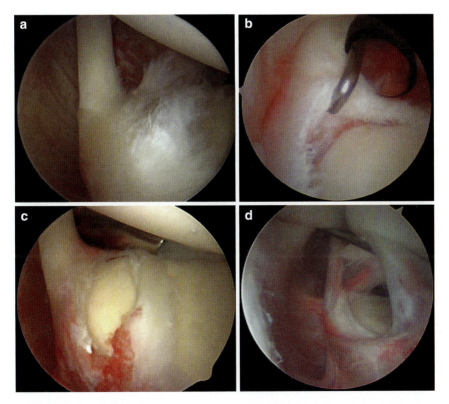

Fig. 11.1 SLAP lesion types I-IV. (**a**) Type I SLAP lesion with degenerative fraying of the superior labrum and biceps anchor. (**b**) Type II SLAP lesion with complete detachment of the biceps anchor from the superior glenoid. (**c**) Type III SLAP lesion with a bucket-handle tear of the superior labrum. (**d**) Type IV SLAP lesion with a bucket-handle tear of the superior labrum that extends into the biceps tendon

athletes and may occur by a peel-back mechanism.[22,26] These patients also possessed a drive-through sign that corrected after repair. Morgan et al. felt these SLAP lesions created a posterosuperior instability or laxity that may lead to additional injuries such as posterior partial thickness rotator cuff tears.[22]

Additional SLAP types have been added describing various extensions of the superior labral tear.[23,27] The SLAP tear may continue anteroinferiorly into a Bankart lesion, posteriorly, circumferentially or into the middle glenohumeral ligament.[23,27]

Diagnosis

History

The diagnosis of SLAP tears can be difficult since it is often associated with additional shoulder pathologies. The history can be nonspecific with patients reporting prolonged, vague shoulder pain, or disability that does not improve with conservative management and is exacerbated with overhead activity.[1] They may complain of mechanical symptoms if a torn fragment is trapped between the humerus and glenoid.[1] Snyder et al. reported 49% of patients noted mechanical catching or grinding.[2] SLAP tears have a high incidence of associated shoulder pathologies including instability, rotator cuff tears, and ganglion cyst formation complicating diagnosis.[1] One large series reported 40% of SLAP lesions were associated with either full or partial thickness rotator cuff tears, while 22% of lesions were associated with Bankart lesions.[2] Only 28% of SLAP lesions were isolated lesions.[2]

The typical patient is a young male that either describes a traumatic origin or one associated with chronic overhead activity. Snyder et al. reported an average age of 38 years with 91% of the patients being male.[1-3] Traumatic injuries often occur with either a compressive injury such as a fall onto an outstretched arm or a traction mechanism of injury from a sudden pull on the arm.[1,23,28-30] Cadaveric models have confirmed reproducible creation of SLAP tears with these traumatic mechanisms.[29,30] Patients with SLAP tears associated with overhead activity may present a distinct group with different characteristics. The "dead arm" symptom or the sudden painful inability to throw a ball with usual velocity may be a result of SLAP lesions.[31] Morgan et al. reported patients with throwers' SLAP tears or posterior SLAP lesions were younger with an average age of 24 years. It is hypothesized their tears occurred with a peel-back phenomenon as the labrum undergoes pathological torsion in the abducted externally rotated throwing motion.[22]

Physical Exam

The physical diagnosis of SLAP tears can be also difficult and nonspecific. No test or combination of tests appears specific for a superior labral injury.[1,2,25,27,28] Patients also often have positive signs because of associated pathologies.[2] Snyder et al. reported that 47% of patients had positive impingement signs, 39% had rotator cuff signs, 16% had anterior instability, and 15% had acromioclavicular signs.[2]

Multiple tests have been reported with varying degrees of accuracy.[27,28,32-36] Tests commonly used to diagnose SLAP tests include Speed's test, O'Brien's test, compression-rotation test, Kibler's anterior slide test, crank test, and Kim's biceps load tests.[1,2,27,28,32-37] Snyder et al. originally reported that the Speed's test and the compression-rotation test may be helpful in diagnosis of SLAP tears.[1] Although Speed's test is used to test the biceps tendon, an unstable biceps origin will also illicit symptoms. The patient resists downward pressure with the arm in 90° forward flexion, full elbow extension, and the forearm supinated. The compression rotation test is performed with compressing or loading the glenohumeral joint axially and rotating the humerus to trap loose labrum within the joint. A painful clunk may be noted with a tear.[1,25] The literature reports good results with O'Brien's test and this may be useful.[22,25,32] With the arm in 90° forward flexion and 10° adduction, downward pressure is applied with the patient resisting with the forearm pronated and the forearm supinated. A positive test occurs when pain is reported deep in the shoulder with the forearm pronated and relieved with the forearm supinated.[32] Kim's biceps load test may also be useful for SLAP diagnosis.[33] The patient's arm is abducted 120°, maximally externally rotated with the elbow in 90° flexion and full forearm supination. The patient flexes the elbow against the examiner. The test is positive with pain production. A variation of this test may also be useful in patients with concomitant anterior instability.[34]

Morgan et al. reported that anterior SLAP tears could be distinguished from posterior SLAP tears with different physical exam tests.[22] Speed's and O'Brien's tests were accurate for anterior lesions, while Jobe's relocation test was sensitive and specific for posterior lesions.[22]

It is important to examine for signs of associated pathology. In addition to instability, impingement, and rotator cuff tear signs, careful observation and inspection of shoulder musculature and strength testing may reveal weakness and atrophy associated with suprascapular nerve impingement from ganglion cysts associated with labral tears.[18,25]

Imaging

MRI is currently the best imaging modality for diagnosing SLAP tears. A glenohumeral injection of gadolinium for an MR arthrogram improves diagnostic accuracy.[38,39] However, MR detection of SLAP tears is not without some difficulty. In 1995, Snyder et al. reported the radiologic diagnosis of SLAP tears as inconsistent with only 26% of MRI radiology readings suggestive of SLAP tears.[2] MR technology and detection of SLAP tears has improved, with the current literature reporting a sensitivity of 75–98% and a specificity of 69–99%[40] for MRI/MR arthrograms. However, the MR detection of the community radiologist for a SLAP tear may be lower with an overall accuracy of 51%.[40] The superior labrum has a unique anatomy with a number of normal anatomic variants that can be diagnostically challenging. In addition, there is some controversy in the radiology literature on accurate signs for distinguishing normal anatomy from a pathological SLAP tear.[13,41-43]

The normal labrum is characterized by a low signal on all MR pulse sequences. It is usually triangular or rounded in shape.[39] The superior labrum is best visualized on coronal oblique images while the anterior and posterior labrum is most easily seen on axial images.[39] A SLAP tear can be best visualized on the coronal oblique images with T2, gradient echo or T1 weighted imaging after intraarticular gadolinium injection.[38,39]

The normal sublabral recess of the superior glenoid-labral complex can be confused for a SLAP tear on MRI. The superior labrum may be meniscoid or possess a sublabral recess in 73% of shoulders. This sublabral recess can be deeper than 5 mm in 27% of shoulders.[13] It often appears as a thin, linear signal that follows the normal contour of the glenoid or extends medially. The sublabral recess may exist throughout the superior glenoid-labral complex or exist posterior to the biceps anchor. Any superior signal posterior to the biceps anchor is not necessarily pathological.[41-43] The inferior labrum tends to be more rounded and inserts directly onto the glenoid without a recess.

Signal direction, morphology, and width help distinguish a normal sublabral recess signal from a SLAP tear. A SLAP tear is characterized by a wide (≥3 mm), ragged signal that extends laterally (Fig. 11.2). The SLAP tear would have indistinct or fuzzy borders because of torn fibers and be wider than the crisp linear normal sublabral recess as fluid or contrast fills the pathologic void. However, following the direction of the signal on coronal oblique pulse sequences appears to be one of the better signs for a SLAP tear.[42] This lateral signal direction sign has a sensitivity, specificity, and positive predictive value of 81%, 53%, and 50%.[42]

This pathological signal can extend partially through the superior labrum as a partial tear or propagate full thickness dividing the labrum into a bucket handle tear.[39] A type II SLAP tear or full detachment may also be noted when the superior labrum is completely separated from the glenoid. Jin et al. report concomitant

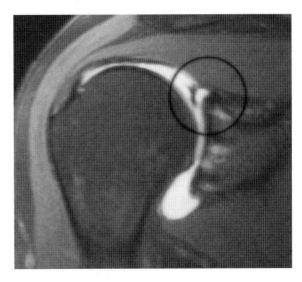

Fig. 11.2 MR arthrogram coronal image with a type II SLAP lesion. The *circle* denotes the wide signal with lateral extension characteristic of a SLAP lesion

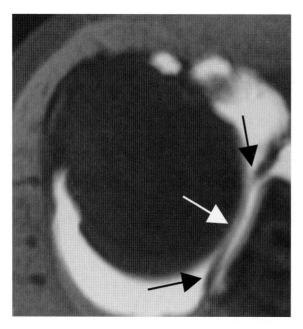

Fig. 11.3 MR arthrogram axial image with a type III SLAP lesion

anterosuperior labral tears and axial images that are able to detect a signal anterior and posterior to the biceps are also helpful in distinguishing a SLAP from a normal sublabral recess (Fig. 11.3).[42]

The anterosuperior labral normal variants can also be confused with a SLAP tear. Carefully evaluating the suspected tear on sequential MRI images will help identify the location of the signal in question. Evaluating the morphology of the signal in conjunction with location will help distinguish normal variant from SLAP tear. Tears will often have wider signals with ragged borders. The sublabral foramen will demonstrate a smooth narrow signal that is localized to the anterosuperior glenoid with labrum that is firmly attached superiorly and at the midglenoid notch. A Buford complex will show a localized absence of labral tissue in the anterosuperior glenoid with normal cartilage and a robust cord-like middle glenohumeral ligament (Fig. 11.4).

Ganglion cysts have also been associated with labral tears and most commonly with SLAP lesions.[44,45] Spinoglenoid cysts visualized on coronal or sagittal T2 weighted images should prompt an evaluation for a SLAP tear (Fig. 11.5). Westerheide et al. reported on 14 patients with spinoglenoid cysts treated arthroscopically.

Eighty-six percent of these cysts were found to be associated with labral pathology.[44]

MR arthrography is the best imaging modality for SLAP diagnosis but its accuracy is dependent on a number of factors, especially in the community setting. Knowledge of normal anatomy, normal anatomic variants, and carefully evaluating signal direction, width, and morphology will help correctly identify SLAP tears.

Arthroscopic Diagnosis of SLAP Tears

Arthroscopy is the gold standard for diagnosing SLAP tears. History and physical examination are nonspecific and MRI can be helpful but often misleading. A thorough systematic inspection of the glenohumeral joint anteriorly and posteriorly is ultimately necessary to diagnose a SLAP tear. A probe or grasper must be used to physically examine the superior labrum for any detachment. An unstable biceps anchor will displace when pulled and arch away from the superior glenoid 5 mm or more.[25] The glenoid articular cartilage normally extends medially over the superior glenoid through a sublabral recess. Hemorrhage, fraying, granulation tissue, or an unusually deep cleft may be signs of a SLAP tear.[25] Normal sublabral holes, cord-like middle glenohumeral ligaments and Buford complexes will similarly appear without significant fraying or hemorrhage. Repair of these normal variants will result in stiff painful shoulders limiting elevation and external rotation. If pulling on the biceps anchor tensions the anterosuperior labrum, superior or middle glenohumeral ligaments, or Buford complex, then a SLAP tear is possible. In addition, posterior SLAP tear subtypes may displace with a peelback maneuver if the arm is taken into abduction and external rotation.[22,26] A positive "drive-through sign" or being able to move the arthroscope from superiorly to inferiorly, may also indicate laxity of the ligament support function from a SLAP tear.[46]

History of Repairs

Type II SLAP lesions were initially treated with simple debridement and abrasion of the bone in an attempt to

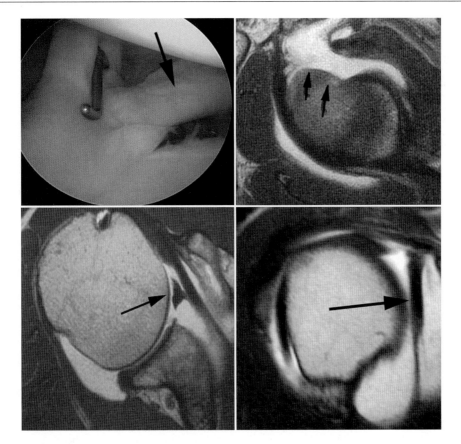

Fig. 11.4 Buford complex with complete absence of anterosuperior labral tissue (*double arrows*) and a robust cordlike middle glenohumeral ligament (*single arrows*)

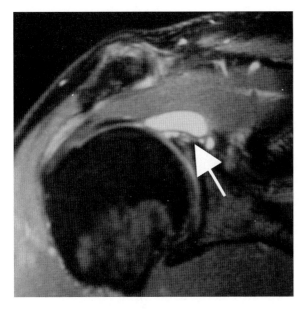

Fig. 11.5 MRI coronal image with arrow highlighting a ganglion cyst that is associated with a SLAP lesion

promote bony healing of the labrum. On second look arthroscopy of five of these abrasion treated lesions, 40% had not healed.[2] Subsequently, a number of different fixation techniques were developed including staples, transosseus sutures, cannulated screw fixation, and bioabsorbable tacks.[2,10,47,48] However, these different techniques often required additional surgery for prominent hardware removal or loose bioabsorbable fragments. These problems begat the development of screw-in suture anchors.[2] Treatment of Type II SLAP lesions has evolved currently utilizing small suture anchors that are double loaded. Because the bone is dense, a small threaded suture anchor provides adequate purchase without being too prominent in a small target area within the biceps anchor origin. One suture limb fixes the biceps anchor anteriorly, while the other is tied posteriorly, providing secure central fixation (Fig. 11.6). Biomechanical data with this repair technique called the "stitch of Burns" revealed significant improvement in strain failure (>2 mm displacement)

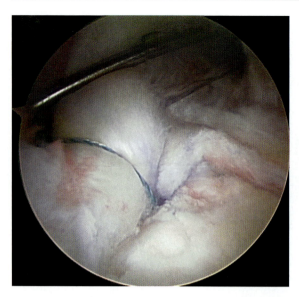

Fig. 11.6 SLAP repair with one central anchor that is double loaded. One suture is anterior and one is tied posterior to the biceps anchor

compared with a 2 anchor repair with an anchor anterior and one posterior to the biceps origin.[49] Central anchor placement for biceps fixation is key. A double loaded anchor will then provide adequate anterior and posterior biceps anchor security with one pass.

SCOI Repair Technique and Avoiding Complications[50]

Preoperative Discussion

Sometimes the biceps tendon is very degenerative at the attachment to the superior labrum. Fixing a detached anchor will still leave this pathology. It is prudent to discuss with the patient preoperatively the possibility of needing to perform either a tenodesis or tenotomy if this situation is encountered. Any significant fraying of the tendon should be considered for tenodesis or tenotomy. If the labrum is repaired, the biceps tendon may continue to be painful.

Single Anchor with Double Suture SLAP Repair

Establishment of Portals

With the arthroscope in the standard posterior portal, the anterior superior portal (ASP) is created with an outside-in technique. Use a spinal needle to determine the ideal location. Insert it approximately 2 cm from the anterolateral corner of the acromion so that it enters the joint in the superior edge of the rotator interval behind the biceps tendon. Insure that the needle can readily reach the superior neck of the glenoid when passing posterior to the biceps (Fig. 11.7). Portal location is critical for proper anchor placement while avoiding injury to the anterior edge of the supraspinatus tendon. After making an incision using a #11 blade in Langer's lines, insert a clear, smooth, plastic 6-mm operating cannula along the chosen path.

Care must be taken when inserting the anterior superior portal. Only the smallest possible cannula should be used that will permit passing the Crescent suture hook (Linvatec Inc, Largo, FL). One should never pass the cannula through the rotator cuff as has been suggested in some studies.

Next, create an anterior midglenoid portal (AMG) with the same outside-in technique as above, entering through the midpoint of the rotator interval above the subscapularis tendon.

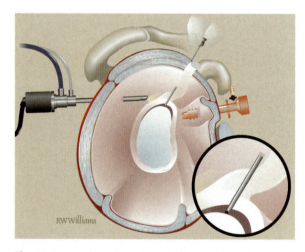

Fig. 11.7 Anterior superior portal placement is critical. Use a spinal needle to confirm access to the biceps anchor origin on the superior glenoid

Prepare the Labrum/Glenoid and Cyst Decompression

Debride any remaining soft tissue off the superior glenoid below the detached labrum/biceps anchor and trim any fraying of the labrum using a 4.2 mm motorized shaver (Fig. 11.8). The posterior portion of the lesion and glenoid is best trimmed with the shaver in the posterior portal and the arthroscope anteriorly. The superior glenoid rim and neck are only slightly decorticated, taking care not to remove excessive bone. The bone here is often relatively soft and use of a burr is seldom necessary.

If any associated spinoglenoid cysts are present, they may likewise be decompressed at this time. The portals dictated for SLAP repair are sufficient for cyst access. Visualization through the ASP and careful attention to the posterosuperior glenoid will help identify the capsular prominence of a cyst. The orifice to the cyst may be also identified under the labrum. We prefer to marsupialize these cysts by opening up the superior capsule adjacent to the labrum. This area is typically posterior to the biceps tendon at the 10:30 or 1:30 o'clock position and delineated by the MRI. Use a shaver with low suction strength or an electrosurgical instrument to open the capsule and gently remove enough wall to prevent closure and recurrence. Amber fluid will spill into the joint upon cyst entry. Cyst wall excision should be performed within a safety margin of approximately 1.5 cm medially from the glenoid rim. The infraspinatus branch of the suprascapular nerve lies 1.8-2.1 cm from the glenoid rim near the scapular spine.[51,52] Aggressive exploration and debridement of the cyst under the labrum may endanger the residual biceps anchor and may not allow sufficient decompression.

Anchor Placement

Insert a 2 mm Revo® punch into the ASP, passing posterior to the biceps tendon to create a pilot hole for the 4 mm Big Eye Revo® anchor loaded with two #2 polyethylene sutures (Linvatec Inc, Largo, FL). The punch must penetrate the superior glenoid exactly at the center of the biceps anchor just below the edge of the cartilage at an angle of 45° relative to the glenoid surface. Extreme caution must be exercised to insure the punch is completely within the bone (Fig. 11.9). If the starter punch is not aligned at the proper angle to the superior glenoid surface, it can very easily skive off into the superior glenoid recess or breach the posterior superior glenoid cortex or pass under the articular cartilage. The punch is carefully advanced under direct vision until the pilot hole is completed. The anchor must follow the pilot hole exactly and be carefully observed once it is seated. The biceps origin is not large and will not tolerate multiple attempts. One anchor is typically enough for type II SLAP lesions.

A titanium 4×12 mm^2 screw anchor or similar small double loaded absorbable anchor is preferred.

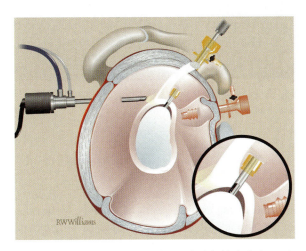

Fig. 11.8 The superior glenoid is gently debrided. A shaver is sufficient and a burr is not necessary because the bone is often relatively soft

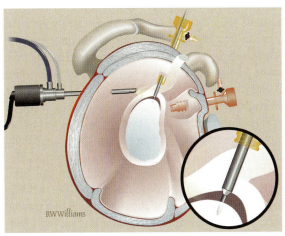

Fig. 11.9 Pass the punch posterior to the biceps at the center of the biceps origin under direct visualization

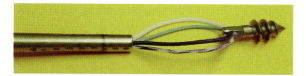

Fig. 11.10 Big Eye Revo (Linvatec Inc, Largo, Fl) metal suture anchor that is double loaded with #2 braided sutures. Half of each suture has been colored purple denoting the limb to be used as the post on the labral side away from the glenohumeral joint

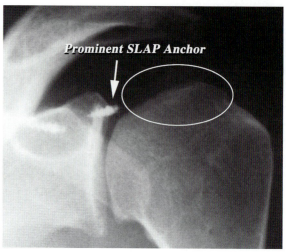

Fig. 11.12 An anterior-posterior radiograph showing a proud metal SLAP anchor. The *circle* highlights the subsequent iatrogenic chondral and humeral head injury

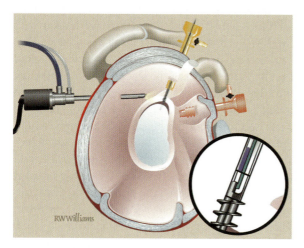

Fig. 11.11 A double loaded suture anchor is placed at the biceps origin

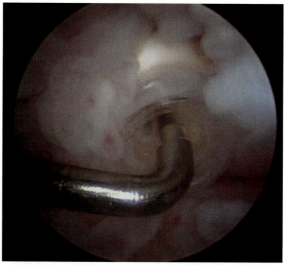

Fig. 11.13 A probe is placed on a proud bioabsorbable SLAP tack resulting in painful synovitis

If a bioabsorbable anchor is used, all steps for the implant (punching, drilling, tapping, etc.) should be fully carried out to ensure smooth implantation without implant breakage. The vertically oriented eyelet is first loaded with two strands of nonabsorbable #2 polyethylene suture in a very specific manner (Fig. 11.10). One suture is white and the other is dark green. By convention, the green suture is located at the upper end of the eyelet, and the white suture is at the lower portion of the eyelet closer to the screw threads. To facilitate suture management, half of each suture limb is colored purple with a surgical marking pen. The anchor is then loaded on the inserter such that the purple suture ends exit on the same side of the eyelet (Fig. 11.11). The anchor is then inserted into the pilot hole until the horizontal seating line is below bone and the purple limbs of the suture are toward the biceps tendon. Seating the anchor so that the opening of the eyelet is toward the biceps allows easier sliding of suture. The screwdriver is removed and the sutures are tested for security by gently pulling on them from outside the ASP.

It is important to ensure the anchor is properly inserted to the correct depth or entirely within the glenoid bone. Attention to the specific instrument markings will prevent proud anchors, either metal or bioabsorbable, that will result in chondral injury (Fig. 11.12) and painful synovitis (Fig. 11.13).

Suture Management

Use a crochet hook to retrieve the two nonpurple sutures into of the AMG portal (Fig. 11.14). Place the sutures outside the cannula using a switching rod. Next retrieve the two purple-dyed suture limbs into the AMG portal (Fig. 11.15).

Labrum Fixation

Insert a Spectrum (Linvatec Inc, Largo, FL) medium-sized crescent hook loaded with a Shuttle Relay Suture Passer® (Linvatec Inc, Largo, FL) or #1 monofilament suture through the AS cannula (Fig. 11.16). Using a penetrating-grasping tool to retrieve the suture can damage the biceps and labrum because of the large puncture size of the tool and is not recommended. Puncture the superior labrum on the posterior edge of the *center* of the biceps attachment at the level of the glenoid. *If the needle passes through the biceps too far lateral it will pull the biceps down medial when the sutures are tied adding abnormal excess tension to the repair.* Pass the needle through the root of the biceps and under the labrum directly in line with the anchor. The Shuttle Relay® is advanced into the joint, retrieved with a grasper, and carried into the AMG cannula. The two purple suture limbs inside the cannula are loaded into the Shuttle® eyelet and carried through the superior labrum into the ASP (Fig. 11.17).

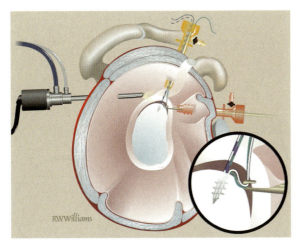

Fig. 11.14 A crochet hook is used to retrieve the *nonpurple* suture limbs, which are placed outside the AMG cannula

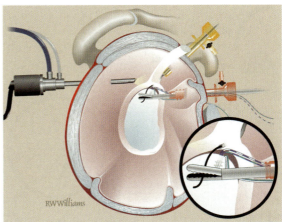

Fig. 11.16 A Spectrum (Linvatec Inc, Largo, FL) medium-sized crescent is used to puncture the biceps origin centrally and pass a shuttle that is retrieved from the AMG cannula

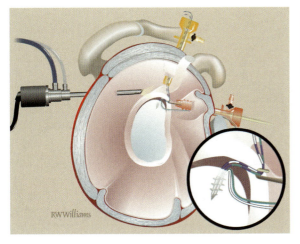

Fig. 11.15 The *purple* suture limbs are then retrieved and left in the AMG cannula

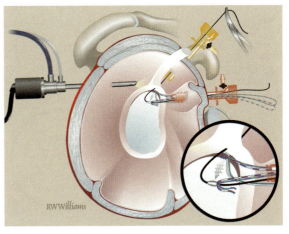

Fig. 11.17 The shuttle carries the *purple* suture limbs from the AMG cannula into the ASP cannula

Next, the purple-white suture is removed from the ASP into the AMG cannula with a crochet hook *anterior* to biceps tendon. This will avoid tangling the white purple suture when tying the green sutures. Retrieve the green-green suture into the ASP posterior to the biceps tendon using a crochet hook (Fig. 11.18). Pull the purple-green suture (the one through the labral tissue) to make it the shorter limb, and use it as the initial post strand. Tie the green suture using a sliding/locking knot and three alternating half-hitches (Fig. 11.19).

When tying the sutures, it is important not to use too much force. Strong suture material will not likely break but the anchor can be pulled out and the labral tissue can be damaged or strangled. Moderate tension that is adequate to hold the labrum to the prepared bone is all that is needed.

The purple color scheme facilitates suture management and proper knot tying. The purple sutures are on the tissue or glenoid-labrum side while the nonpurple sutures are toward the glenohumeral joint side. *The purple sutures are used as the posts for knot tying, ensuring that the knots will be behind the labrum and not located near the glenohumeral joint preventing any cartilage irritation.*

Retrieve both limbs of the white suture anterior to the biceps into the AS cannula using a crochet hook (Fig. 11.20). Pull the suture so that the purple-white strand is the shorter limb and tie it using a sliding knot and alternating half-hitches. Evaluate the repair by pulling on the biceps tendon with a probe checking for tension and stability (Fig. 11.21).

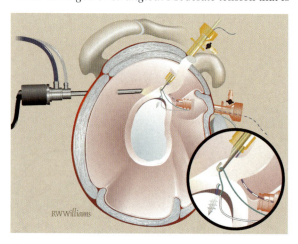

Fig. 11.18 A crochet hook has passed the *purple-white* suture into the AMG portal while the *green* suture limb is retrieved posterior to the biceps into the ASP cannula

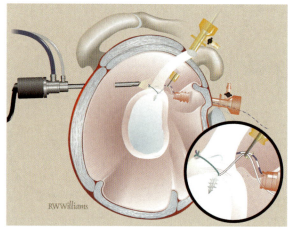

Fig. 11.20 The *white* sutures are then retrieved anteriorly to the biceps anchor and tied

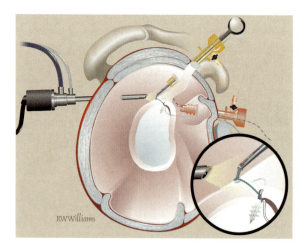

Fig. 11.19 The posterior or green sutures are tied securing the biceps anchor to the glenoid posteriorly. The *purple-green* suture should be the post

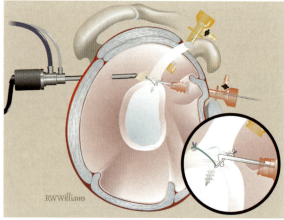

Fig. 11.21 The final SLAP repair has a firmly secured biceps anchor that should be tested with a probe

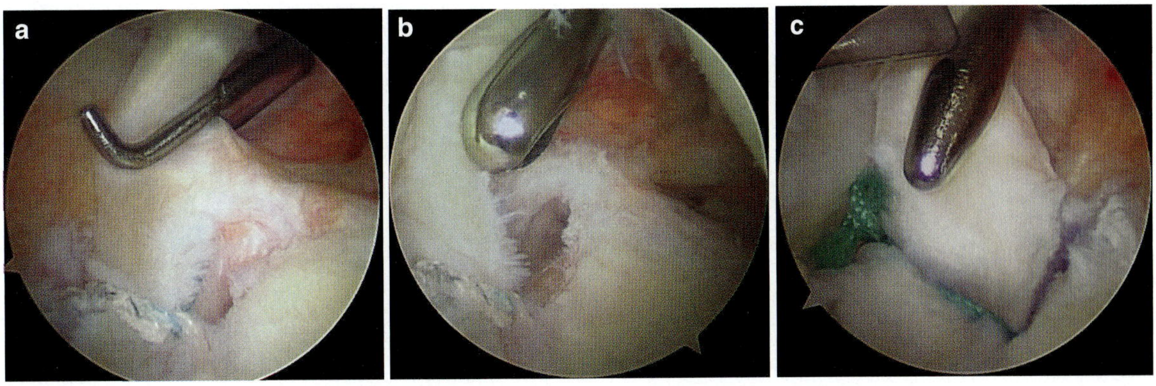

Fig. 11.22 A painful failed SLAP repair and subsequent revision. (**a**) One suture anchor was previously placed posterior to the biceps anchor origin at an outside institution. (**b**) The SLAP repair is inadequate and does not firmly secure the biceps anchor. (**c**) A new double loaded anchor was placed anterior to the previous anchor at the biceps origin and firmly secures the biceps anchor

Improper anchor placement or anchors that are too anterior or too posterior will not provide central fixation of the biceps anchor to the glenoid. These repairs will often continue to be problematic for patients and need to be revised. The biceps anchor continues to be unstable and is painfully tethered (Fig. 11.22). Proper anchor placement is dependent on portal placement and punch orientation.

Closure

The portals are closed with a single 3-0 subcutaneous stitch supplemented with a Steri-strip. A sterile dressing is applied.

Immobilization

The arm is supported in an UltraSling in 15° external rotation and slight abduction (DJ Orthopedics, Carlsbad, CA). *This position has been useful for preventing the complication of internal rotation contracture and stiffness that previously often resulted from the standard internal rotation brace or sling.* The arm can be removed for elbow, wrist, and hand exercises throughout the day, and pendulum exercises are encouraged three times a day for 4 weeks. Physical therapy begins at 4 weeks and progresses to full activities after 4 months.

Intraoperative Complications and Revision Surgery

The most important aspect for dealing with complications is avoidance of them in the first place. Following the outline above will insure that the lesion is properly secured to bone using the least number of anchors needed (Fig. 11.23). Occasionally, things do go wrong

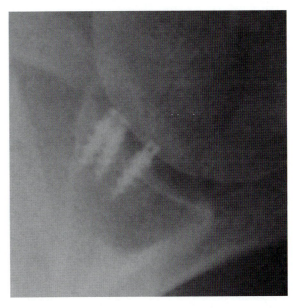

Fig. 11.23 An axillary radiograph revealing multiple, ineffective, anteriorly placed anchors for a SLAP repair. One double loaded anchor correctly placed at the biceps origin is sufficient for a type II SLAP repair

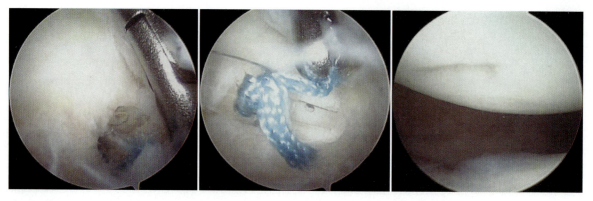

Fig. 11.24 A proud, failed SLAP anchor is removed with a grasper. Note the chondral damage on the humeral head

and the surgeon must be prepared to deal with the situations when they arise.

Sutures unloading or breaking before knots are tied: if a 4 mm metal anchor is used as described above, it can be removed by reloading the remaining suture (if present) into the screw driver and following the suture to the anchor. The orientation seating line on the driver must be aligned with the anchor eyelet and carefully seated over the anchor hub. The anchor can be removed simply by unscrewing it and retrieving it into the AS cannula. If both sutures are broken, it is advised to use an anchor retriever. This is a sheath made by the Linvatec (Largo, Fl) company that has an internal reverse thread. The screwdriver is passed inside the retriever, and the anchor is unscrewed and locks into the thread of the retriever. If no retriever is available for the anchor, great care must be taken not to dislodge the loose anchor and lose it in the joint. In that case it should be loosened only half way and the screw driver removed. An arthroscopic grasper can be inserted into the AS cannula and used to complete the removal (Fig. 11.24).

In some cases, the SLAP lesion fails to heal and the anchor is too tightly in-grown in the bone to be readily removed. The bone anterior and posterior to the anchor can be debrided, and two additional single suture anchors can be inserted on either side. Simple loop stitches are passed around the corners of the biceps and labrum shoulders and tied. It is difficult to remove an old anchor unless one has access to the Shoulder Rescue Plug® system from OBI/S&N. (Smith and Nephew, Andover, MA.) This product has a coring tool that can remove the anchor leaving a clean socket in the bone. A synthetic bone dowel of OBI material (Smith and Nephew, Andover, MA) can be inserted to fill the socket and another anchor then inserted adjacent to the plug.

Additional SLAP Repair Thoughts

There are reports in the literature regarding single portal SLAP repair techniques.[53,54] Single portal SLAP repair is possible with one ASP. However, these techniques can easily lead to suture tangling. One author reports percutaneous spinal needle retrieval of 1 set of sutures, which acts essentially as a "mini" AMG portal.[54] However, we feel that creation of a standard AMG portal greatly facilitates suture management and subsequently prevents tangling, minimizes operative time with minimal morbidity, especially for the arthroscopic surgeon who infrequently performs these surgeries.

Type II SLAP lesions are treated as above. SLAP type III and IVs are typically debrided. If these lesions have unstable biceps anchors, then the bucket handle tear is removed and the anchor fixed as above. We have on occasion repaired the bucket handle if the torn labrum may have functional importance. This occasionally occurs in instability patients with a middle glenohumeral ligament that originates from the superior labrum (Fig. 11.25). In these instances, we have removed the posterior bucket handle tear and fixed the residual anterior labrum with associated middle glenohumeral ligament back to the glenoid.

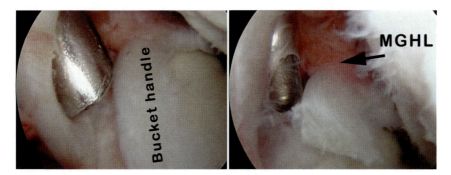

Fig. 11.25 A type III SLAP tear with bucket handle component. The middle glenohumeral ligament originates from the anterior labrum which was retained and fixed to the glenoid in this instability patient

Postoperative Considerations and Rehabilitation

A common problem early in the course of SLAP treatment has been postoperative capsular adhesions. SLAP repair fixes the loose superior labrum along with its superior and middle glenohumeral ligament attachments. If the arm is held in a regular sling or shoulder immobilizer in a position of internal rotation, these tissues along with the traumatized rotator interval tissues will scar, thereby restricting external rotation. It is now possible to avoid this problem by treating the shoulder in an external rotation brace. The brace is worn for 3 weeks but the patient has to remove it for gentle pendulum exercises, and elbow, wrist, and hand exercises, immediately postoperatively. The shoulder should be protected from excess stress on the biceps tendon for 12 weeks. Progressive resistance exercises are allowed at 6 weeks. *Aggressive postoperative rehabilitation too early can result in repair failure*. Vigorous throwing or strenuous lifting is allowed after 4 months if there are no limitations on motion and the patient is asymptomatic.

References

1. Snyder S, Karzel R, Del Pizzo W et al (1990) SLAP lesions of the shoulder. Arthroscopy 6:274-49
2. Snyder S, Banas M, Karzel R (1995) An analysis of 140 injuries to the superior glenoid labrum. J Shoulder Elbow Surg. 4:243-8
3. Handelberg F, Willems S, Shahabpour M et al (1998) SLAP lesions: A retrospective multicenter study. Arthroscopy. 14:856-62
4. Andrews J, Carson W Jr, McLeod W (1985) Glenoid labrum tears related to the long head of the biceps. Am J Sports Med. 13:337-41
5. Kumar V, Satku K, Balasubramaniam P (1989) The role of the long head of biceps brachii in the stabilization of the head of the humerus. Clin Orthop Relat Res. 244:172-5
6. Itoi E, Kuechle D, Newman S et al (1993 Jul) Stabilising function of the biceps in stable and unstable shoulders. J Bone Joint Surg Br 75(4):546-50
7. Gowan I, Jobe F, Tibone J et al (1987) A comparative electromyographic analysis of the shoulder during pitching. Professional versus amateur pitchers. Am J Sports Med. 15:586-90
8. Glousman R, Jobe F, Tibone J et al (1988) Dynamic electromyographic analysis of the throwing shoulder with glenohumeral instability. J Bone Joint Surg Am. 70:220-26
9. Rodosky M, Harner C, Fu F (1994) The role of the long head of the biceps muscle and superior glenoid labrum in anterior stability of the shoulder. Am J Sports Med. 22:121-30
10. Pagnani M, Deng X, Warren R et al (1995) Effect of lesions of the superior portion of the glenoid labrum on glenohumeral translation. J Bone Joint Surg Am. 77:1003-10
11. Mileski R, Snyder S (1998) Superior labral lesions in the shoulder: pathoanatomy and surgical management. J Am Acad Orthop Surg. 6:121-31
12. Prodromos C, Ferry J, Schiller A et al (1990) Histological studies of the glenoid labrum from fetal life to old age. J Bone Joint Surg Am. 72:1344-48
13. Smith D, Chopp T, Aufdemorte T et al (1996) Sublabral recess of the superior glenoid labrum: study of cadavers with conventional nonenhanced MR imaging, MR arthrography, anatomic dissection, and limited histologic examination. Radiology 201:251-6
14. Cooper D, Arnoczky S, O'Brien S et al (1992) Anatomy, histology, and vascularity of the glenoid labrum. An anatomical study. J Bone Joint Surg Am. 74:46-52

15. Huber W, Putz R (1997) Periarticular fiber system of the shoulder joint. Arthroscopy 13:680-91
16. Pal G, Bhatt R, Patel V (1991) Relationship between the tendon of the long head of biceps brachii and the glenoidal labrum in humans. Anat Rec. 229:278-80
17. Vangsness C Jr, Jorgenson S, Watson T et al (1994) The origin of the long head of the biceps from the scapula and glenoid labrum. An anatomical study of 100 shoulders. J Bone Joint Surg Br 76:951-4
18. Snyder S (2003) Superior labrum, anterior to posterior lesions of the shoulder. In: Snyder SJ (ed) Shoulder Arthroscopy. Lippincott Williams and Wilkins, Philadelphia, pp 147-65
19. Williams M, Snyder S, Buford D Jr (1994) The Buford complex-the "cord-like" middle glenohumeral ligament and absent anterosuperior labrum complex: A normal anatomic capsulolabral variant. Arthroscopy 10:241-7
20. Rao A, Kim T, Chronopoulos E et al (2003) Anatomical variants in the anterosuperior aspect of the glenoid labrum: A statistical analysis of seventy-three cases. J Bone Joint Surg Am. 85:653-9
21. Panossian V, Mihata T, Tibone J et al (2005) Biomechanical analysis of isolated type II SLAP lesions and repair. J Shoulder Elbow Surg. 14:529-34
22. Morgan C, Burkhart S, Palmeri M et al (1998) Type II SLAP lesions: three subtypes and their relationships to superior instability and rotator cuff tears. Arthroscopy 14:553-65
23. Maffet M, Gartsman G, Moseley B (1995) Superior labrum-biceps tendon complex lesions of the shoulder. Am J Sports Med. 23:93-8
24. Barber A, Field L, Ryu R (2007) Biceps tendon and superior labrum injuries: decision-marking. J Bone Joint Surg Am. 89:1844-55
25. Nam E, Snyder S (2003) The diagnosis and treatment of superior labrum, anterior and posterior (SLAP) lesions. Am J Sports Med. 31:798-810
26. Burkhart S, Morgan C (1998) The peel-back mechanism: Its role in producing and extending posterior type II SLAP lesions and its effect on SLAP repair rehabilitation. Arthroscopy. 14:637-40
27. Powell S, Nord K, Ryu R (2004) The diagnosis, classification, and treatment of SLAP lesions. Oper Tech Sports Med. 12:99-110
28. McFarland E, Kim T, Savino R (2002) Clinical assessment of three common tests for superior labral anterior-posterior lesions. Am J Sports Med. 30:810-5
29. Bey M, Elders G, Huston L et al (1998) The mechanism of creation of superior labrum, anterior, and posterior lesions in a dynamic biomechanical model of the shoulder: The role of inferior subluxation. J Shoulder Elbow Surg. 7:397-401
30. Clavert P, Bonnomet F, Kempf J, Clavert P, Bonnomet F, Kempf J et al (2004) Contribution to the study of the pathogenesis of type II superior labrum anteroposterior lesions: a cadaveric model of a fall on the outstretched hand. J Shoulder Elbow Surg 13:45-50
31. Burkhart S, Morgan C, Kibler W (2003) The disabled throwing shoulder: spectrum of pathology Part I: pathoanatomy and biomechanics. Arthroscopy. 19:404-20
32. O'rien S, Pagnani M, Fealy S et al (1998) The active compression test: a new and effective test for diagnosing labral tears and acromioclavicular joint abnormality. Am J Sports Med. 26:610-13
33. Kim S, Ha K, Ahn J et al (2001) Biceps load test II: A clinical test for SLAP lesions of the shoulder. Arthroscopy. 17:160-4
34. Kim S, Ha K, Han K (1999) Biceps load test: A clinical test for superior labrum anterior and posterior lesions in shoulders with recurrent anterior dislocations. Am J Sports Med. 27:300-3
35. Stetson W, Templin K (2002) The crank test, the O'Brien test, and routine magnetic resonance imaging scans in the diagnosis of labral tears. Am J Sports Med. 30:806-9
36. Kibler W (1995) Specificity and sensitivity of the anterior slide test in throwing athletes with superior glenoid labral tears. Arthroscopy. 11:296-300
37. Liu S, Henry M, Nuccion S (1996) A prospective evaluation of a new physical examination in predicting glenoid labral tears. Am J Sports Med. 24:721-5
38. Jee W, McCauley T, Katz L et al (2001) Superior labral anterior posterior (SLAP) lesions of the glenoid labrum: Reliability and accuracy of MR arthrography for diagnosis. Radiology. 218:127-32
39. Kaplan P, Helms C, Dussault R et al (2001) Shoulder. In: Kaplan PA, Helms CA, Dussault R, Anderson MW, Major NM (eds) Musculoskeletal MRI. WB Saunders, Philadelphia, pp 175-223
40. Reuss B, Schwartzberg R, Zlatkin M et al (2006) Magnetic resonance imaging accuracy for the diagnosis of superior labrum anterior-posterior lesions in the community setting: Eighty-three arthroscopically confirmed cases. J Shoulder Elbow Surg. 15:580-5
41. Tuite M, Cirillo R, De Smet A et al (2000) Superior labrum anterior-posterior (SLAP) tears: Evaluation of three MR signs on T2-weighted images. Radiology. 215:841-5
42. Jin W, Ryu K, Kwon S et al (2006) MR arthrography in the differential diagnosis of type II superior labral anteroposterior lesion and sublabral recess. AJR Am J Roentgenol. 187:887-93
43. Bencardino J, Beltran J, Rosenberg ZS et al (2000) Superior labrum anterior-posterior lesions: diagnosis with MR arthrography of the shoulder. Radiology. 214:267-71
44. Westerheide K, Dopirak R, Karzel R et al (006) J Suprascapular nerve palsy secondary to spinoglenoid cysts: Results of arthroscopic treatment. Arthroscopy 22:721-7
45. Westerheide K, Karzel R (2003) Ganglion cysts of the shoulder: technique or arthroscopic decompression and fixation of associated type II superior labral anterior to posterior lesions. Orthop Clin North Am. 34:521-8
46. Burkhart S, Morgan C, Kibler W (2003) The disabled throwing shoulder: Spectrum of pathology Part II: Evaluation and treatment of SLAP lesions in throwers. Arthroscopy 19:531-9

47. Yoneda M, Hirooka A, Saito S et al (1991) Arthroscopic stapling for detached superior glenoid labrum. J Bone Joint Surg Br. 73:746-50
48. Field L, Savoie FIII (1993) Arthroscopic suture repair of superior labral detachment lesions of the shoulder. Am J Sports Med. 21:783-90
49. Burbank S, Snyder S (2007). Biomechanical analysis of SLAP repair techniques and meta-analysis of literature. Hospital for Special Surgery and Southern California Orthopedic Institute. Unpublished data.
50. Tyorkin M, Snyder S (2008) Arthroscopic Repair of SLAP lesions by the single anchor double suture technique. In: Cole B, Cole B, Sekiya M (eds) Surgical techniques of the shoulder, elbow and knee in sports medicine. Elsevier, New York
51. Bigliani L, Dalsey R, McCann P et al (1990) An anatomical study of the suprascapular nerve. Arthroscopy. 6:301-5
52. Warner J, Krushell R, Masquelet A et al (1992) Anatomy and relationships of the suprascapular nerve: Anatomical constraints to mobilization of the supraspinatus and infraspinatus muscles in the management of massive rotator-cuff tears. J Bone Joint Surg Am. 74:36-45
53. Buess E, Schneider C (2006) Simplified single-portal V-shaped SLAP repair. Arthroscopy 22(680):e1-4
54. Kim K, Rhee K, Shin H et al (2008) Modified single-portal type II SLAP repair. Arch Orthop Trauma Surg 128(11):1251-4

Editors' Comments (Slap Repairs)

A single anterosuperior portal can be utilized if one is comfortable with using a "crabclaw" type device to untangle sutures that will inevitably tangle.

If a suture breaks while tying and a plastic or bioabsorbable anchor has been used, the same pilot hole may be utilized and redrilled with placement of the same sized anchor. If the anchor then pulls out upon insertion, be prepared to have a larger anchor available for insertion. Thus, for a 3 mm suture anchor that pulls out, a 4.5 mm anchor can be utilized as a bail out.

There seems to be more emphasis of late on reducing the peel back phenomenon of SLAP tears by ensuring that the posterosuperior aspect of the SLAP is addressed.

Examine for associated anteroinferior and/or posteroinferior labral pathology.

Chapter 12
Avoiding and Managing Complications of Arthroscopic Biceps Tenodesis

Michael S. Bahk, Joseph P. Burns, and Stephen J. Snyder

Top 10 Pearls

- Biceps pathology is a common and potentially underestimated source of shoulder pain, even without subacromial impingement or rotator cuff pathology
- Tenotomy may be associated with cosmetic deformity, residual cramping and weakness, thus is often reserved for older, less active patients.
- Various biceps tenodesis techniques exist and can be tailored for the specific patient and associated pathologies present at the time of surgery.
- Subpectoral biceps tenodesis is the gold-standard for biceps tenodesis and removes the possibility of residual tendon pain within the biceps groove.
- For the subpectoral technique, careful marking of the natural resting tone of the biceps prior to tenotomy will prevent restriction of the biceps or undertensioning. This is performed by tenotomizing 99% of the biceps tendon initially within the glenohumeral joint.
- If the tendon is prematurely released, a rough approximation we have noticed is that the biceps musculotendinous junction corresponds to the inferior border of the pectoralis muscle as it crosses the humerus.
- Carefully placed 90° bent Hohmann retractors are helpful for exposure in subpectoral tenodesis, allowing for a very small incision.
- A small Spectrum (Linvatec Inc, Largo, FL) crescent suture hook helps feed the PDS shuttle retrograde through the humeral canal in subpectoral tenodesis.
- Excision of rotator interval tissue and internal rotation of the arm will help visualize the bicipital groove opening for arthroscopic glenohumeral suture anchor fixation.
- A small push-in anchor along with a suture control cannula are helpful for all intraarticular biceps arthroscopic glenohumeral suture anchor fixation.

Introduction and Background

There have been a number of changes in the management of lesions of the tendon of the long head of the biceps brachii over the past century.[1,2] Various biceps tenodesis techniques were popularized as a means of managing shoulder pain historically.[2–9] Neer emphasized impingement syndrome and rotator cuff disease as a major source of shoulder pain in 1972. He recommended anterior acromioplasty and warned against blind biceps tenodesis.[1,10] Preservation of the biceps for shoulder function was felt to be important.[3,10–12] Recently, there has been increased recognition of the diseased biceps as a source of continued pain.[13–15] However, there is some controversy in the literature as to the importance of the long head of the biceps in shoulder function. Currently, it is felt that the long head of the biceps does have some functional importance in shoulder function, but it may be more important as a clinical source of pain if a diseased biceps tendon is left untreated.

M.S. Bahk (✉)
Southern California Orthopedic Institute, Van Nuys, CA, USA
e-mail: mbahk@scoi.com

J.P. Burns
Southern California Orthopedic Institute, Van Nuys, CAlifornia , USA

S.J. Snyder
Southern California Orthopedic Institute, Van Nuys, CAlifornia, USA

Pertinent Biceps Anatomy

The biceps brachii muscle has a long head and a short head. The short head tendon originates from the coracoid process, while the long head originates from the glenoid or superior labrum,[16] travels intra-articularly and exits through the bicipital groove.

The tendon of the long head of the biceps is on average 102 mm in length (range 89-146 mm) and tends to be larger in males than females.[17] It has a larger cross sectional area proximally and tapers distally. Near its glenoid-labrum origin, the tendon has a cross-sectional area of 8.4×3.4 mm^2, tapers to 5.1×2.7 mm^2 at the proximal bicipital groove and is smallest after it exits the groove distally at 4.5×2.1 mm^2.[17] The distal groove is also the narrowest portion of the bicipital groove.[17] The tendon may appear to be flattened in shoulders with associated rotator cuff tears.[17,18] A study of 104 cadaveric shoulders also found degenerative changes occurred primarily at the distal bicipital groove and near the glenoid-labrum origin.[17] Tenodesis of the biceps proximal to the distal bicipital groove may retain diseased biceps tendon. However, it is unclear if this is clinically important.

The Biceps in Shoulder Function

The significance of the biceps in shoulder function is controversial. A number of studies report that the long head of the biceps contributes significantly to glenohumeral stability,[19–25] while others report little biceps activity with isolated shoulder motion.[26,27] The long head of the biceps is reported to act as a humeral head depressor or as a counterbalance to proximal migration of the humeral head with biceps short head contraction.[19] Other investigators report that biceps contraction in the abducted, externally rotated arm helps reduce anterior displacement of the humerus.[20] Electromyography (EMG) studies also seem to suggest an anterior stabilizing function of the biceps.[24,25] Cadaveric studies have reported increased superoinferior and anteroposterior translation with proximal biceps-labral lesions.[21,22] Others have reported proximal biceps injury leading to decreased torsional rigidity and increased inferior glenohumeral strain in the vulnerable, overhead arm positions.[23] However, some investigators have reported little biceps activity with shoulder motion when the elbow is controlled.[26,27] Most likely, the biceps has some role in shoulder stability and function; however, a retained biceps may be more important clinically as a source of pain.

Important Clinical Source of Pain

Especially in patients with associated shoulder pathology, biceps pathology may be an underestimated source of pain.[28,29] Arthroscopic evaluation identifying diseased biceps tendons underestimated the extent of extra-articular disease lying within the bicipital groove distally in 49% of cases.[28] In other words, the biceps tendon is an important source of pain that cannot be fully evaluated with standard arthroscopic technique and may be particularly overlooked in patients with additional shoulder pathology such as rotator cuff tear and glenohumeral arthritis.[30] Walch noted that patients with chronic rotator cuff tears often experienced relief after spontaneous ruptures of the long head of the biceps. He subsequently reported that patients with irreparable rotator cuff tears who underwent biceps tenotomy had significant clinical improvement.[30]

Treating the Structurally Diseased Biceps Tendons

With structural disease of the biceps tendon, definitive surgical management of the biceps tendon with tenotomy or tenodesis may have more positive clinical benefits than any negative functional loss caused by these procedures.[1,13,30–33] Any significant tearing, hypertrophy, subluxation or intrasubstance degeneration of the tendon may be considered as a possible source of pain that requires tenodesis or tenotomy. Some authors have suggested that >25% partial tearing is significant.[1,3,27] There is some controversy regarding the incidence and treatment of primary biceps tendonitis or simple inflammation of the tendon without structural changes. We feel that tenodesis and tenotomy should be reserved primarily for those patients with symptomatic anterior shoulder pain, corresponding physical exam, and visible structural changes. On rare occasions, however, biceps subluxation or refractory tenosynovitis requires surgical intervention for biceps with otherwise normal intraarticular appearance.

Biceps Tenotomy

Biceps tenotomy has the advantages of being technically easy to perform with clinical relief of pain.[32,34] Some authors have reported no difference in residual pain,[32] cosmesis,[35] or strength[36] between patients with tenodesis and tenotomy. However, tenotomy may have the disadvantages of cosmetic "popeye" deformity,[32,33,37,38] residual cramping pain,[33,38,39] and loss of elbow flexion and supination strength.[37] A Popeye sign was present in 70% of tenotomy patients, while residual biceps fatigue soreness was reported in 38% of patients.[38] Mariani et al. reported a 21% loss of supination strength and an 8% loss of elbow flexion strength in patients with proximal tendon rupture of the biceps tendon.[37] Sixty-seven percent of these patients reported subjective weakness with 30% of patients reported being unable to return to work at full capacity because of weakness.[37] In general, because of the possible functional and cosmetic disadvantages, most surgeons prefer to reserve biceps tenotomy for older, less active patients.

Tenotomy can be easily performed with a biting basket or an electrosurgical instrument. We prefer to tenotomize the tendon at its glenoid-labral origin leaving a normal appearing superior labrum with no residual stump. A shaver can be used to remove any remnant that may become a mechanical issue. If a tenotomy is performed, it is important to confirm full release and distalization of the tendon. A hypertrophic proximal biceps tendon may have an hourglass deformity and become incarcerated at the bicipital groove, becoming a mechanical block that has been reported to prevent a return of full shoulder motion.[40] In these cases, excision of the hypertrophic tendon and release of the proximal groove may be necessary.

Biceps Tenodesis

Tenodesis is technically more challenging to perform. We typically perform tenodesis in younger, more active patients, hoping to maintain the muscle length-tension relationship, maximize elbow flexion/supination strength, and preserve normal cosmesis. There are a number of techniques in performing biceps tenodesis. It may be arthroscopically performed in the glenohumeral joint or within the subacromial space. These techniques can be performed with soft tissue suture fixation,[41,42] suture anchor fixation, or with interference screws.[43-47] Biceps tenodesis may also be performed in a mini-open fashion with a small subpectoral incision.[48-51]

Arthroscopic Soft Tissue Suture Fixation

If an arthroscopic biceps tenodesis is desired in a lower-demand patient, suture fixation of the biceps to the adjacent soft tissues can be performed. We prefer to use the rotator interval for fixation while other surgeons utilize the adjacent rotator cuff.[42,50,52] This technique is relatively simple and quick and can be performed with an intact rotator cuff. The downside of this technique is the initial fixation of tendon to soft tissue and not to bone. However, some authors have reported only a 3% clinical failure of fixation and resultant biceps deformity with similar techniques.[42,52]

After a full diagnostic arthroscopy of the shoulder, the biceps is pulled into the joint with a grasper and pierced in its midsubstance with a percutaneous spinal

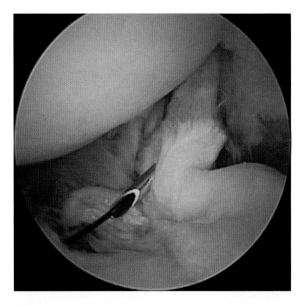

Fig. 12.1 A pinching grasper pulls the biceps into the glenohumeral joint while a percutaneous spinal needle pierces the biceps tendon

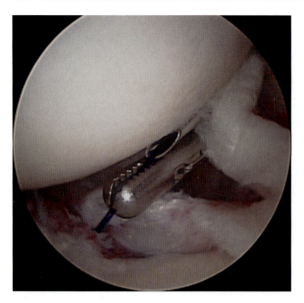

Fig. 12.2 A grasper retrieves the monofilament suture shuttle from the anterior cannula

needle placed through the rotator interval (Fig. 12.1). A monofilament no. 1 suture is fed through the spinal needle and brought out the anterior midglenoid (AMG) cannula (Fig. 12.2). This suture is then used to pass a strong Mehalik Hitch around and through the biceps in the following fashion: through the anterior cannula a high-strength braided No. 2 suture is looped around the biceps and both ends are brought back out the cannula. We prefer to create a rosette of suture in the grasper such that it is easy to "dump" several inches of suture around the biceps at once (Fig. 12.3). If the suture "dump" is performed inferior to the biceps tendon, the grasper retrieves a suture end superior to the biceps, creating a loop (Fig. 12.4). Both braided suture ends are then tied to the monofilament suture end outside the anterior cannula. The percutaneous end of the monofilament suture is then used to shuttle the braided sutures through the biceps midsubstance, then out the shoulder through the rotator interval. The Mehalik Hitch thus passes around and through the biceps, giving excellent hold (Fig. 12.5). To create a bridge of rotator interval tissue between braided sutures, one braided limb can then be brought out the anterior cannula and shuttled back through a different place in the rotator interval (~1 cm away) using another pass of the monofilament suture through a percutaneously placed spinal needle.

The tendon may then be released with an electrosurgical instrument or biting basket 5 mm proximal to the hitch. The remaining proximal biceps tendon may then be incised near the glenoid-labral origin with a biting basket or electrocautery device and then subsequently removed. The natural resting tension of the biceps is retained if the biceps and rotator interval are penetrated at their natural meeting point near the proximal bicipital groove. To stabilize the construct, the two ends of the braided suture are then identified in

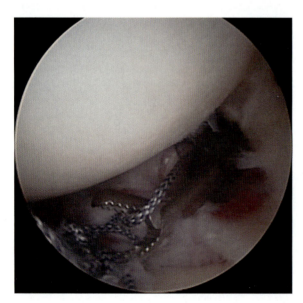

Fig. 12.3 A grasper "dumps" several inches of suture into the glenohumeral joint inferior to the biceps tendon

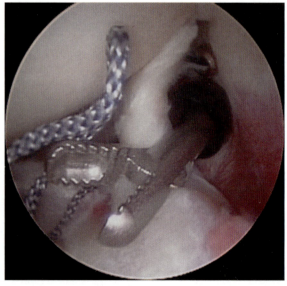

Fig. 12.4 The grasper is then maneuvered superior to the biceps to retrieve the suture out the anterior cannula creating a loop around the biceps tendon

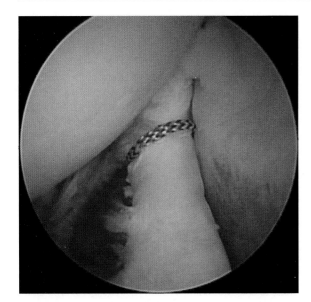

Fig. 12.5 The monofilament is tied around both ends of the high-strength braided suture which is then shuttled through the biceps tendon completing the Mehalik hitch

the subacromial space and tied together over the rotator interval soft tissue bridge.

Arthroscopic Suture Anchor Fixation

Suture anchor fixation of the biceps tendon may provide more secure fixation, tendon to bone healing, and can be easily performed with a rotator cuff repair in the subacromial space. We more often perform this fixation technique when a rotator cuff tear is present and in the higher demand patient. It can also be performed in the glenohumeral joint when a rotator cuff tear is not present. We prefer the intra-articular glenohumeral technique in younger more active patients with an intact rotator cuff who may require stronger fixation than soft tissue suture fixation may provide.

Subacromial Arthroscopic Suture Anchor Fixation

When the shoulder is first examined within the glenohumeral joint and the decision is made to perform a tenodesis, the biceps can be tenodesed with a separate anchor or it can be fixed with a rotator cuff repair anchor. If the tendon will be incorporated into the rotator cuff repair, the above soft tissue fixation technique is employed with a spinal needle creating a Mehalik hitch over a soft tissue rotator cuff/rotator interval bridge.

A shaver is used to expose the rotator cuff footprint and prepare the proximal bicipital groove for tenodesis. We will usually use one suture from a multiple loaded suture anchor for additional biceps fixation and a second suture for rotator cuff fixation. Spectrum suture hooks (Linvatec Inc, Largo, FL) are typically used for tendon or rotator cuff purchase. Because of the biceps, there are a few important technical points. First, the anterior anchor may be more anterior than usual to accommodate for the biceps tendodesis portion of the case. This may require the anchor to be placed through the anterior cannula. Second, full visualization of the anterior shoulder may require the arm to be placed in more abduction and external rotation than the traditional bursal position. Third, performing the biceps tenodesis before the rotator cuff repair will allow better visualization of the biceps and bicipital groove.

If a separate anchor is used for biceps tenodesis, we prefer to use a push-in, smaller, double-loaded suture anchor such as a Mitek G4 anchor (Depuy Mitek, Raynham, MA) placed in the bicipital groove. This smaller anchor will prevent any hardware interference with the rotator cuff anchors. The Mehalik hitch is not tied over a suture bridge but retrieved into the subacromial space through the cuff tear. Viewing from the lateral portal in the bursal position, the proximal bone of the bicipital groove is prepared with a shaver. A spinal needle is used to localize skin entry for the push-in anchor and the proper location of tenodesis near the bicipital groove opening. A small skin incision is made. A mini-Revo (Linvatec Inc, Largo, FL) punch is used to create a tract through the soft tissue and confirm proper access and location of the tenodesis anchor. A pinching grasper retrieves one limb of the Mehalik hitch, which is passed though the Mitek G4 anchor eyelet (Depuy Mitek, Raynham, MA) outside the shoulder. These push-in anchors are typically double-loaded, but to accommodate the suture from the Mehalik Hitch, one suture is removed from the eyelet. The anchor is passed through the skin and tapped into bone. The Mehalik hitch sutures can then be tied together, stabilizing the biceps to the anchor site. Backup fixation can be achieved with the second suture from the anchor. Using a suture hook and standard shuttling technique, the second suture can be passed through and then tied to the biceps.

SCOI Arthroscopic Glenohumeral Suture Anchor Fixation

For younger or more active patients and an intact rotator cuff, we have been performing an arthroscopic biceps tenodesis in the glenohumeral joint. It requires an AMG working portal, a posterior viewing portal, and a separate stab incision to pass the sutures.

Rotator Interval and Bone Preparation

After the biceps has been evaluated (Fig. 12.6), the rotator interval tissue is removed with a shaver to allow access to the proximal aspect of the bicipital groove (Fig. 12.7). The shaver or ball burr can then be used to abrade the bone in the proximal bicipital groove. Visualization of this fairly anterior area can be facilitated by internally rotating the arm or using a 70° scope (Fig. 12.8).

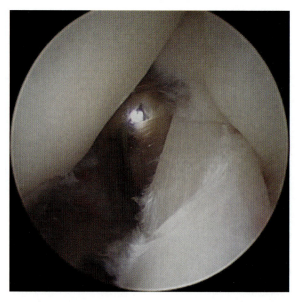

Fig. 12.7 A shaver through the anterior cannula removes rotator interval tissue allowing access to the bicipital groove opening

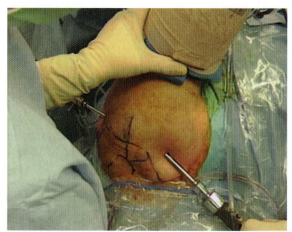

Fig. 12.8 Internal rotation of the arm aids in access to the anterior part of the humerus

Biceps Tendon Hitch

A grasper or pinching instrument can then pull the biceps into the glenohumeral joint, exposing the tendon for a 17-gauge 6-in. epidural needle to puncture the biceps tendon. The needle is percutaneously placed off the anterolateral acromion, and the entry of the epidural needle roughly corresponds to the natural resting position of the intact biceps tendon (Fig. 12.9). Once the correct needle position has been identified, a small

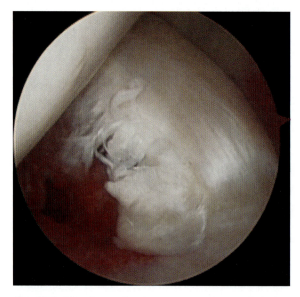

Fig. 12.6 Glenohumeral arthroscopy reveals a pathological biceps tendon

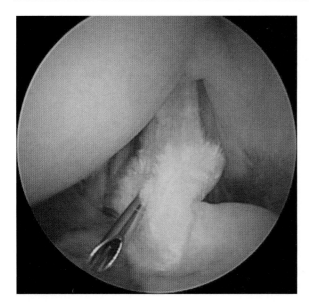

Fig. 12.9 An epidural needle percutaneously punctures the biceps tendon

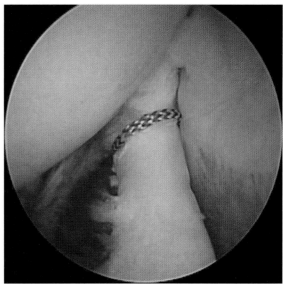

Fig. 12.11 A Mehalik hitch or a loop of suture is placed around and through the tendon

stab incision is made and a "suture control cannula" or SCC is passed into the glenohumeral joint (Fig. 12.10). This SCC cannula is a 5 in. thin metal cannulated tube that has a smooth beveled tip. The epidural needle passes freely within the suture control cannula, which protects and manages the sutures. A no. 1 PDS shuttle suture is passed through the biceps tendon and retrieved

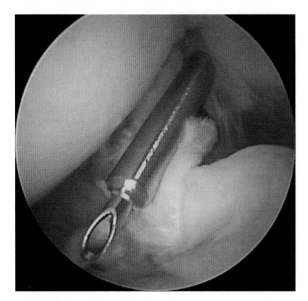

Fig. 12.10 A suture control cannula is percutaneously placed over the epidural needle and will aid in suture management and delivery

out the AMG portal. A Mehalik hitch is subsequently performed as described previously. A rosette of a no. 2 polyethylene braided suture is placed inferior to the tendon and retrieved superiorly placing a loop around the tendon (Fig. 12.11). The two free ends of the polyethylene braided suture are then tied with the PDS shuttle, the needle is removed, and the sutures are carried through the suture control cannula externally. A clamp is used to keep tension on the sutures on the end of the suture control cannula.

Anchor Placement

A small double loaded push-in anchor like the Mitek G4 (Depuy Mitek, Raynham, MA) will be used for suture anchor fixation. One suture from the anchor is removed to accept one suture from the previously prepared Mehalik hitch. The anterior midglenoid cannula is directed toward or placed against the humeral bone near the bicipital groove. A pilot hole is drilled in the bone through the anterior cannula near the medial edge of the biceps groove (Figs. 12.12 and 12.13). A mini-Revo (Linvatec Inc, Largo, FL) punch painted with purple dye is then used to mark the hole to facilitate later identification. One end of the Mehalik hitch is carried out the AMG portal. The suture control cannula can help deliver the sutures into the joint for easier

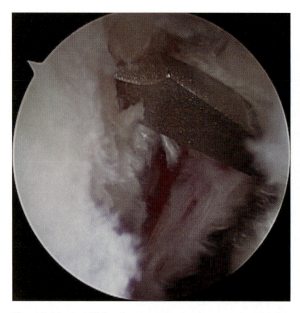

Fig. 12.12 A drill is placed on the humerus at the bicipital groove opening for anchor preparation

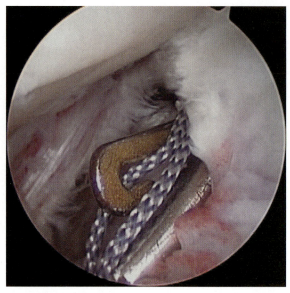

Fig. 12.14 The suture control cannula helps deliver the Mehalik hitch into the glenohumeral joint

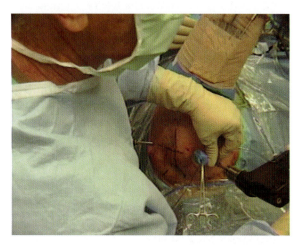

Fig. 12.13 The drilling is performed through the anterior cannula

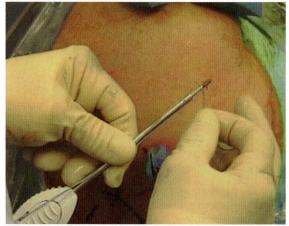

Fig. 12.15 The retrieved end is loaded into the anchor eyelet

retrieval (Fig. 12.14). The retrieved end of the Mehalik hitch is then placed through the eyelet of the anchor (Fig. 12.15). The anchor is then passed though the AMG cannula and subsequently tapped into the bone (Fig. 12.16). The anchor is tested for adequate fixation (Fig. 12.17). The second loaded suture is then retrieved with a crochet hook and placed outside the AMG cannula for later use. The partner of the Mehalik hitch is retrieved and brought into the AMG cannula with the aid of the suture control cannula (Fig. 12.18). A pinching instrument is used to strip the suture to ensure there are no twists. A nonsliding knot such as modified Revo knot is then tied, securing the biceps to the anchor (Fig. 12.19).

Second Biceps Tendon Hitch

The other set of sutures, loaded with the anchor, are then retrieved from outside the cannula and brought into the AMG cannula. The epidural needle is then used to puncture the biceps again,

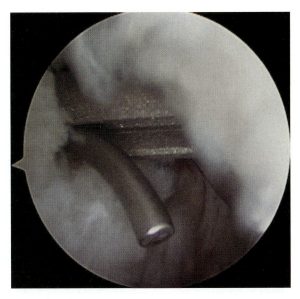

Fig. 12.16 The anchor is placed over the predrilled humeral hole

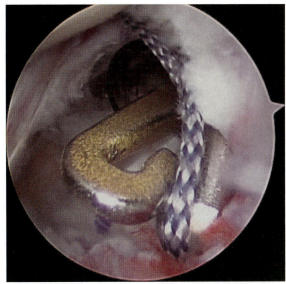

Fig. 12.18 The other end of the Mehalik hitch is retrieved with the aid of the suture control cannula

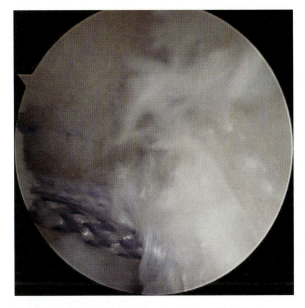

Fig. 12.17 The double loaded anchor is tapped into the humerus and tested

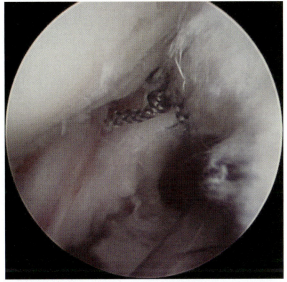

Fig. 12.19 A nonsliding knot is tied securing the tendon to the humerus

proximal to the first knot. A no. 1 PDS shuttle is passed and retrieved out the AMG as before followed by another Mehalik hitch. A second Mehalik hitch is then performed and tied as above with a nonsliding knot. This second stitch is tied further securing the biceps (Fig. 12.20).

Biceps Release and Labrum Final Preparation

A biting basket is used to release the biceps tendon (Fig. 12.21). There should be no biceps retraction as two sutures have been tied (Fig. 12.22). A shaver is then used to ensure there are no loose fragments in the joint.

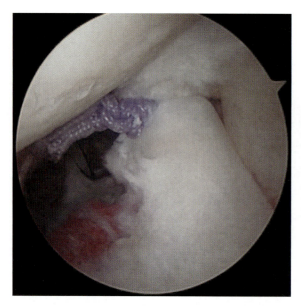

Fig. 12.20 The Mehalik hitch is repeated and a second nonsliding knot is tied providing additional tenodesis security

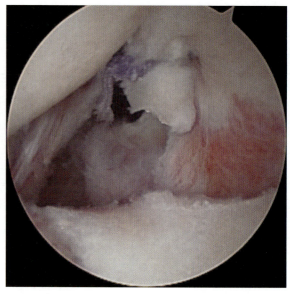

Fig. 12.22 An arthroscopic biceps tenodesis is performed within the glenohumeral joint with a push-in suture anchor and two suture hitches

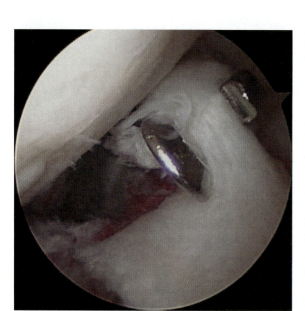

Fig. 12.21 The biceps is tenotomized with a biting basket

Arthroscopic Interference Screw Fixation

Another technique for biceps tendon is arthroscopic interference screw fixation. This has the advantage of more tendon to bone apposition with typically greater pull-out strength.[53] However, some authors have discontinued using this technique because of residual pain[51] either from the retained biceps in the bicipital groove or due to breakdown of the bioabsorbable screw.

Within the glenohumeral joint, a spinal needle is percutaneously passed off the anterolateral acromion to place a no. 1 PDS suture through the biceps tendon. A simple pass can be performed as it aids in subacromial identification in the later parts of the surgery. A biting basket or electrosurgical instrument can be used to divide the tendon. The rest of the procedure is performed in the subacromial space.

The lateral viewing portal is positioned more anteriorly to aid in visualization of the anterior shoulder. It is placed between the anterolateral corner of the acromion and the midpoint of the acromion.[54] The subacromial bursa is debrided with a shaver and the PDS is identified. An electrosurgical device can then be used to open the biceps sheath and expose the tendon. Once the tendon has been sufficiently released, an anterolateral incision can be made to externalize the tendon with a clamp. Twenty millimeter of tendon is excised and a running locking stitch is placed in 15 mm of tendon. These measurements will allow for proper tension restoration.[54] An anterolateral cannula can be placed in this incision and drilling can be performed through the cannula. Subsequently, a 7-8 mm bioabsorbable interference screw can be placed through the anterolateral skin incision to secure the tendon to bone.[47,54]

Subpectoral Biceps Tenodesis

The subpectoral biceps techniques provide immediate secure fixation, tendon to bone apposition, excises all pathological biceps tissue and avoids the possibility of any residual pain with bicipital groove involvement. It is also avoids the need for any additional hardware. We feel it is the gold standard for biceps tenodesis. However, it requires the conversion from an arthroscopic procedure to a small open procedure. The incision used is small, lies within Langer's lines near the axilla and is nearly unnoticeable. In addition, it is the salvage procedure for any previous biceps surgery that needs to be revised. For a previously performed biceps tenodesis that continues to be painful, this technique can be easily performed to resolve the pain. For a tenodesis that failed to hold fixation or for a failed tenotomy, this technique can be performed for a salvage procedure. The retracted tendon can be often identified with this incision.

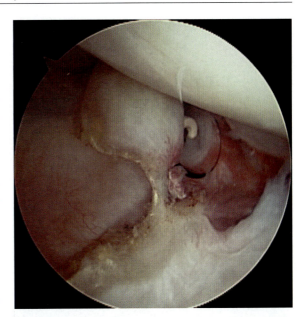

Fig. 12.23 The biceps tenotomy is nearly completed. A few fibers are left in place to hold biceps tension for the mini-open procedure

SCOI Subpectoral Biceps Tenodesis Technique

Arthroscopic Identification and Release

The patient is placed in the usual lateral decubitus position and a systematic glenohumeral arthroscopic examination is performed with the standard posterior and AMG portals. The biceps tendon is examined with a grasping tool and pulled into the glenohumeral joint to maximize visualization of the tendon. If significant pathology is present and the decision to perform a tenodesis is made, the biceps tendon is then partially released. Ninety-nine percent of the fibers are taken down with electrocautery or with a biting basket near the tendon labral origin (Fig. 12.23). A few fibers are left remaining to maintain normal biceps length-tension relationship, prevent distal retraction, and facilitate open identification. During the open part of the procedure, by pulling the tendon into the wound, the tenotomy will then be easily completed.

Repositioning

After the arthroscopic portion has been performed, the arm is taken out of the Shoulder Traction and Rotation (STaR) Sleeve (Arthrex, Inc, Naples, FL) and a sterile stockinette is placed over the arm. The beanbag is then deflated and the patient is tilted further posteriorly 30° to gain access to the arm and axilla. When adequate access has been determined with the surgeon standing between the abducted arm and the patient's body, the beanbag is reinflated holding the position. We typically reprepare the arm with betadine for the open portion of the procedure.

Incision and Tendon Preparation

With the arm abducted, the inferior border of the pectoralis major muscle can be palpated and outlined with a marking pen. Next the anterior axillary crease is marked out in Langer's lines perpendicular to the inferior margin of the pectoralis major muscle (Fig. 12.24). The incision is approximately 3-4 cm in length. The skin is incised 1 cm above the inferior pectoralis major border and extended for 2-3 cm below the inferior border into the axilla. Small skin flaps are raised and the

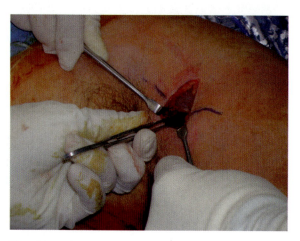

Fig. 12.24 The inferior border of the pectoralis major muscle and the anterior axillary crease are marked out

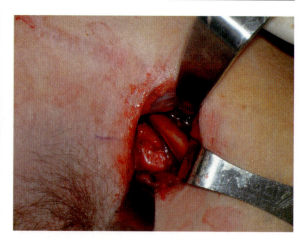

Fig. 12.26 The biceps tendon is well visualized with the aid of bent human retractors

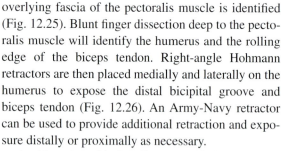

Fig. 12.25 The inferior border of the pectoralis major muscle is identified

overlying fascia of the pectoralis muscle is identified (Fig. 12.25). Blunt finger dissection deep to the pectoralis muscle will identify the humerus and the rolling edge of the biceps tendon. Right-angle Hohmann retractors are then placed medially and laterally on the humerus to expose the distal bicipital groove and biceps tendon (Fig. 12.26). An Army-Navy retractor can be used to provide additional retraction and exposure distally or proximally as necessary.

At this point with the elbow extended, the natural resting position of the biceps tendon within the groove can be noted. The tendon has not been fully tenotomized yet. Electrocautery is used to mark the bone at the distal bicipital groove, and a stitch of high-strength no. 2 or no. 5 suture is placed through the tendon at the same level (Fig. 12.27). The tendon is then pulled easily out of the wound completing the tenotomy (Fig. 12.28). The tendon is then sutured proximally for 1.5 cm with a locking stitch, and the excess proximal tendon is excised (Fig. 12.29). The tendon can then be sized and is typically 5 mm in diameter at this point. It is interesting to note that there is often significant pathological tendinopathy throughout the proximal tendon, particularly in the distal groove and near the origin.

If the natural resting position of the tendon cannot be identified, it can be approximated by noting that the biceps musculotendinous junction tends to correspond with the level of the inferior border of the pectoralis.

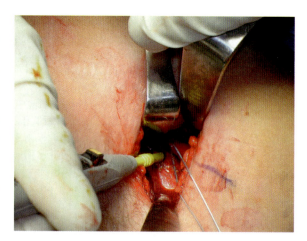

Fig. 12.27 An electrocautery mark on the humerus with a corresponding suture in the tendon helps to denote the natural position of the biceps

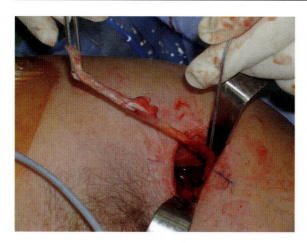

Fig. 12.28 The whole biceps is easily pulled into the wound completing the tenotomy

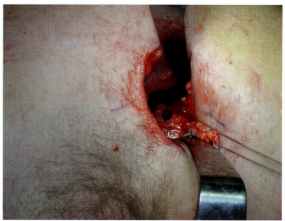

Fig. 12.30 The proximal hole is drilled at the original electrocautery mark at the distal bicipital groove

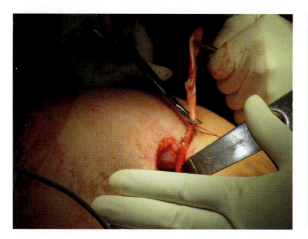

Fig. 12.29 After a running locking stitch is performed, the promixal diseased tendon is excised

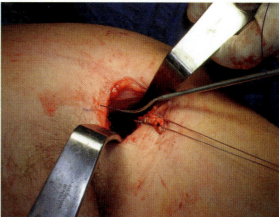

Fig. 12.31 A crescentic suture hook helps feed a monofilament shuttle retrograde through the humeral canal

Humeral Drilling and Tendon Passing

A guide pin is then placed at the electrocautery mark centered on the humerus. This marks the level of tendon fixation. The proximal drill site should be at the inferior edge of the biceps groove and not in the cortical bone. The pin is then overdrilled unicortically between 5 and 7 mm, depending on the size of the tendon (Fig. 12.30). Cannulated "acorn" type reamers are preferable. A second small unicortical hole approximately 2-3 mm in diameter is then placed 1.5 cm distally. The distance between drill holes should be equal to the length the tendon has been sutured proximally (1.5 cm). A small Spectrum (Linvatec Inc, Largo, FL) crescent suture passer is placed into the distal drill hole and a PDS suture acting as a shuttle is fed proximally up the canal of the humerus (Fig. 12.31). The shuttle is retrieved from the larger proximal hole with a clamp (Fig. 12.32). The PDS stitch is then tied around the composite suture, which is then shuttled out the distal humeral hole (Fig. 12.33).

Final Fixation and Closure

With the arm fully extended and the forearm supinated, the sutures are pulled, reducing the tendon into the humeral drill hole (Fig. 12.34), and stopping at the natural resting point: the 1.5 cm of proximal sutured

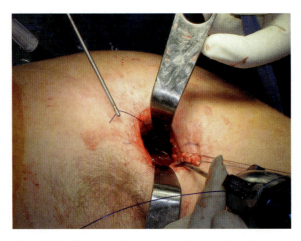

Fig. 12.32 The monofilament shuttle is retrieved with a grasper

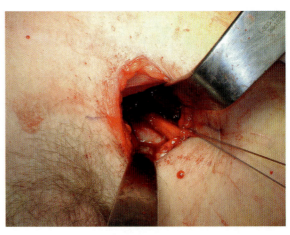

Fig. 12.35 The tendon has been fully delivered into the proximal drill hole and down the humeral canal

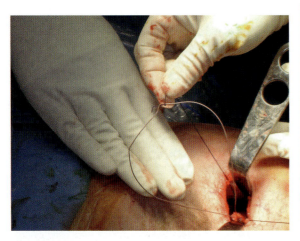

Fig. 12.33 The tendon suture is tied and shuttled with the monofilament

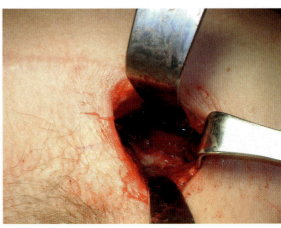

Fig. 12.36 The sutures are tied around the biceps securing the tenodesis

tendon is now within the humerus, lying in the 1.5 cm between drill holes (Fig. 12.35). This measuring technique ensures restoration of the natural tendon length and tension. The sutures are then placed around or through the tendon and tied securely at the distal humeral drill hole (Fig. 12.36). The wound is irrigated and closed leaving a small incision that heals well within Langer's lines and is typically out of sight (Fig. 12.37).

Conclusion

The tendon of the long head of the biceps does have functional importance, although the extent of its clinical relevance is still unclear. However, it is certainly an

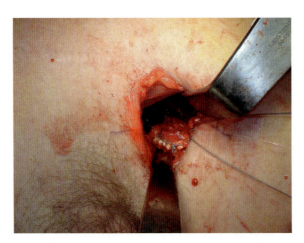

Fig. 12.34 The tendon has entered the proximal drill hole

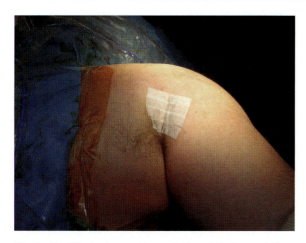

Fig. 12.37 The final wound is small, lies within Langer's lines and heals well

important and common source of shoulder pain. Surgical treatment of the tendon usually includes either tenotomy or tenodesis. Good to excellent function can be maintained with either procedure, as has been shown in the literature. Various arthroscopic tenodesis techniques exist and can be technically more challenging. For experienced surgeons, however, the arthroscopic technique can be a relatively easy, cosmetic, and safe way of providing excellent fixation by detensioning and decreasing painful motion and friction of the biceps within the bicipital groove. A mini-open procedure may provide a stronger construct, increased bone-to-bone healing potential, and excision of all pathologic tissue within the bicipital groove. It does require a small incision located near the axilla, which may be at increased risk for infection or iatrogenic soft tissue injury. Tenotomy is certainly the easiest procedure to do, but does affect strength and cosmesis. Although the indications for one procedure vs. the other are still a subject of debate, the choice for either treatment should be tailored to each patient and especially to each surgeon's comfort level.

References

1. Ball C, Galatz L, Yamaguchi K (2001) Tenodesis or tenotomy of the biceps tendon: Why and when to do it. Techn Shoulder Elbow Surg 2:140-52
2. Becker D, Cofield R (1989) Tenodesis of the long head of the biceps brachii for chronic bicipital tendinitis. Long-term results. J Bone Joint Surg Am 71:376-81
3. Sethi N, Wright R, Yamaguchi K (1999) Disorders of the long head of the biceps tendon. J Shoulder Elbow Surg 8:644-54
4. Gilcreest E (1936) Dislocation and elongation of the long head of the biceps brachii. An analysis of six cases. Ann Surg 104:118-38
5. Abbott L, Saunders J (1939) Acute traumatic dislocation of the tendon of the long head of the biceps brachii. A report of six cases with operative findings. Surgery 6:817-40
6. Hitchcock H, Bechtol C (1948) Painful shoulder Observations on the role of the tendon of the long head of the biceps brachii in its causation. J Bone Joint Surg Am 30:263-73
7. DePalma A, Callery G (1954) Bicipital tenosynovitis. Clin Orthop 3:69-85
8. Michele A (1960) Bicipital tenosynovitis. Clin Orthop 18:261-7
9. Foimson A, Oh I (1975) Keyhole tenodesis of biceps origin at the shoulder. Clin Orthop 112:245-9
10. Neer CII (1972) Anterior acromioplasty for the chronic impingement syndrome in the shoulder A preliminary report. Bone Joint Surg Am 54:41-50
11. Rockwood C, Lyons F (1993) Shoulder impingement syndrome: Diagnosis, radiographic evaluation, and treatment with a modified Neer acromioplasty. J Bone Joint Surg Am 75:409-24
12. Warner J, McMahon P (1995) The role of the long head of the biceps brachii in superior stability of the glenohumeral joint. J Bone Joint Surg Am 77:366-72
13. Berlemann U, Bayley I (1995) Tenodesis of the long head of biceps brachii in the painful shoulder: improving results in the long term. J Shoulder Elbow Surg 4:429-35
14. Walch G, Nové-Josserand L, Boileau P, Levigne C (1998) Subluxations and dislocations of the tendon of the long head of the biceps. J Shoulder Elbow Surg 7:100-8
15. Pfahler M, Branner S, Refior H (1999) The role of the bicipital groove in tendopathy of the long biceps tendon. J Shoulder Elbow Surg 8:419-24
16. Vangsness C Jr, Jorgenson S, Watson T et al (1994) The origin of the long head of the biceps from the scapula and glenoid labrum. An anatomical study of 100 shoulders. J Bone Joint Surg Br 76:951-4
17. Refior H, Sowa D (1995) Long tendon of the biceps brachii: Sites of predilection for degenerative lesions. J Shoulder Elbow Surg 4:436-40
18. Erickson S, Fitzgerald S, Quinn S et al (1992) Long bicipital tendon of the shoulder: Normal anatomy and pathologic findings on MR imaging. AJR 158:1091-6
19. Kumar VP, Satku K, Balasubramaniam P (1989) The role of the long head of biceps brachii in the stabilization of the head of the humerus. Clin Orthop Relat Res 244:172-5
20. Itoi E, Kuechle D, Newman S et al (1993 Jul) Stabilising function of the biceps in stable and unstable shoulders. J Bone Joint Surg Br 75(4):546-50
21. Pagnani M, Deng X, Warren R et al (1995) Effect of lesions of the superior portion of the glenoid labrum on glenohumeral translation. J Bone Joint Surg Am 77:1003-10
22. Panossian V, Mihata T, Tibone J et al (2005) Biomechanical analysis of isolated type II SLAP lesions and repair. J Shoulder Elbow Surg 14:529-34

23. Rodosky M, Harner C, Fu F (1994) The role of the long head of the biceps muscle and superior glenoid labrum in anterior stability of the shoulder. Am J Sports Med 22:121-30
24. Gowan I, Jobe F, Tibone J et al (1987) A comparative electromyographic analysis of the shoulder during pitching professional versus amateur pitchers. Am J Sports Med 15:586-90
25. Glousman R, Jobe F, Tibone J et al (1988) Dynamic electromyographic analysis of the throwing shoulder with glenohumeral instability. J Bone Joint Surg Am 70:220-6
26. Levy A, Kelly B, Lintner S et al (2001) Function of the long head of the biceps at the shoulder: electromyographic analysis. J Shoulder Elbow Surg 10:250-5
27. Yamaguchi K, Riew K, Galatz L et al (1997) Biceps activity during shoulder motion: An electromyographic analysis. Clin Orthop Relat Res 336:122-9
28. Murthi A, Vosburgh C, Neviaser T (2000) The incidence of pathologic changes of the long head of the biceps tendon. J Shoulder Elbow Surg 9:382-5
29. Walch G, Nové-Josserand L, Boileau P et al (1998) Subluxations and dislocations of the tendon of the long head of the biceps. J Shoulder Elbow Surg 7:100-8
30. Walch G, Edwards T, Boulahia A et al (2005) Arthroscopic tenotomy of the long head of the biceps in the treatment of rotator cuff tears: Clinical and radiographic results of 307 cases. J Shoulder Elbow Surg 14:238-46
31. Neviaser T, Neviaser R, Neviaser J et al (1982) The four-in-one arthroplasty for the painful arc syndrome. Clin Orthop Relat Res 163:107-12
32. Edwards T, Walch G (2003) Biceps tendonitis: classification and treatment with tenotomy. Operat Tech Sports Med 11:2-5
33. Boileau P, Baqué F, Valerio L et al (2007) Isolated arthroscopic biceps tenotomy or tenodesis improves symptoms in patients with massive irreparable rotator cuff tears. J Bone Joint Surg Am 89:747-57
34. Gill T, McIrvin E, Mair S et al (2001) Results of biceps tenotomy for treatment of pathology of the long head of the biceps brachii. J Shoulder Elbow Surg 10:247-9
35. Osbahr D, Diamond A, Speer K (2002) The cosmetic appearance of the biceps muscle after long-head tenotomy versus tenodesis. Arthroscopy 18:483-7
36. Hawkins R, Shank J, Kissenberth M et al (2007) A comparison of forearm supination and alebow flexion strength in patients with either long head of the biceps tenotomy or tenodesis. J Shoulder Elbow Surg 16:e64
37. Mariani E, Cofield R, Askew L et al (1988) Rupture of the tendon of the long head of the biceps brachii Surgical versus nonsurgical treatment. Clin Orthop Relat Res 228:233-39
38. Kelly A, Drakos M, Fealy S et al (2005) Arthroscopic release of the long head of the biceps tendon: functional outcome and clinical results. Am J Sports Med 33:208-13
39. Barber F, Byrd J, Wolf E et al (2001 Jul) How would you treat the partially torn biceps tendon? Arthroscopy 17:636-9
40. Boileau P, Ahrens P, Hatzidakis A (2004) Entrapment of the long head of the biceps tendon: The hourglass biceps-a cause of pain and locking of the shoulder. J Shoulder Elbow Surg. 13:249-57
41. Gartsman G, Hammerman S (2000) Arthroscopic biceps tenodesis: Operative technique. Arthroscopy 16:550-2
42. Castagna A, Conti M, Mouhsine E et al (2006) Arthroscopic biceps tendon tenodesis: The anchorage technical note. Knee Surg Sports Traumatol Arthrosc 14:581-5
43. Boileau P, Krishnan S, Coste J et al (2001) Arthroscopic biceps tenodesis: A new technique using bioabsorbable interference screw fixation. Tech Shoulder Elbow Surg 2:153-65
44. Boileau P, Krishnan S, Coste J et al (2002) Arthroscopic biceps tenodesis: A new technique using bioabsorbable interference screw fixation. Arthroscopy 18:1002-12
45. Klepps S, Hazrati Y, Flatow E (2002) Arthroscopic biceps tenodesis. Arthroscopy 18:1040-5
46. Romeo A, Mazzocca A, Tauro J (2004) Arthroscopic biceps tenodesis. Arthroscopy 20:206-13
47. Kim S, Yoo J (2005) Arthroscopic biceps tenodesis using interference screw: End-tunnel technique. Arthroscopy 21:1405
48. Weber S (1993) Arthroscopic "mini-open" technique in the treatment of ruptures of the long head of the biceps [abstract]. Arthroscopy 9:365
49. Wiley W, Meyers J, Weber S et al (2004) Arthroscopic assisted mini-open biceps tenodesis: Surgical technique. Arthroscopy 20:444-6
50 Snyder S (2003) Biceps tendon. In: Snyder SJ (ed) Shoulder Arthroscopy. Lippincott Williams and Wilkins, Philadelphia, pp 74-96
51. Mazzocca A, Cote M, Arciero C, Mazzocca A, Cote M, Arciero C et al (2008) Clinical outcomes following subpectoral biceps tenodesis with an interference screw. Am J Sports Med 36(10):1922-9
52. Castagna A, Garofalo R, Conti M et al (2008) Biceps soft tissue tenodesis. In: Abrams JS, Bell RH (eds) Arthroscopic rotator cuff surgery. Springer Science and Business Media, LLC, New York, NY, pp 276-89
53. Richards D, Burkhart S (2005) A biomechanical analysis of two biceps tenodesis fixation techniques. Arthroscopy. 21:861-66
54. Romeo A, Mazzocca A, Tauro J (2004) Arthroscopic biceps tenodesis. Arthroscopy 20:206-13

Editors' Comments (Biceps Tenodesis)

Interference Screw Technique

There are many potential pitfalls to this technique. Patients who are obese, very muscular, or if there has been fluid extravasation present a challenge to the surgeon as there may be very little working tendon length once the tendon is retrieved through the working anterolateral portal. If this occurs, one can consider either an arthroscopic suture anchor technique or an open approach. Another alternative is to leave the tendon long (i.e., do not excise any tissue), place the whipstich, and then use a deeper tunnel to recess the tendon into the proximal humerus and thus recreate proper biceps tendon tension.

If one does not have the Arthrex Biotenodesis set available, but wishes to utilize an interference screw tenodesis technique, it can easily be performed with a Beath pin passed through the humerus out posteriorly, taking care to avoid the area of the axillary nerve. The sutures are passed through the eyelet of the Beath pin, and fixation is performed with a standard bioabsorbable interference screw.

Another easy technique for biceps tenodesis from a glenohumeral approach is to pass a screw-in anchor from an anterior cannula, directly through the tendon. This saves a step, since all sutures are thus already through the tendon with at least once pass, and additional passes can be made as desired. We have also found it useful when performing a glenohumeral biceps tenodesis approach to reposition the arm in more forward flexion, and to occassionally utilize a medially placed posterior portal to allow improved visualization directly down the biceps groove.

When performing a tenodesis with the patient in the lateral decubitus position, we have found it easier to walk around the head of the patient standing anteriorly rather than repositioning the patient and standing in the axilla. This in effect puts the surgeon somewhat upside down, but in effect makes the approach quite easy without any need to adjust the bean bag or the arm traction.

Finally, we have had recent success using a knotless locking anchor for our tenodesis, which saves time and ensures proper suture tension.

Chapter 13
Avoiding and Managing Complications of Arthroscopic Rotator Cuff Repair

John Trantalis and Ian K.Y. Lo

Top 10 Pearls

- Always optimize your view at every step
- Perform a complete bursectomy
- Understand the tear pattern
- Plan and mentally visualize the repair
- Use traction sutures to assist in reduction and suture placement
- Rapid and reproducible suture management
- Make the first suture pass count
- Keep the repair tension low
- Perform releases when necessary
- Practice, practice, practice

Introduction and Background

Techniques of arthroscopic rotator cuff repair continue to evolve. In addition to advances in arthroscopic equipment and fixation devices, our increased understanding of tear mobility, tear patterns, margin convergence, and interval releases has expanded the boundaries as to what is considered reparable.

Although the vast majority of rotator cuff tears may be repaired arthroscopically from a technical perspective, whenever offering treatment, foremost in our decision-making process is the concept *"Primum non nocere"* or "First do no harm." Despite the fact that arthroscopic rotator cuff repair is considered "minimally invasive surgery," it too has a wide range of potential complications.

Since arthroscopic rotator cuff repair is a relatively new operative procedure, most reports in the literature on complications of rotator cuff repair are based on open or mini-open techniques. In 1997, Mansat et al.[1] reported on 116 open rotator cuff repairs and reported a complication in 44 cases (38%), with 38 (33%) of these being surgical complications and 14 are early medical complications. Nineteen shoulders (16%) had a major complication affecting the final result. The most common complication was failure of tendon healing, followed by stiffness, infection, and dislocation. Four shoulders (3.4%) required subsequent surgical treatment. The literature was reviewed in the same report, and a total of 310 complications were reported in 2,948 rotator cuff repairs (10.5%) with a revision rate of 3%.

In 2007, Brislin et al.[2] specifically reported on complications after arthroscopic rotator cuff repair. Out of 263 patients, 28 (10.6%) sustained a complication. By far the most common complication was postoperative stiffness, which comprised 23 out of the 28 complications. The remaining five complications were failure of healing, reflex sympathetic dystrophy, infection, deep venous thrombosis, and death. Their conclusion was that complications after arthroscopic rotator cuff repair are similar to results published for open rotator cuff repair.

In 2002, Weber et al.[3] reviewed the literature on complications associated with any type of arthroscopic shoulder surgery, and reported a complication rate of 5.8–9.5%. While this rate may be generally accepted, the definition of a complication (e.g., stiffness, failure of repair) has varied widely in the literature making interpretation between reports difficult. In addition, studies using diagnostic imaging to assess re-tear rates often report higher re-tear rates when compared to

J. Trantalis
Division of Orthopaedics, Department of Surgery,
The University of Calgary, Calgary, AB, Canada
e-mail: john@trantalis.com.au

Ian K.Y. Lo (✉)
Surgery, University of Calgary, Calgary, Alberta, AB, Canada
e-mail: ikylo@ucalgary.ca

studies using clinical criteria of a re-tear. For example, using postoperative ultrasound Galatz et al.[4] reported a re-tear in 17 out of 18 (94%) arthroscopic repairs of large and massive rotator cuff tears. Similarly, Bishop et al.[5] reported a re-tear rate of 76% of arthroscopic repairs in tears >3 cm in size. However, re-tears or persistent defects following rotator cuff repair can be relatively asymptomatic,[6] and thus defining a "complication" can be difficult and has commonly been at the discretion of the surgeon.

Complications after arthroscopic rotator cuff repair can be generally classified into general and specific complications. General complications include those associated with any type of arthroscopic surgery encompassing a wide range of adverse events including, but not limited to death, myocardial infarction / ischemia, pulmonary events, and cerebral ischemic events. A thorough preoperative work-up and appropriate medical consultation is mandatory to minimize general complications. In particular, hypotensive ischemic events are potentially more at risk during arthroscopic rotator cuff surgery,[7] due to the preference of hypotensive anesthesia during repair to limit bleeding and improve visualization.

This chapter will focus primarily on complications specific to arthroscopic rotator cuff repair, which can be further classified into intraoperative and postoperative complications. In addition, the technique segments of this chapter have been limited to repair of the rotator cuff. Arthroscopic techniques for managing the long head of biceps, acromioclavicular joint, and subacromial decompression are beyond the scope of this chapter.

Functional Anatomy at Risk

Although arthroscopic rotator cuff repair is a relatively safe procedure, knowledge of the surrounding anatomic structures is essential in preventing iatrogenic injury. Neurologic injury after any type of shoulder arthroscopy has been reported to be as prevalent as 30%.[8] Although most of these injuries are transient neuropraxias, permanent neurologic injury has been reported.[9] Direct nerve injury, excessive traction, swelling, and tourniquet effects of limb wrapping are potential mechanisms of injury.[10]

Of particular concern is the potential for damage to neurovascular structures. The brachial artery and plexus are in close proximity medial to the coracoid process. These structures may be at risk during placement of anterior cannulas and during advanced reconstruction and release of chronic subscapularis tendon tears. In a cadaveric anatomic study, Lo et al.[11] found that the shortest average distance from the anteromedial portion of the coracoid tip to the axillary nerve, the musculocutaneous nerve, the lateral cord, and the axillary artery was 30.3 ± 3.9 mm, 33.0 ± 6.2 mm, 28.5 ± 4.4 mm, and 36.8 ± 6.1 mm, respectively, and the shortest distance from the anteromedial aspect of the base of the coracoid to the axillary nerve, the musculocutaneous nerve, the lateral cord, and the axillary artery was 29.3 ± 5.6 mm, 36.5 ± 6.1 mm, 36.6 ± 6.2 mm, and 42.7 ± 7.3 mm, respectively. In order to minimize the chance of catastrophic injury to these structures, procedures around the coracoid tip and coracoid base must remain lateral to the coracoid. Subcoracoid decompression, subscapularis repair, and anterior interval release can all be performed safely provided the surgeon remains lateral to the coracoid process.

The axillary nerve is potentially at risk during arthroscopic surgery around the shoulder. Its proximity to the capsule of the inferior recess has been reported by Price et al.[12] to be an average of 2.5 mm from the inferior glenohumeral ligament and 12.4 from the glenoid rim in cadaveric dissections. The potential for injury to the axillary nerve is greatest in procedures within the inferior recess (e.g., arthroscopic stabilizations, capsular releases). However, its position is important when performing releases during subscapularis tendon repair. When performing releases of a contracted subscapularis tendon, superior, posterior, and anterior surfaces may be carefully released. However, the inferior border should generally be avoided to minimize the chance of damage to the axillary nerve and is usually not required to obtain sufficient mobilization for repair.

The suprascapular neurovascular bundle is also potentially at risk during arthroscopic rotator cuff repair. After passing through the suprascapular notch and giving off a motor branch to supraspinatus, the suprascapular nerve winds laterally around the base of the spine of the scapula, before innervating the infraspinatus. The suprascapular nerve is at risk when performing intra-articular capsular releases for retracted rotator cuff tears. To avoid injury, intra-articular releases should not extend >2 cm medial to the rim of the glenoid.[13] In more complex releases including posterior interval slides, the suprascapular nerve is vulnerable to injury as it winds laterally around the base of the spine of the scapula. To minimize the chance of injury to the suprascapular nerve during posterior interval slides, angled long blade arthroscopic scissors can allow careful step-by-step dissection and release of the posterior interval, with the release continued until the surrounding "fat pad" is visualized adjacent to the scapular spine, heralding proximity to the suprascapular neurovascular bundle.

Other more remote organs around the shoulder have been reported to be at risk in the literature. Pneumothorax,[14] tracheal compression,[15] and skin necrosis[16] have all been reported. Finally, the acute angles involved in subscapularis repair can put the head, and in particular the eyes at risk of blunt trauma from the surgical procedure. The surgeon must be constantly vigilant to prevent such trauma. However, the eyes can be protected with specifically designed adhesive goggles.

Preventing Complications

As with any surgical procedure, meticulous planning and preparation is the key to not only optimizing the efficiency and success of the operation but also avoiding complications. Multiple possible techniques exist at almost every step for achieving a successful arthroscopic rotator cuff repair. Recently, there has been an explosion of interest and popularity of various suture anchor constructs and repair configurations which are beyond the scope of this chapter. In the following paragraphs, we briefly describe our preferred setup and technique for arthroscopic rotator cuff repair with emphasis on its rationale and the avoidance of complications.

Set-up

The patient is positioned in the lateral decubitus position. A bean bag and taping is used to secure the patient. The arm is positioned in a hydraulic arm positioner (Spider Arm Positioner, Tenet Medical, Canada) allowing hands-free positioning and traction on the arm (Fig. 13.1). The entire arm is prepped and the arm positioner draped allowing full access to the shoulder and arm.

The senior author prefers the patient's head to be in a slightly dependent position (i.e., lower than the

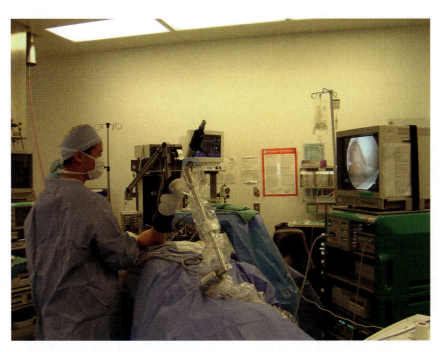

Fig. 13.1 Photo demonstrating intraoperative positioning for arthroscopic rotator cuff repair. The surgeon and the assistant stand behind the patient with the monitor, pump, shaver, and electrocautery unit on the opposite side. The arm is placed in a pneumatic arm positioner (Spider, Tenet Medical, Calgary, Alberta) allowing hands free for traction and positioning

shoulder) to maximize the gravitational effect of blood flow to the central nervous system and hence minimize the chance of an adverse neurological event. Pohl et al.[7] recently described four cases of ischemic brain and spinal cord injury after shoulder surgery in the beach chair position, and came to the conclusion that "the sitting position and the head position create specific physiological conditions that may be conducive to cerebral and spinal cord ischemia during this type of surgery." Autoregulation of cerebral perfusion may be hindered in this relatively older population making positioning particularly relevant when combined with hypotensive anesthesia.

Although beach chair positioning is widely accepted, particularly for transitioning from mini-open to all arthroscopic rotator cuff repair, lateral positioning may be easier for combined procedures (e.g., instability (particularly posterior instability) with rotator cuff tears), subscapularis tendon repair, access to particular portals (e.g., modified Neviaser portal), and areas of the joint (e.g., posterior capsule/rotator cuff).

Standard arthroscopic equipment is used and is positioned across from the operating surgeon. The arthroscopic fluid pump maintains pressure at 60 mmHg (pressure setting 60 mmHg). In addition to an arthroscopic shaver (5.5-mm Gator, Linvatec, Conmed., Largo, FL), a 90° arthroscopic electrocautery ablation device (Arthrocare, Inc., Austin, TX) is used for hemostasis and clearing of the subacromial bursa. A burr (6.0-mm oval burr, Linvatec Conmed, Largo, FL) is used to prepare the bony beds of repair sites. A single 8.25 mm × 70 mm clear cannula (Arthrex, Inc., Naples, FL) is used for most arthroscopic repairs.

Rotator Cuff Repair Principles

Like most orthopedic procedures, arthroscopic rotator cuff repair can be fraught with potential complications at each step. While a detailed description of the technical aspect of rotator cuff repair or the multitude of repair constructs and configurations is beyond the scope of this chapter, having a step-wise plan and adhering to various principles can lead to effective, efficient, and complication-free rotator cuff repair. It should be noted however, that rotator cuff repair is a "relatively" timed procedure. That is, prolonged operative time can lead to excessive swelling of the deltoid/subacromial space, obscuring visualization, and making repair extremely difficult.

Steps Involved in an Arthroscopic Rotator Cuff Repair

Step 1: Define the entire extent of the rotator cuff tear

Following diagnostic arthroscopy, the rotator cuff insertions both intra-articularly and subacromially are evaluated. In particular, the confluence of the leading edge of the supraspinatus tendon, the long head of the biceps, the medial sling, and the subscapularis tendon are carefully palpated and evaluated. Partial thickness tears and full thickness upper subscapularis tendon tears are commonly missed if not specifically evaluated. By placing the arm in abduction, traction, and internal rotation the oblique fibers of the subscapularis tendon are lifted away from the humeral head revealing its insertion (Fig. 13.2a, b).

Attention is then turned to the subacromial space, which must be thoroughly cleared of bursal and soft tissue. A complete bursectomy must be performed to remove the lateral and posterior reflections of the bursa to allow complete visualization of the bursal side of the rotator cuff. Inadequate removal of the overlying bursa not only obscures visualization of the margins of the rotator cuff, but also can lead to underestimation of tear size, inappropriate repair of the bursa, and can obliterate subacromial visualization, particularly as swelling progresses, making rotator cuff repair a difficult and frustrating procedure (Fig. 13.3). While performing a bursectomy, care is taken to not violate the inner deltoid fascia, which can accelerate deltoid swelling and lead to herniation of the deltoid muscle fibers into the subacromial/subdeltoid space.

Step 2: Determine the Mobility of the Tear

Once the tear has been fully exposed, the next step is to assess the mobility of the tear in order to plan the repair. The tear mobility must be assessed in a medial to lateral direction and in an anterior to posterior direction. A tendon grasper is used through the lateral, anterior, and

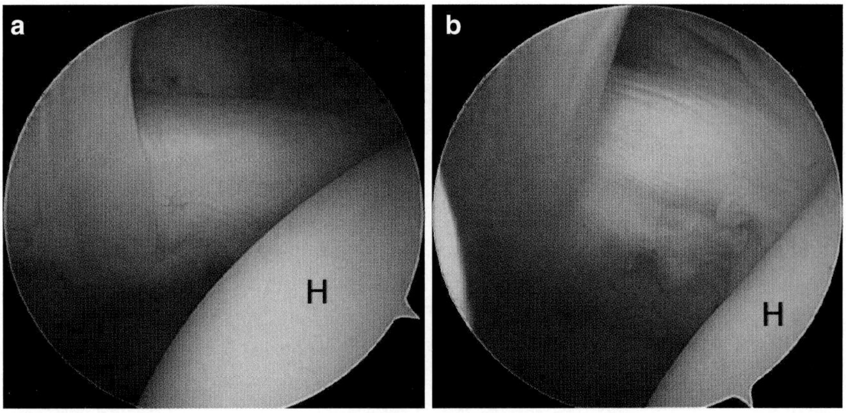

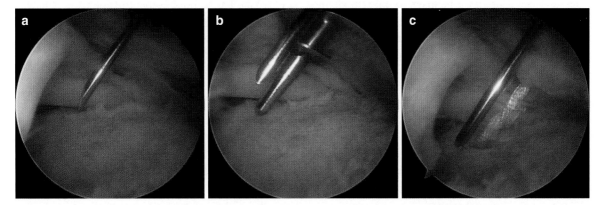

Fig. 13.2 Arthroscopic photo from a posterior glenohumeral portal of a right shoulder demonstrating the subscapularis insertion in: (**a**) neutral position and (**b**) internal rotation. Note how internal rotation slackens the fibers of the subscapularis tendon revealing its insertion. *H* Humeral head. Note: All arthroscopic photos are oriented in the beach chair position

Fig. 13.3 Arthroscopic view through a posterior subacromial portal of a right shoulder demonstrating anchor insertion. (**a**) A spinal needle is used as a guide to ensure the correct angle of approach for a proper deadmans angle. (**b**) Using the spinal needle as a guide, the bone is punched and tapped. (**c**) The spinal needle is kept in place while the anchor is inserted. It is removed only after the anchor is seated, so that it can serve as a guide for the entire procedure of anchor insertion. *RC* Rotator cuff, *GT* Greater tuberosity, and *BT* Biceps tendon

posterior portals to grasp each leaflet and assess its mobility. By assessing which leaflets have the greatest mobility, the surgeon is able to plan for a tension-free repair, a critical element in repair longevity. Overtensioning or inappropriate tensioning (i.e., in an inappropriate direction) of a repair will lead to repair failure, pain, and loss of function.

As described by Burkhart et al.,[17] tears of the posterosuperior cuff can be generally classified as follows:

1. Crescent
2. U-shaped tear
3. L-shaped and reverse L-shaped tear
4. Massive contracted immobile tears

While a discussion on each individual repair pattern chosen is beyond the scope of this chapter,[17] a number of key elements should be emphasized. Determining tear mobility and thus tear pattern is a critical step and its importance cannot be overemphasized. Care must be taken in evaluating the mobility of essentially all margins of the rotator cuff in all directions. With this in mind, it should be noted, however, that very few tears are pure crescent tears. That is, although the tear may at first appear mobile from a straight medial to lateral direction, there is usually even more mobility from a posteromedial to an anterolateral direction which allows complete reduction of the tendon to the bone bed in a tension-free manner.

Similarly, U-shaped tears imply equal mobility of the anterior and posterior margins of the rotator cuff. However, more likely, one of the leafs (commonly the posterior leaf) is more mobile, and its apex must be determined similar to an L-shaped tear.

Interval releases are infrequently performed (less than 10% of *massive* tears) and reserved for tear patterns with minimal or no mobility from a medial to lateral and anterior to posterior direction.

Step 3: Preparing the Bony Bed

In order to optimize the healing response, the bony footprint is prepared with a 6.0-mm tapered burr allowing *access* of bone marrow elements to the tendon-bone interface. Care must be taken to not remove the entire cortex of the greater tuberosity which can decrease pull-out strength of suture anchor constructs, particularly those which rely on cortical fixation.

Step 4: Suture-Anchor Insertion and Suture Management

To maximize pull-out strength, suture anchors should be generally inserted at a 45° deadman's angle. To ensure an adequate angle and placement of suture anchors, a spinal needle is used to act as a guide for insertion of the anchor. We prefer to leave the spinal needle in situ during bone punching and tapping, so that the needle will serve as a guide for the entire procedure of anchor insertion (Fig. 13.3). This can be very helpful when placing anchors with limited visualization or while viewing from the lateral subacromial portal.

Furthermore, when performing arthroscopic rotator cuff repair it is not uncommon to have 5 anchors, or 10 sutures, and therefore 20 limbs of suture to repair a rotator cuff. This can make suture management extremely difficult and time consuming when using one portal or cannula to place all suture anchors. We prefer to use small separate 2-3 mm stab incisions for each suture anchor. This ensures an adequate angle of approach to the bone bed and we create a pattern of suture-anchor portals on the skin which reflects their arrangement on the bony bed (i.e., The Mirror Method) (Fig. 13.4). This simplifies identification and management of the sutures. The key to this technique is after suture passage and before placement of the next anchor; the sutures are retrieved back out from the skin puncture wound used for inserting the corresponding suture anchor. This organizes the sutures together with the corresponding anchor and simplifies retrieving sutures during knot tying.

Step 5: Passing Sutures and Tying Knots

Recently, there has been explosion of methods and instrumentation for passing sutures arthroscopically. These include antegrade passing instruments

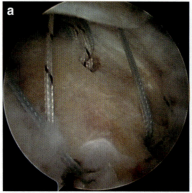
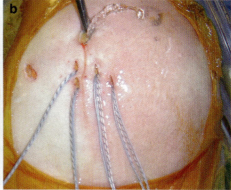

Fig. 13.4 Mirror method of suture management. (**a**) Arthroscopic view of right shoulder from a lateral subacromial portal demonstrating two medial and two lateral anchors. (**b**) External view of the same shoulder demonstrating the skin puncture wounds which were used to insert the anchors, with two medial and two lateral puncture wounds mirroring the footprint created. Following suture passage, the sutures are retrieved through the corresponding anchor portal simplifying suture management

(e.g., Scorpion, Arthrex, Inc., Naples, FL), retrograde passing instruments (e.g., Penetrator, Arthrex, Inc., Naples, FL), and shuttling techniques (e.g., Banana Lasso, Arthrex, Inc., Naples, FL). Although, each technique has its own inherent advantages and disadvantages, since one technique is not universally applicable to all situations, it is important to become facile with all methods.

Similarly, there are literally dozens of arthroscopic knots that have been described for tissue fixation to bone. These include sliding (e.g., Duncan loop, SMC knot, Roeder knot, Weston knot) and nonsliding knots (e.g., Revo knot, Surgeons knot). Although knotless technology has recently gained popularity, the surgeon will still be called upon to tie an arthroscopic knot (e.g., side-to-side margin convergence sutures). While many of these knots are sufficient for use during arthroscopic rotator cuff repair, we prefer to tie a Surgeon's knot (Fig. 13.5) using a Surgeon's Sixth Finger double diameter knot pusher (Arthrex, Naples, FL) (Fig. 13.6). This static knot has the theoretical advantage of limiting abrasion of the suture, and limiting abrasion of the suture against the tendon, and has been demonstrated to have superior loop security and knot security under biomechanical testing.[18] Although knot tying can initially be a very frustrating portion of the procedure with practice (practice and practice), knot tying should become the least daunting portion of the procedure.

Step 6: Repair Constructs

For most repairs of the rotator cuff a double row construct is utilized. Although the majority of evidence supporting double row repair is theoretical or mechanical in nature, double row repairs more closely reproduce the footprint of the rotator cuff[19] and have generally demonstrated superior biomechanical characteristics compared to single row repairs.[20,21] Our preference currently is to use a double row construct with cross and bridging sutures maximizing repair strength, and footprint contact.

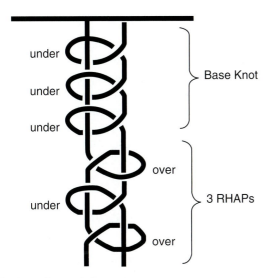

Fig. 13.5 Surgeon's knot

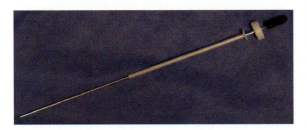

Fig. 13.6 Surgeon's sixth finger double diameter knot pusher

Specific Intraoperative Complications

I Can't See!

The key to performing a successful operative procedure is adequate visualization. Just as in open surgery, adequate exposure and visualization is critical. Taking the time to optimize the view and gain the best perspective on the pathology maximizes the chance of a successful repair. This may involve creating another portal for an improved angle of visualization, utilizing an alternative angle arthroscope (e.g., 70° vs. 30° arthroscope) (Fig. 13.7) or removing obscuring soft tissue.

Bleeding, however, is probably the primary intraoperative factor limiting visualization. To limit bleeding, hypotensive anesthesia is generally employed. In the absence of medical contraindications, a systolic blood pressure of 100 mmHg or less should be maintained. Developing a good professional relationship with an experienced anesthesiologist is important in achieving the goals of arthroscopic rotator cuff repair. We generally set the arthroscopic pump pressure at 60 mmHg and only occasionally increase the pump pressure transiently to help achieve hemostasis. Attempting

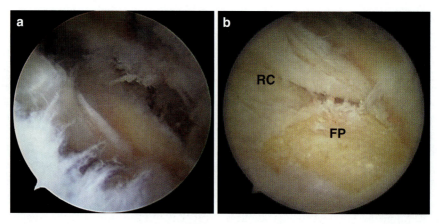

Fig. 13.7 Arthroscopic view through a posterior subacromial portal of a right shoulder with an anterior leading edge, partial thickness bursal surface supraspinatus tear. The arm is in maximal external rotation. (**a**) 30° arthroscope. Note: It is difficult to completely see the tear, particularly along the medial aspect of the footprint. (**b**) 70° arthroscope. Note: The 70° arthroscope provides an expanded view of the rotator cuff tear, including the medial footprint, allowing easy debridement and repair of the rotator cuff. *RC* Rotator cuff and *FP* Footprint

to control bleeding with high pump pressures for a prolonged period of time is not advisable as tissue swelling can rapidly increase making completion of the surgical procedure technically demanding.

When bleeding is encountered, the temptation is to increase outflow in order to flush the blood-stained fluid out of the joint. This, however, is rarely effective and usually increases bleeding via the Bernoulli effect. The Bernoulli effect, simply stated, is the negative pressure gradient created by a stream of fluid to surrounding structures and effectively sucks blood out of bleeding vessels thereby increasing the bleeding. In contrast, by decreasing outflow (e.g., obstructing portals where fluid is leaking) bleeding from vessels will slow allowing them to be identified and cauterized with an electrocautery ablation device. Turbulence control can be an extremely effective method of improving visualization, particularly when bleeding appears to be occurring from all directions (Fig. 13.8).

The use of electrocautery devices (e.g., UltraVac 90, Arthrocare Sportsmedicine, Sunnyvale, CA) can also be extremely useful during subacromial decompression, debridement and dissection of the rotator cuff, and for maintaining hemostasis. In areas such as the acromial insertion of the coracoacromial ligament, the medial subacromial bursa, the scapular spine region, and the pericoracoid region, bleeding is consistently encountered and electrocautery dissection helpful. When bleeding is encountered and other parameters have been optimized, it can sometimes be difficult to locate the source of the bleeding due to the "red-out" or limited vision secondary to the bleeding. In this scenario, the bleeding vessel is easily identified by "zeroing in" on the general area of bleeding with the camera. The flow from the tip of the camera clears blood in the immediate vicinity of the cannula tip, allowing the fresh stream of bleeding to be visualized as it pulses out of the vessel. Once localized with this technique it can be easily cauterized.

It should be noted, however, that by controlling the aforementioned parameters (e.g., turbulence, blood pressure), the surgeon will tend to rely less and less on isolated cauterization to control bleeding.

I Just Pulled An Anchor Out!

Optimal placement of the suture anchors requires adequate visualization and planning. Although viewing from a posterior subacromial portal is usually sufficient for visualization during anchor insertion, visualization can be obscured when placing anchors in the posterior medial aspect of the footprint. Optimal visualization can be achieved by viewing through a lateral or posterolateral portal or by using a 70° arthroscope. One must have an unobstructed view of the punch, tap, and anchor insertion into the bone bed. As previously stated, anchors should be placed at an angle of 45° or less in keeping with the "deadman" concept.[22]

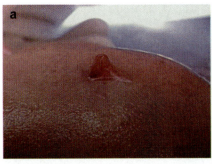
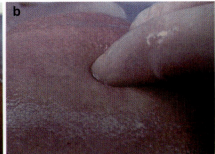

Fig. 13.8 Turbulence control. (**a**) Egress of fluid from noncannulated portals creates a negative pressure gradient which draws blood into the subacromial space from bleeding vessels. (**b**) Digital pressure is applied to stop the flow of fluid eliminating the negative pressure gradient

Although the majority of new anchors systems (e.g., 5.5-mm BioCorkscrew FT, Arthrex, Inc., Naples, FL) will obtain sufficient fixation even in osteoporotic bone, on occasion anchor fixation will be inadequate. One option is to place a larger anchor (e.g., 6.5-mm BioCorkscrew, Naples, FL). This is easiest when poor bone quality has been recognized during punching and tapping. However, if an anchor has already been placed, rather than pulling the anchor forcibly out of the bone (which usually leads to further bone damage) it is better to employ the "buddy system." This involves pushing the initial anchor back to just below the bone surface and placing a second anchor next to it creating a press-fit compressive wedge between the two anchors and bone (Fig. 13.9). In this situation, a bone punch is used to create a small pilot only adjacent to the first anchor. As the second anchor is being inserted, in order to prevent the first anchor from migrating into the bone, light traction is applied to the sutures of the first anchor, ensuring the anchors are placed adjacent to each other creating an interference fit.

I Just Unloaded An Anchor!

Unloading an anchor usually occurs when retrieving sutures limbs for suture passage or knot tying. The simplest method of avoiding this complication is to consistently visualize the anchor eyelet as the suture is being pulled. As long as the suture is not pulling through the eyelet, the anchor will not unload. If the "wrong limb" of the suture loop is being pulled (which would lead to unloading of the anchor), then the suture

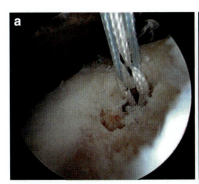
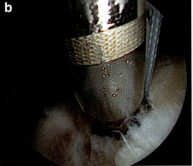
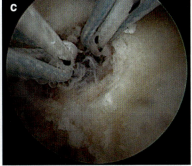

Fig. 13.9 Arthroscopic view through a posterior subacromial portal of a left shoulder demonstrating the method of interference fixation of an anchor against an anchor in poor bone. (**a**) A 5.0-mm BioCorkscrew (Arthrex, Inc., Naples, FL) suture anchor has been inserted into poor bone and, when tested, pulls out beyond the bone bed. (**b**) A second 5.0-mm BioCorkscrew suture anchor is inserted adjacent to the original 5.0-mm BioCorksrew suture anchor securing both anchors together and to the bone bed via an interference fit. Light traction is applied to the sutures of the first anchor during insertion of the second anchor. (**c**) The double anchor configuration provides four pairs of sutures for fixation

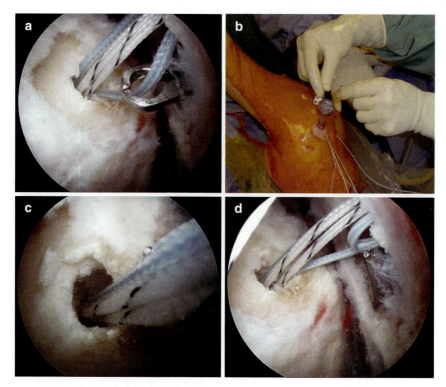

Fig. 13.10 Retrieving suture limbs - avoiding unloading anchors. (**a**) A lateral portal has been established and one limb of the suture is retrieved and pulled out the lateral cannula. Arthroscopic view of a right shoulder through a posterior subacromial portal. (**b**) After the suture has been retrieved, an assistant grasps each side of the suture loop with separate hands. (**c**) Arthroscopic view through a posterior subacromial portal using a 70° arthroscope. As the assistant alternatively pulls each side of the loop, the arthroscopist views the suture eyelet. Pulling on the incorrect side of the loop will cause the suture to run through the eyelet, potentially unloading the anchor. (**d**) Pulling on the correct side of the loop will not move the suture through the eyelet but will pull the correct limb into the cannula

will be seen to "run" through the eyelet leading to unloading of the anchor (Fig. 13.10).

If one limb of a double-loaded suture anchor has been unloaded, then it may be possible to reload a second suture through the anchor eyelet even if the anchor has been deployed. This is particularly relevant when using anchors which have a suture loop eyelet (i.e., 5.0-mm BioCorkscrew, Arthrex, Inc., Naples, FL). Reloading double loaded anchors can be performed using the suture weave technique, which utilizes the remaining suture as a suture shuttle (Fig. 13.11). In this situation, retrieve the remaining suture out of the cannula so that most of the suture is extracorporeal. A suture needle is then used to penetrate the remaining suture and passing a second (different colored) suture through it. The original suture is then used to shuttle the suture through the eyelet and the second suture is then disengaged from the original suture.

I've got a suture "jungle"!

When a suture "jungle" does occur, it can be very difficult determining which suture limbs match each other for knot tying. This scenario is generally rare when using the "mirror" method which organizes but spreads out sutures for easier retrieval. The easiest method to match sutures is first to retrieve one limb (usually the anchor limb is easiest) without unloading the anchor (see the section "I Just Unloaded An Anchor!"). To find the matching limb, the retrieved suture is then pulled, allowing a small amount of the suture to run through the anchor eyelet. However, this will also pull on the matching limb and then the suture limb that has moved can be identified and retrieved.

When retrieving sutures, commonly many of the suture limbs will be overlapped and twisted upon

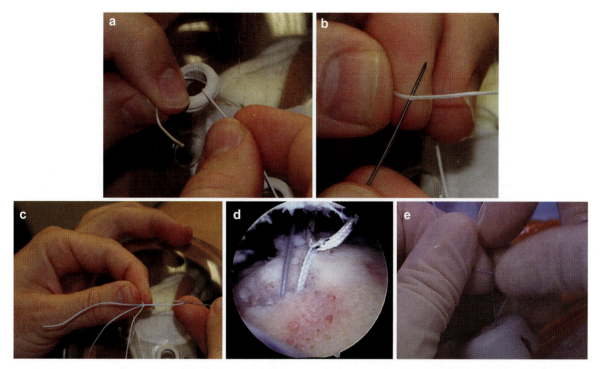

Fig. 13.11 Suture weave technique: The method of reloading an anchor using the remaining (loaded) suture as a suture shuttle. (**a**) The remaining suture is retrieved out the cannula so that most of the suture is extracorporeal. (**b**) A suture needle is used to penetrate the remaining suture and pass a second differently colored suture through it (**c**). (**d**) Arthroscopic view through a posterior portal of a left shoulder. The original suture is pulled and thereby shuttles the second suture through the anchor eyelet and out a second portal. (**e**) The second suture is then disengaged from the original suture

one another. However, one can retrieve the sutures and untangle the limbs all in a single, simple step. The key is to retrieve the suture limbs as close to its exit from the rotator cuff or anchor eyelet as possible (Fig. 13.12). Furthermore by retrieving both matching suture limbs simultaneously, it creates an unobstructed pathway for subsequent knot tying. If a suture knot is inadvertently created, then one may have to use a suture retriever to untangle the knot. Care must be taken during this procedure, however, not to damage the suture.

I've Lost My Suture!

Occasionally when swelling becomes extreme in the subacromial space, the bursa and fibrofatty tissue can obstruct visualization of some of the suture limbs. This most commonly occurs with suture limbs exiting the posterior portal or modified Neviaser portal. Despite

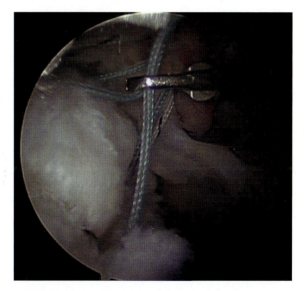

Fig. 13.12 Arthroscopic view through a posterior subacromial portal of a right shoulder. Clearing a path for knot tying. When retrieving sutures for knot tying, each suture limb should be retrieved simultaneously as close to the tendon (soft tissue limb) and anchors (free limb) as possible without crossing over any sutures. This creates an unobstructed path for knot tying

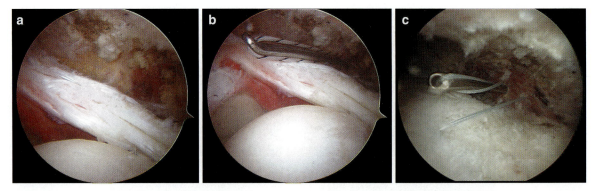

Fig. 13.13 Arthroscopic view through a lateral subacromial portal of a right shoulder looking toward the posterior leaf of the rotator cuff (**a**). The suture limb cannot be identified in the fat overlying the posterior leaf of the rotator cuff because during retrograde suture passage, the suture passer did not exit the fat before entering the tendon. (**b**) A single-diameter knot pusher is used to push the suture limb into the field of view and the matching suture can now be retrieved (**c**) Arthroscopic view through a lateral subacromial portal of a right shoulder, looking toward the posterior cuff. It is important to recreate the same angle of approach and the same soft tissue tunnel; otherwise a soft tissue bridge of deltoid muscle will be created as seen in this arthroscopic photo. The soft tissue bridge will bind the deltoid muscle to the rotator cuff.

careful debridement of overlying fatty tissue, the suture limb may be difficult to identify. In this case, one can use a single diameter (or standard) knot pusher and thread the "lost" limb extracorporeally through the knot pusher (Fig. 13.13). The knot pusher (and suture limb) is then pushed back into the subacromial space until the suture limb is identified and retrieved. When performing this technique, it is important to reproduce the same angle of approach and to use the same established soft tissue tunnel, otherwise a bridge of tissue will become trapped within the suture loop. This will bind the deltoid against the rotator cuff. This is important to recognize and one should either attempt to reproduce the correct soft tissue tunnel again, debride the intervening soft tissue, or if the suture limb can be seen exiting the rotator cuff now, it can be retrieved adjacent to the cuff and will "untangle" itself from the tissue bridge and knot pusher (see the section "I've got a suture 'jungle'!").

The Sutures Are Pulling Through the Cuff

Poor quality rotator cuff tissue is in fact relatively rare. The majority of patients with poor quality tissue can be identified preoperatively. This includes patients with massive tears of the rotator cuff with chronic changes including extreme fatty infiltration and muscular atrophy. Many will also have proximal migration of the humerus, narrowing of the acromial humeral interval and secondary acromial or humeral changes. Although the surgeon may chose to operate on the described patient, one should generally never be "surprised" by poor quality tissue.

Usually, in the absence of the above, the most common reason for poor quality rotator cuff tendon tissue is misidentifying the margins of the rotator cuff. It is not uncommon to initially confuse a thickened, hypertrophied bursa as the margin of the rotator cuff. This is particularly relevant in the posterior margin of a massive rotator cuff tear (Fig. 13.14). It is important to recognize, however, that bursal leaders insert laterally into the deltoid muscle fascia, while rotator cuff tissue inserts into the bone. Rotating the arm can also help to determine whether the tissue is rotator cuff tissue or fibrofatty bursal leader. Debridement of the bursa to true intact rotator cuff tissue will usually lead to thicker more robust tissue.

The second most common reason for suture pull through rotator cuff is tension overload. Tension overload usually occurs due to misinterpretation of the direction of mobility (and therefore classification) of the rotator cuff tendon tear, or less commonly as a result of inadequate releases. It is important to reassess the mobility of the margins of the rotator cuff from medial-to-lateral and from anterior-to-posterior. Attempting to repair a U-shaped tear in a crescent

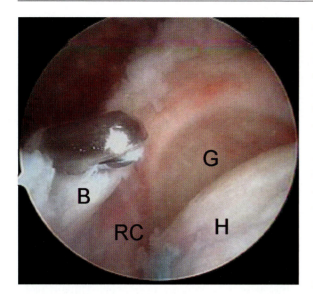

Fig. 13.14 Arthroscopic photo from a lateral subacromial portal of a right shoulder demonstrating the posterior bursal leader (B), which when thickened can obscure and be confused with the true margin of the rotator cuff (RC). *H* Humeral head and *G* Glenoid

preventing dog-ears. When performing techniques such as the suture-bridge technique with crossing-limbs, it is important to preserve all the medial sutures (after tying) so that all medial suture limbs are available for crossing sutures not only to compress the rotator cuff against the footprint but also to eliminate dog-ears.

If a dog-ear does occur (and all suture limbs are tied or used) and if the dog-ear is small, then they may be left alone. Larger dog-ears may be lightly debrided or can be eliminated by passing a stitch through the dog-ear and pulling it down to a lateral anchor (e.g., Pushlok anchor, Arthrex, Inc., Naples, FL).

My Knots Are Loose!

Assuming you are very facile with knot tying normally both in the lab and in the operating room, this should generally be a very rare experience. If fact, most knot tying complications can be avoided if there is a clear view and path for knot tying. Occasionally, however, swelling may be so severe and the subacromial space so tight that visualization can be difficult. In this case, tying the knot within a clear cannula can expand the working space and allow adequate visualization (Fig. 13.15). It can, however, be sometimes difficult to tie a

fashion or vice versa, even if you are able to reduce it to the bone bed will undoubtedly lead to structural failure postoperatively. As a corollary then, suture anchor placement and suture passage through the cuff must therefore reflect this inherent tear mobility. Suture passage should obtain deep and wide "bites" of the rotator cuff using which ever technique is optimal (i.e., antegrade, retrograde, suture shuttle). Occasionally, however, the cuff tissue may be of extremely poor quality and a simple stitch configuration may be inadequate. In this scenario, a modified construct may be used, for example the MAC stitch,[23] which serves to dissipate suture-tendon tension through a transverse suture limb. In some cases, releases (e.g., intra-articular, anterior interval, posterior interval) may improve tendon mobility allowing a lower tension repair.

I've Got a Dog-Ear!

With careful planning and assessment of tear mobility with a tendon grasper, so-called "dog-ears" or out-foldings of rotator cuff can be avoided. Suture placement and adequate suture "spread" is important to

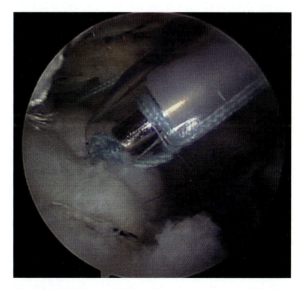

Fig. 13.15 Arthroscopic view through a posterior subacromial portal demonstrating knot tying completely within a clear 7.0-mm cannula that has been placed through a lateral portal

knot with good loop security (e.g., a tight suture loop) if the tissue is under tension. A Surgeons Sixth Finger Double Diameter Knot Pusher (Arthrex, Inc., Naples, FL) is our preferred choice for tying knots during rotator cuff repair, since it has the ability to tie knots with superior knot security and loop security even when tissues are under tension.[32] However, tension during tying can be reduced when tying any knot by helping to reduce the rotator cuff margin to the bone bed by using traction sutures (or tendon grasper), or by reducing the bone to the rotator cuff by manipulation of the arm.

Postoperative Complications

Adverse outcomes occur ubiquitously throughout all surgical specialties, and the field of arthroscopic rotator cuff repair is not unique in this respect. The complication rate depends entirely on what is defined as a complication (e.g., what range of motion is acceptable at 3 months postoperatively). In general, the literature reports complication rates from shoulder arthroscopic procedures varying from 4.8 to 10.6%.[2,3,8,24–29] Brislin et al.[2] performed a retrospective study examining the complication rate specifically after arthroscopic rotator cuff repair, and found a complication rate of 10.6%.

A wide range of failures or complications have the potential to develop during the postoperative period. The three postoperative complications that will be discussed in this chapter are stiffness, infection, and failure of repair.

Stiffness

Stiffness or postoperative adhesive capsulitis is an uncommon complication after arthroscopic rotator cuff repair. Most patients with rotator cuff tears have some degree of loss of passive range of motion, especially internal rotation in adduction consistent with a posterior capsular contracture. Apart from the trauma of the surgical insult, the reattachment of a potentially shortened rotator cuff serves to provide a further restraint to passive motion. Finally, some form of restriction on postoperative motion at least in the first 6 weeks is necessary to protect the repair. All these factors contribute to the development of postoperative stiffness.

The rates of postoperative stiffness will vary depending at what stage postoperatively the patient is assessed and what range of motion is considered unacceptable Brislin et al.[2] defined postoperative stiffness when one or more of the following persisted for 90 days postoperatively: total passive external rotation with the arm at the side of less than 10°, total passive external rotation with the arm in 90° abduction of less than 30°, or total passive forward flexion of less than 100°. Using these criteria, postoperative stiffness was diagnosed in 23 out of 263 (8.7%) patients, and was easily the most common complication. Twenty-one out of these 23 patients were treated successfully with physiotherapy, with 14 patients having resolved their stiffness by 5 months postoperatively. Three patients underwent a subacromial steroid injection, and two patients were recommended to have an arthroscopic capsular release.

Thus, most patients will respond to a modification of the physiotherapy program. A thorough program of physiotherapy is therefore essential, and the use of subacromial steroid injections may be beneficial in selected cases. When a patient has not responded to the above measures, then consideration may be given to arthroscopic capsular release. In addition to addressing the thickened contracted capsule and rotator interval, attention should also be given to releasing adhesions within the subacromial space, or the so-called "captured shoulder."[30]

Infection

Infection after arthroscopic rotator cuff repair is uncommon. In a review of the literature in 1997, McFarland et al.[8] reported an infection rate of 0.04–0.23% after open and mini-open rotator cuff repair. Most reports of infection after rotator cuff repair involve series using open or mini-open repair techniques, possibly reflecting the relative shorter history of arthroscopic rotator cuff repair. With the minimally invasive nature of arthroscopic rotator cuff repair, and with the technique involving continual irrigation of the joint with normal saline, it may be assumed that infection rates would be even lower when compared to other repair techniques. In 2007, Brislin et al.[2] reported one deep infection in their retrospective review of 263 arthroscopic rotator cuff repairs.

Pain, erythema, increased temperature, swelling, and ongoing discharge from skin portals are all possible clinical presentations of infection after shoulder arthroscopy. Kwon et al.[31] had an average interval of 3 weeks between the rotator cuff repair and diagnosis of infection. *Proprionibacterium acnes*, *Staphylococcus aureus*, and coagulase-negative *Staphylococcus* are among the more common organisms. In addition to a high index of suspicion, laboratory investigations can aid in the diagnosis. A raised C-Reactive protein (CRP), erythrocyte sedimentation rate (ESR), and leukocyte count can all raise suspicion of a diagnosis of infection. However, it is important to note that they can be normal in the presence of infection, which may be related to the nature of the infecting organism. Athwal et al.[32] reported a raised CRP in only 50% of cases, and ESR in 60%.

Proprionibacterium is one of the more common organisms causing infection after rotator cuff repair. Herrera et al.[33] reported *P. acnes* as the causative organism in six out of seven (86%) infections after rotator cuff repair. *Propionibacterium* is a slow-growing fastidious organism that requires prolonged culture of at least 7-10 days to isolate it.[32] Knowledge of this culture characteristic is critical to forewarn microbiology departments of the need for an extended culture period and to maintain alertness. *Propionibacterium* is the most common anaerobic bacteria isolated from skin flora, particularly the axilla.

Herrera et al.[33] reported on 360 shoulder arthroscopies and mini-open rotator cuff repairs, seven of whom (1.9%) developed postoperative infections. They noted that these infections were noted only to occur in arthroscopically assisted rotator cuff repairs, and recommended that a second skin preparation and draping be instituted as routine. In their subsequent 200 mini-open repairs, no cases of infection were reported. Re-prepping the skin, and application of an adhesive antimicrobial drape (Ioban: 3M, St. Paul, MN) should be given serious consideration when converting a rotator cuff repair from an arthroscopic to a mini-open or open procedure.

Early diagnosis and aggressive treatment is the key to optimizing outcomes in patients with infections after arthroscopic rotator cuff repair. After appropriate deep culture specimens are obtained and sent for prolonged culture, aggressive lavage, and debridement, in addition to appropriate antimicrobial therapy (in consultation with Infectious Diseases) are the first steps in management. Most patients require more than one operative debridement. Setteceri et al.[34] reported that an average of 3.5 procedures was required to eradicate infection after rotator cuff repair in their series. At debridement, the question as to whether to "take down" the repair and remove all foreign bodies can be only answered by the treating surgeon. Most reports in the literature do report that patients are usually left with residual rotator cuff defects after treatment.[33,34] Rotator cuff repair in this scenario falls into the realm of revision rotator cuff repair, and will be discussed later in the chapter.

Failure of the Rotator Cuff Repair

Any repair has the potential to fail. The surgeon can minimize the chance of failure by careful selection of patients, optimizing the repair construct at the time of operation, appropriately treating any coexisting pathology, and prescribing a postoperative physiotherapy program that minimizes tension on the repair construct but maximizes gliding at the movement interface.

Patient factors that are associated with failed rotator cuff repair are age,[35,36] gender,[35,37] smoking,[38] larger tear size,[39,40] compensation status,[41,42] poor tendon quality,[40] and lower patient expectations.[43] Most of these factors are beyond the control of the surgeon, however, knowledge of the associations with poorer outcomes after rotator cuff repair aids in decision making and patient counseling.

Treating coexistent pathology is important in optimizing outcomes after rotator cuff repair. In particular, the long head of biceps can commonly be associated with rotator cuff tears, and must be addressed appropriately. In addition, lesions of the superior labrum are not uncommon in the patient with a rotator cuff repair, and should also be treated appropriately. In a recent study by Franceschi et al.,[44] in patients over the age of 50 years undergoing arthroscopic rotator cuff repair with concomitant type II SLAP lesions, improved clinical outcomes were observed when tenotomy was performed compared with SLAP repair. Finally, the acromioclavicular joint and subacromial space must also be assessed and treated accordingly.

Failure of the rotator cuff repair construct is not uncommon and has a number of potential mechanisms of failure. First, the suture anchor may loosen in its bony bed,[45,46] particularly in osteoporotic bone. Second, the suture may fail at the eyelet of the anchor.[47,48] Third, the repair may failure at the knot, with loosening and potentially gap formation.[18,49,50] However, with current suture anchor design and arthroscopic knot tying techniques, the "weakest link" in the repair construct remains the suture tendon interface.[51] In a study of revisions of open suture anchor rotator cuff repairs in 2003, Cummins et al.[52] reported on 22 revision rotator cuff tears, and found that the predominant mode of failure was tendon pulling through sutures (19 out of 22 cases).

The patient who has ongoing symptoms after rotator cuff repair despite optimization of further nonoperative modalities warrants further investigation and treatment. Our preference is to perform magnetic resonance arthrography, which provides the greatest detail as to the integrity of the repair, existence of full thickness rotator cuff lesions, and details relevant to surrounding anatomic structures. It must be noted that rotator cuff defects detected by MR after rotator cuff surgery can be present in asymptomatic patients. Spielmann et al.[6] in a study on 15 asymptomatic patients postrotator cuff repair found that six had full thickness rotator cuff defects. Also, MRA performed after rotator cuff repair is technically more difficult to read correctly than in a shoulder that has not undergone any surgery due to the presence of postsurgical changes,[53] including suture anchors and suture indentation of tendon. For these reasons, careful correlation of the clinical and imaging findings is crucial in the decision-making process.

Revision Rotator Cuff Repair

The techniques and principles involved in arthroscopic revision rotator cuff repair are similar to those discussed for primary arthroscopic repair. In a revision situation, however, the surgeon is faced with a number of challenging situations not frequently encountered during primary repair. First, massive scarring and adhesions may be present, particularly following open or mini-open rotator cuff repair which can obscure the anatomy at hand. Second, suture anchors may be present within the greater tuberosity, making further suture anchor insertion more challenging. Third, large cavities or cysts may exist where previous suture anchors had been inserted and have either been removed or reabsorbed. Each of these scenarios can be seen in isolation or in combination with each other, however, with a careful well-executed plan, arthroscopic revision rotator cuff repair can lead to excellent results.

Excavating the Adhesed Rotator Cuff

Following mini-open or open rotator cuff repair, massive scarring of the rotator cuff is common with obliteration of the margins. In this scenario, the true margin of the rotator cuff is commonly scarred to the undersurface of the acromion and the inner deltoid fascia. In many cases, it can first appear as if there is no rotator cuff to repair. In this scenario, the margins of the rotator cuff tear are identified easiest first medially at the apex of the tear where there is a consistent fibrofatty layer which separates the rotator cuff below from the acromion above.

To locate this layer, while viewing through a lateral subacromial portal, an electrocautery ablation or shaver device is introduced from a posterior portal. However, the instrument is not introduced into the glenohumeral joint. Instead, the posterior instrument (e.g., electrocautery, shaver) is directed beneath the medial acromion and posterior to the AC joint in the fibrofatty layer between rotator cuff (below) and acromion (above). This maneuver is performed "blind" since you cannot actually visualize where the instrument is located (although many times you can observe a soft tissue bulge). It is easiest to perform this maneuver by palpating the posterior border of the acromion with the instrument and sliding just underneath it. The rotator cuff (along with a bursal leader) is then peeled off the acromion and inner deltoid fascia working laterally, anteriorly, and posteriorly (Figs. 13.16 and 13.17). After the rotator cuff and bursal leader have been released from the overlying acromion and inner deltoid fascia, the bursal leader is debrided as described in the section "The Sutures Are Pulling Through The Cuff".

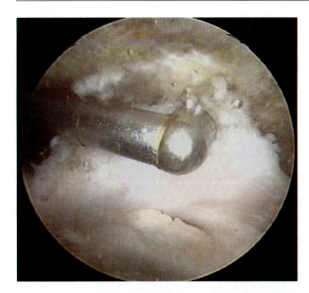

Fig. 13.16 Arthroscopic view through a lateral portal of a right shoulder during rotator cuff mobilization in a revision rotator cuff repair. The rotator cuff is initially dissected beneath the medial acromion and the fibrofatty layer is identified above the rotator cuff. This fibrofatty layer identifies the plane between the rotator cuff and acromion

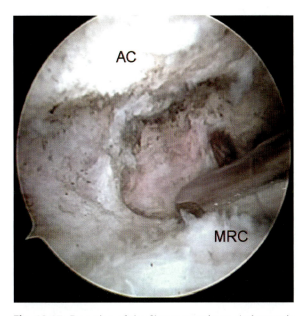

Fig. 13.17 Resection of the fibrous scar tissue. Arthroscopic views from a posterior portal of a right shoulder. The medial rotator cuff is bound by overlying fibrous scar tissue. The scar tissue is resected using a shaver until the typical yellowish fat is demonstrated overlying the muscular fibers of the rotator cuff. *MRC* Medial rotator cuff and *AC* Acromion

Dealing with Residual Metal Anchors

In a revision situation, metal anchors may be present in the greater tuberosity. In this scenario, the easiest option is to ignore the anchor and work around it. However, sometimes this is not possible particularly if the anchor location is specifically required of if the anchor is seated above the bone surface of the greater tuberosity. A thorough preoperative assessment can be critical (including a prior operative report) since some anchors may have specific inserters/extractors which if available may make the process of extraction efficacious. If not available or if the anchor is broken making use of an inserter or extractor impossible, the anchor can be removed using the OATS harvesting tube (Osteochondral Autogenous Transfer System, Arthrex, Naples, FL). This technique removes a cylindrical core of bone which includes the anchor (Fig. 13.18).

In this situation, a spinal needle is first used to create a portal in line with the anchor. For most anchors, a 6-mm tube is sufficient to remove the anchor and is impacted over the anchor to a depth of 12-15 mm. The OATS harvester is then turned counterclockwise to remove the anchor and the surrounding core of bone. If the anchor can be removed from the harvested cylinder of bone so that an intact cylinder of bone remains then this extracted bone can be reinserted as its own graft. Otherwise, the defect created is then grafted as described below.

Dealing with Large Bone Cysts or Defects on the Tuberosity: Compaction Bone Grafting

When a large cyst or bone defect is present, it may be filled with autograft or allograft bone and compacted, and an anchor even inserted if desired. Following complete debridement and removal of the cyst, an appropriate sized OATS harvesting tube (usually 6 mm) is packed with bone chips. We generally use allograft cancellous bone chips and pack them into a 6-mm OATS harvesting tube (Fig. 13.19). The OATS harvesting tube is then placed at the mouth of the cyst, and the bone chips delivered into the cyst and compacted into the defect with an impactor. This process is

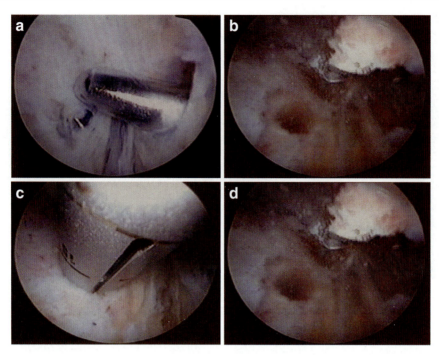

Fig. 13.18 Removing metal anchors using the OATS system. (**a**) The OATS (Arthrex, Inc., Naples, FL) harvester is advanced over the anchor, in line with the axis of the anchor. (**b**) The OATS harvester is impacted into the bone to a depth of 12 mm. (**c**) The screw-in anchor is visible at the base of the OATS harvester as it is removed. Counterclockwise removal of the harvester ensures the screw will withdraw with the bone

repeated until adequate graft density has been created in the defect. If an anchor is to be inserted into the defect, then to achieve even more impaction, the anchor should be inserted without any tapping. Usually adequate fixation may be achieved.

References

1. Mansat P, Cofield R, Kersten T et al (1997) Complications of rotator cuff repair. Orthop Clin North Am 28:205-13
2. Brislin K, Field L, Savoie FIII (2007) Complications after arthroscopic rotator cuff repair. Arthroscopy 23:124-8
3. Weber S, Abrams J, Nottage W (2002) Complications associated with arthroscopic shoulder surgery. Arthroscopy 18:88-95
4. Galatz L, Ball C, Teefey S et al (2004) The outcome and repair integrity of completely arthroscopically repaired large and massive rotator cuff tears. J Bone Joint Surg Am 86-A:219-24
5. Bishop J, Klepps S, Lo I et al (2006) Cuff integrity after arthroscopic versus open rotator cuff repair: a prospective study. J Shoulder Elbow Surg 15:290-9
6. Spielmann A, Forster B, Kokan P et al (1999) Shoulder after rotator cuff repair: MR imaging findings in asymptomatic individuals - initial experience. Radiology 213:705-8
7. Pohl A, Cullen D (2005) Cerebral ischemia during shoulder surgery in the upright position: a case series. J Clin Anesth 17:463-9
8. McFarland E, O'Neill O, Hsu C (1997) Complications of shoulder arthroscopy. J South Orthop Assoc 6:190-6
9. Nottage W (1993) Arthroscopic portals: anatomy at risk. Orthop Clin North Am 24:19-26
10. Rodeo S, Forster R, Weiland A (1993) Neurological complications due to arthroscopy. J Bone Joint Surg Am 75:917-26
11. Lo I, Burkhart S, Parten P (2004) Surgery about the coracoid: neurovascular structures at risk. Arthroscopy 20:591-5
12. Price M, Tillett E, Acland R et al (2004) Determining the relationship of the axillary nerve to the shoulder joint capsule from an arthroscopic perspective. J Bone Joint Surg Am 86-A:2135-42
13. Warner J, Krushell R, Masquelet A et al (1992) Anatomy and relationships of the suprascapular nerve: anatomical constraints to mobilization of the supraspinatus and infraspinatus muscles in the management of massive rotator-cuff tears. J Bone Joint Surg Am 74:36-45
14. Dietzel D, Ciullo J (1996) Spontaneous pneumothorax after shoulder arthroscopy: a report of four cases. Arthroscopy 12:99-102
15. Borgeat A, Bird P, Ekatodramis G et al (2000) Tracheal compression caused by periarticular fluid accumulation: a rare complication of shoulder surgery. J Shoulder Elbow Surg 9:443-5
16. Mohammed K, Hayes M, Saies A (2000) Unusual complications of shoulder arthroscopy. J Shoulder Elbow Surg 9:350-3

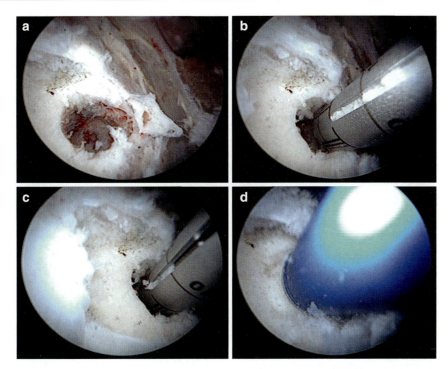

Fig. 13.19 Impaction grafting technique: Arthroscopic views through a lateral subacromial portal of a right shoulder. (**a**) The cyst has been thoroughly debrided and the fibrous capsule removed. (**b**) An OATS (Arthrex, Inc., Naples, FL) harvester tube containing allograft cancellous bone chips is then inserted subacromially into the cyst. (**c**) The cancellous bone chips are then used to fill the cavity. (**d**) A tamp is used to impact the cancellous bone chips into the cyst. Completed compaction bone grafting of a cyst

17. Burkhart S, Lo I, Brady P (2006) Burkhart's View of the Shoulder; A Cowboy's Guide to Advanced Shoulder Arthroscopy. Lippincott Williams & Wilkins, Philadelphia, PA
18. Lo I, Burkhart S, Chan K et al (2004) Arthroscopic knots: determining the optimal balance of loop security and knot security. Arthroscopy 20:489-502
19. Curtis A, Burbank K, Tierney J et al (2006) The insertional footprint of the rotator cuff: an anatomic study. Arthroscopy 22:603.e1-9.e1
20. Milano G, Grasso A, Zarelli D et al (2007) Comparison between single-row and double-row rotator cuff repair: a biomechanical study. Knee Surg Sports Traumatol Arthrosc 16:75-80
21. Kim D, Elattrache N, Tibone J et al (2006) Biomechanical comparison of a single-row versus double-row suture anchor technique for rotator cuff repair. Am J Sports Med 34:407-14
22. Burkhart S (1995) The deadman theory of suture anchors: observations along a south Texas fence line. Arthroscopy 11:119-23
23. MacGillivray J, Ma C (2004) An arthroscopic stitch for massive rotator cuff tears: the Mac stitch. Arthroscopy 20:669-71
24. Shaffer B, Tibone J (1999) Arthroscopic shoulder instability surgery. Complications. Clin Sports Med 18:737-67
25. Berjano P, Gonzalez B, Olmedo J et al (1998) Complications in arthroscopic shoulder surgery. Arthroscopy 14:785-8
26. Small N (1993) Complications in arthroscopic surgery of the knee and shoulder. Orthopedics 16:985-8
27. Brulhart K, Roggo A, Kossmann T et al (1993) Arthroscopy of the shoulder joint. Technique, indications, surgery and complications. Langenbecks Arch Chir 378:200-5
28. Bigliani L, Flatow E, Deliz E (1991) Complications of shoulder arthroscopy. Orthop Rev 20:743-51
29. Small N (1988) Complications in arthroscopic surgery performed by experienced arthroscopists. Arthroscopy 4:215-21
30. Mormino M, Gross R, McCarthy J (1996) Captured shoulder: a complication of rotator cuff surgery. Arthroscopy 12:457-61
31. Kwon Y, Kalainov D, Rose H et al (2005) Management of early deep infection after rotator cuff repair surgery. J Shoulder Elbow Surg 14:1-5
32. Athwal G, Sperling J, Rispoli D et al (2007) Deep infection after rotator cuff repair. J Shoulder Elbow Surg 16:306-11
33. Herrera M, Bauer G, Reynolds F et al (2002) Infection after mini-open rotator cuff repair. J Shoulder Elbow Surg 11:605-8
34. Settecerri J, Pitner M, Rock M et al (1999) Infection after rotator cuff repair. J Shoulder Elbow Surg 8:1-5
35. Cofield R, Parvizi J, Hoffmeyer P et al (2001) Surgical repair of chronic rotator cuff tears. A prospective long-term study. J Bone Joint Surg Am 83-A:71-7
36. Romeo A, Hang D, Bach B Jr et al (1999) Repair of full thickness rotator cuff tears. Gender, age, and other factors affecting outcome. Clin Orthop Relat Res Oct(367): 243-55
37. Gartsman G, Brinker M, Khan M (1998) Early effectiveness of arthroscopic repair for full-thickness tears of the rotator cuff: an outcome analysis. J Bone Joint Surg Am 80:33-40
38. Mallon W, Misamore G, Snead D et al (2004) The impact of preoperative smoking habits on the results of rotator cuff repair. J Shoulder Elbow Surg 13:129-32

39. Hollinshead R, Mohtadi N, Vande Guchte R et al (2000) Two 6-year follow-up studies of large and massive rotator cuff tears: comparison of outcome measures. J Shoulder Elbow Surg 9:373-81
40. Pai V, Lawson D (2001) Rotator cuff repair in a district hospital setting: outcomes and analysis of prognostic factors. J Shoulder Elbow Surg 10:236-41
41. Watson E, Sonnabend D (2002) Outcome of rotator cuff repair. J Shoulder Elbow Surg 11:201-11
42. Shinners T, Noordsij P, Orwin J (2002) Arthroscopically assisted mini-open rotator cuff repair. Arthroscopy 18:21-6
43. Henn RIII, Kang L, Tashjian R et al (2007) Patients' preoperative expectations predict the outcome of rotator cuff repair. J Bone Joint Surg Am 89:1913-9
44. Franceschi F, Longo U, Ruzzini L et al (2008) No advantages in repairing a type II superior labrum anterior and posterior (SLAP) lesion when associated with rotator cuff repair in patients over age 50: A randomized controlled trial. Am J Sports Med 36:247-53
45. Barber F, Coons D, Ruiz-Suarez M (2007) Cyclic load testing of biodegradable suture anchors containing 2 high-strength sutures. Arthroscopy 23:355-60
46. Mahar A, Allred D, Wedemeyer M et al (2006) A biomechanical and radiographic analysis of standard and intracortical suture anchors for arthroscopic rotator cuff repair. Arthroscopy 22:130-5
47. Bynum C, Lee S, Mahar A et al (2005) Failure mode of suture anchors as a function of insertion depth. Am J Sports Med 33:1030-4
48. Bardana D, Burks R, West J et al (2003) The effect of suture anchor design and orientation on suture abrasion: An in vitro study. Arthroscopy 19:274-81
49. Burkhart S, Wirth M, Simonick M et al (1998) Loop security as a determinant of tissue fixation security. Arthroscopy 14:773-6
50. Abbi G, Espinoza L, Odell T et al (2006) Evaluation of 5 knots and 2 suture materials for arthroscopic rotator cuff repair: very strong sutures can still slip. Arthroscopy 22:38-43
51. Burkhart S, Diaz Pagan J, Wirth M et al (1997) Cyclic loading of anchor-based rotator cuff repairs: confirmation of the tension overload phenomenon and comparison of suture anchor fixation with transosseous fixation. Arthroscopy 13:720-4
52. Cummins CA, Murrell GA (2003) Mode of failure for rotator cuff repair with suture anchors identified at revision surgery. J Shoulder Elbow Surg 12:128-33
53. Zanetti M, Hodler J (2006) MR imaging of the shoulder after surgery. Radiol Clin North Am 44:537-51

Editors' Comments (Rotator Cuff)

Pain pumps that have been used in the past for postoperative pain control have been questioned of late as a potential source of chondrolysis in the shoulder. There also exists the potential for the tubing of this device to be a conduit for infection. As such we do not recommend the routine use of a pain pump following rotator cuff surgery.

Tendon augmentation grafts (e.g., Graftjacket, Restore) have been utilized in the revision setting. Performing this technique arthroscopically is extremely demanding so at least on the early phase of the "learning curve" this should be performed through a mini-open approach. Controversy surrounds its efficacy and so should be used judiciously.

Controversy surrounds single row vs. double row techniques, although the literature seems to be trending toward a double row repair when possible. Consider, though, that with a fluid pump a rotator cuff repair should be performed by 2 h to prevent fluid extravasation. If one is still working at the 3-h mark, consideration should be to spend additional time in a "learning center" and/or commit to a mini-open approach. A formal subacromial decompression in the setting of a rotator cuff repair is not always necessary and so will give one additional time for the repair.

As the authors note, interval slides are rarely performed but it is critical to perform a thorough bursectomy. Capsular releases can be performed on occasion to mobilize the tendons.

To avoid capturing the long head of the biceps tendon on side-to-side margin convergence repair, all suture should be passed initially prior to tying. For partial thickness articular sided repairs (PASTA), it is helpful to perform the bursectomy in the subacromial (SA) space prior to passage of the suture anchors. A switching stick can be placed in the glenohumeral (GH) space posterosuperiorly while a second posterosuperior portal can be placed for subacromial work. This allows one to move seamlessly between the GH and SA spaces. View all full thickness repairs in the GH space following repair to ensure that all suture anchors placed along the medial space have not displaced and that the repair is matted down appropriately. In addition, one can ensure that the medially placed anchors have not migrated or dislodged superiorly.

Chapter 14
Avoiding and Managing Complications of Surgery of the Acromioclavicular Joint

Matthew T. Provencher, Lance LeClere, Anthony A. Romeo, and Augustus A. Mazzocca

Top 10 Pearls

- Essential to any successful AC joint surgery is complete and accurate diagnosis of the pathology involved. Concomitant injuries to the shoulder girdle should be ruled out prior to surgery. Coracoid fractures may be overlooked, pectoralis major tendon tears, shoulder instability and dislocations, rotator cuff tears, pulmonary contusions, and pneumothorax should be investigated on physical examination and imaging.
- An understanding of the classification system of AC joint injuries has been shown to dictate treatment, helps guide patient expectations and options, and also emphasizes the various forms of AC injuries to prevent improper recognition and hence improper treatment of an AC injury.
- Surgical treatment of the AC joint should be designed to avoid sacrificing the competence of the superior and posterior AC ligaments, as complications of resultant AC joint instability and subsequent pain have been commonly described when these ligaments are rendered incompetent. The joint capsule also provides restraint to joint translation.
- Understanding the anatomy of insertion of the coracoclavicular ligaments reduces potential for instability and thus continued pain. The mean length from the end of the clavicle, or the acromioclavicular joint, to the coracoclavicular ligaments is 46.3±5 mm; the distance between the trapezoid laterally and conoid medially is 21.4±4.2 mm.
- Abrasions, lacerations, or skin tenting frequently accompany AC joint injuries and may develop local infection. Skin tenting associated with injury may lead to local skin necrosis. Previously, AC joint injuries have been treated with a Kenny-Howard device, but due to a 20% incidence of skin compromise,[1] they are no longer recommended.
- When preparing the coracoid bone tunnel, an intraoperative coracoid fracture may result. This can be fixed with a 3.5 mm screw or anchor device that was temporarily fixed with k-wire(s).
- Inability to pass allograft or autograft under the coracoid process during anatomic coracoclavicular ligament can cause intraoperative frustration. Instrumentation such as a 90° right angle clamp, or commercially available 90° suture passers (akin to a Hewson suture passer) may be utilized to place passing sutures under the coracoid to transmit the graft.
- If too much of the distal clavicle was or is excised resulting in persistent instability despite reconstruction, ensure adequate anterior to posterior repair of the deltotrapezial fascia with #2 Ethibond suture in a "pants over vest" fashion.
- Blowing out posterior or anterior cortical rim of the clavicle when making drill holes or passing graft and/or sutures can be addressed by redrilling in another location. However, this may not reproduce biomechanically

M.T. Provencher (✉)
Division of Orthopaedic Shoulder and Sports Surgery,
Naval Medical Center San Diego, San Diego, CA
e-mail: matthew.provencher@med.navy.mil

L. LeClere
Orthopedic Surgery, Naval Medical Center San Diego,
San Diego, CAlifornia, USA

A.A. Romeo
Department of Orthopedics, Rush University Medical Center,
Chicago, ILlinois, USA

A.A. Mazzocca
Orhthopaedic Surgery, University of Connecticut Health Center,
Frarmington, CTonnecticut, USA

the desired effect of the anatomic reconstruction. Alternatively, pass the graft over the top of the clavicle and affix to the remaining intact drill hole with sutures.
- Hardware migration is one of the most serious complications of AC joint surgery. Frequency of pin migration and seriousness of potential complications have prompted most surgeons to abandon their use, especially the use of smooth pins.

Introduction and Background

Injuries to the acromioclavicular (AC) joint are common, especially in a young, active population. Of all shoulder girdle injuries, approximately 9% involve the AC joint.[2] AC joint injuries are often seen in young, active individuals, especially those participating in sports. Almost half of AC joint injuries occur in patients in their twenties, and there is a five to one male to female ratio.[2] AC joint dislocations represent 12% of all shoulder girdle dislocations, and 8% of all joint dislocations throughout the body.[3,4]

Since injuries to the AC joint are prevalent, complications from both operative and nonoperative treatments have been described. In addition, failure to correctly diagnose the AC joint injury as well as failure to address concomitant shoulder girdle injuries may diminish overall outcomes. There are well over 30 described variations in treating symptomatic AC joint dislocations, owing to the relative inability of one technique to emerge as the "gold-standard." As such, complications encountered during the surgical procedure are varied and commonplace. Not only is it important to understand some common intraoperative "bailout" strategies, but also to understand the clinical examination, anatomy at risk, and associated conditions that may preclude a successful operative outcome.

Diagnosis and Pathophysiology of AC Joint Injuries: Complications Associated with Patient Presentation and Clinical Evaluation

Mechanism of Injury and Associated Injuries

It is important to understand that the vast majority of injuries to the AC joint occur as the result of direct trauma. The direct trauma usually comes in the form of a blow to the lateral aspect of the shoulder, as in a fall, which pushes the acromion away from the distal clavicle.[5] Indirect injury can also cause injury to the AC joint. This can occur via fall on an outstretched hand or elbow, which drives the humeral head into the acromion, or traction on the arm. The force involved in the injury varies. However, it is usually significant enough that additional injuries to the glenohumeral joint and shoulder girdle can occur. Clinical evaluation of AC joint injuries relies on careful history taking and physical examination. Point tenderness, pain at the AC joint with cross-arm adduction, and relief of symptoms with injection of a local anesthetic are indicative of AC joint pathology. The cross-arm adduction test is performed by elevating the arm 90°, flexing the elbow to 90°, and adducting the arm across the chest. The test is considered positive if it produces pain at the AC joint. A careful physical examination should rule-out sternoclavicular injury and dislocation (especially posterior), physeal fracture of the proximal clavicle (especially in those less than 18 years of age), rotator cuff tear, pectoralis major tendon tear (axillary fold present?) and instability injuries. An examination, if focused immediately to the AC deformity that is usually obvious may miss commonly associated injuries.

Classification: Importance of Knowing What Injury Pattern You Have

The classification of AC joint injuries is important to understand as it helps dictate treatment options and helps to avoid complications by failure to recognize the pattern of injury. Cadenat was first to classify AC joint injuries in 1917.[6] Later, Tossy classified AC injuries into three groups.[7] This classification scheme was based on the extent of involvement of the acromioclavicular and coracoclavicular ligaments (Fig. 14.1). In 1984, Rockwood[2] expanded this classification to six types: (table below)

Type I: Force on the shoulder produces a mild strain to the acromioclavicular ligament, which remain in tact. The joint is stable and X-rays remain normal.

Type II: Increased force compared with Type I injuries – enough to rupture the ligaments of the AC joint, but the coracoclavicular ligaments remain in tact. Instability is present in the horizontal plane, but vertical stability is preserved. There may be widening of the

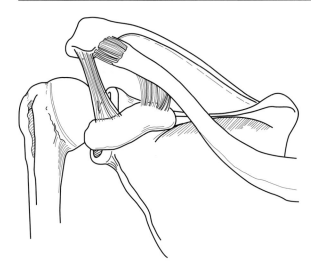

Fig. 14.1 Anatomy of the distal clavicular ligaments. The coracoclavicular (CC), acromioclavicular (AC) and distal clavicle joint capsule are shown

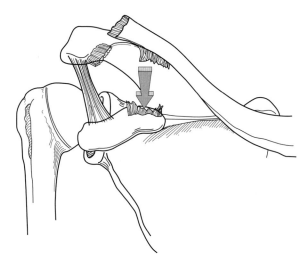

Fig. 14.2 Acromioclavicular separation, type III indicating complete tear of the coracoclavicular and joint capsule

AC joint, or slight relative elevation of the distal clavicle on X-rays.

Type III: Represents an injury involving complete disruption of the acromioclavicular ligaments and the coracoclavicular ligaments. The deltoid and trapezial fascia are not significantly disrupted. The clavicle appears high riding relative to the acromion due to the scapula and acromion drooping inferomedially. On X-ray examination, there is a 25-100% increase in the coracoclavicular space. The clavicle is unstable in the horizontal and vertical planes (Fig. 14.2).

Type IV: Posterior displacement of the distal clavicle into the trapezius. This may result in tenting of the posterior skin. Posterior displacement can be visualized on the axillary X-rays.

Type V: Regarded as a more severe Type III injury, this form results when the distal clavicle has been stripped of all its soft tissue attachments. The result is severe drooping of the scapula and acromion and upward pull of the clavicle by the sternocleidomastoid. X-rays show an increase in the coracoclavicular distance of 100-300% (Fig. 14.3).

Type VI: This injury is very rare, and is an inferior dislocation of the distal clavicle. This type of injury is seen in a severe trauma setting, and is associated with multiple injuries. The proposed mechanism is severe hyperabduction and external rotation of the arm combined with retraction of the scapula. The clavicle becomes lodged behind the intact conjoined tendon.

An understanding of this well-known classification system has been shown to dictate treatment, helps guide patient expectations and options, and also emphasizes the various forms of AC injuries to prevent improper recognition and hence improper treatment of an AC injury.

Imaging: The Importance of Adequate Studies to Confirm the Diagnosis

Radiographic evaluation of the AC joint includes anteroposterior and axillary views. Comparison views of the contralateral sides can provide helpful relative normals. If radiographs of the shoulder are obtained, there may be overpenetration of the AC joint. For this reason, specific AC joint radiographs (Zanca view) should be obtained. This requires one third to one half of the radiographic penetration. Additionally, stress views may be performed with 5 pound weights placed on the wrist of the affected side. However, these are not necessary and rarely change treatment guidelines. Most feel that stress radiographs are unnecessary,[8] and may add cost, patient discomfort, and time while having limited utility in management. If a fracture of the distal clavicle is suspected (Figs. 14.4-14.6), the AP view can be tilted cephelad 10-15° for better visualization.[5] Additional radiographs should be ordered if there is clinical suspicion of a sternoclavicular injury, with careful attention to the under 18 population that may present in this area with a physeal fracture. If there is any doubt as to whether additional injuries to the glenohumeral joint have

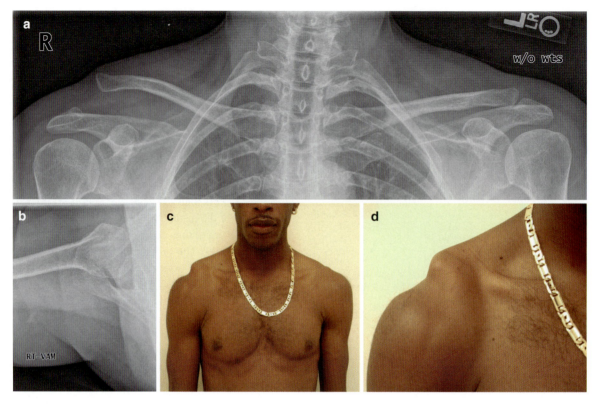

Fig. 14.3 Type V acromioclavicular separation demonstrated on bilateral AP views (**a**) lateral (**b**), and clinical photos which show the severity of the injury (**c** and **d**)

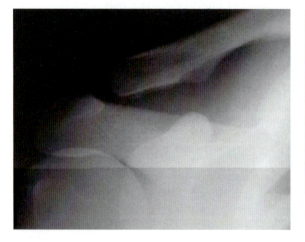

Fig. 14.4 Periosteal sleeve avulsion of the distal clavicle

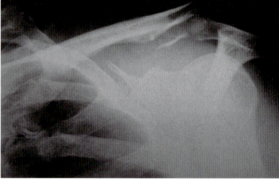

Fig. 14.5 Example of a distal clavicle fracture, left shoulder

occurred, magnetic resonance imaging is useful to help confirm clinical suspicions of additional glenohumeral injuries. It is important to realize that the imaging should be utilized to confirm clinical diagnosis and does not supplant a careful physical examination. Management complications, both operative and nonoperative are prevented with a thorough patient work-up, and exclusion of concomitant injuries.

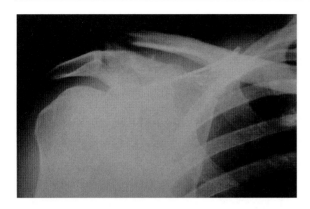

Fig. 14.6 Example of a distal clavicle fracture, right shoulder

Treatment: Avoiding Complications by Offering the Optimal Evidence-Based Treatment for an AC Injured Patient

The main goals of treatment are to achieve a pain-free shoulder with full range of motion, full strength, and full activity. It should be kept in mind that each patient places different demands on his or her shoulder. Athletes that participate in contact sports, for example, have a high risk of reinjury and may be more likely to receive nonoperative treatment.[2]

Most authors agree that Type I and II AC joint injuries should be treated nonoperatively. Treatment consists of sling immobilization for 3-7 days, ice, and rest. Likewise, most authors agree on operative treatment of Types IV, V, and VI injuries due to the extensive soft tissue disruption and significant morbidity associated with persistently dislocated joints.

It is the Type III injury that remains controversial. The current trend is toward nonoperative treatment initially, with supportive meta-analysis data.[9] In a review of over 1,100 patients, the rate of successful outcomes in operative and nonoperative treatment was 88% and 87%, respectively. On the basis of the complication rates including the need for further surgery (59% operative vs. 6% non-operative), infection (6% vs. 1%), and deformity (3% vs. 37%), the authors recommended nonoperative treatment for Type III injuries in young patients. Of note, pain and range of motion were not significantly affected in either group. Although Type III AC injuries remain controversial, Type V injuries (elevation of 100-300%) are usually surgical, and although Type IV and VI injuries are rare, it is generally recommended that surgical treatment be offered.[4,9-12]

Functional Anatomy at Risk

It is important to understand the function and important anatomical structures of the AC joint to avoid treatment complications. The AC joint is a diarthrodial joint that interfaces the lateral aspect of the clavicle and the medial acromion. It is the one true connection between the appendicular and axial skeleton. Within the joint lies a hyaline cartilage articular surface and a meniscal-like structure. The actual function of this intra-articular structure appears to be minimal. DePalma, Petersson, and Salter have shown that beyond the fourth decade, it is no longer functional due to degeneration.[13-15] The AC joint is surrounded by a joint capsule and synovium.

Static and dynamic stabilizers contribute to AC joint stability. Static stabilizers include acromioclavicular ligaments, coracoclavicular ligaments, and the coracoacromial ligament. The acromioclavicular ligaments consist of superior, inferior, anterior, and posterior ligaments. The trapezoid and the conoid comprise the coracoclavicular ligaments. The deltoid and trapezius muscles provide dynamic stability to the AC joint. When the trapezius and deltoid flex, the fascia of these muscles that are blended with the superior acromioclavicular ligament provide added stability.

One of the critical aspects of the AC joint that has been consistently demonstrated is the importance of the AC joint capsule and superior AC ligaments. The primary restraints to anterior and posterior translation of the AC joint are the joint capsule and the capsular ligaments.[16] On average, these ligaments insert 16.7 mm posterior-superior on the capsule, and 12.8 mm anterior-superior. The maximum average distance from the joint line was 16.1 mm with a maximum of 20 mm. These numbers are of significant importance when performing a distal clavicle resection. If these restraints of horizontal motion are not in tact, posterior translation of the distal end of the clavicle can occur. This results in abutment of the posterolateral clavicle on the spine of the scapula.[17] Serial sectioning of the AC joint showed that the superior ligament contributed 56% of the posterior translational resistance, with the posterior ligament contributing 25%.[17] Thus surgical treatment of the AC joint should be designed to avoid sacrificing the competence of the superior and posterior ligaments, as complications of resultant AC joint instability and subsequent pain have been commonly described.

Vertical stability comes primarily from the coracoclavicular (CC) ligament. The two structures that make up the coracoclavicular ligament, the trapezoid and conoid, prevent superior and inferior translation of the clavicle. The trapezoid and conoid reside posteriorly to the pectoralis minor's attachment on the coracoid. The trapezoid is anterior and lateral to the conoid. While the conoid's insertion on the clavicle is variable, the trapezoid inserts approximately 15 mm from the distal clavicle.[18] By attaching the clavicle to the scapula, the coracoclavicular ligaments mediate synchronous scapulohumeral motion. Additionally, they act to strengthen the acromioclavicular articulation. By reinforcing or reconstructing the anatomic relationship of the CC ligaments, complications may be avoided by restoring AC joint kinematics to as normal as possible.[19]

As stated earlier, the distance from the coracoid to the clavicle is important in determining the classification of AC joint injury present, thus factoring into treatment algorithms. If a distance greater than the average range of 1.1-1.3 cm[20] is evident on radiographs, then there is likely injury to the AC joint. Of course, comparison to the contralateral side aids in diagnosis.

Reportedly, the primary stabilizer of superior translation changes with the amount of displacement. With small displacements, the acromioclavicular ligaments are 68% of the restraints to superior translation (as well as 89% of posterior translation).[21] With large displacements, the acromioclavicular ligaments remain the primary restraint for posterior translation, but the primary stabilizer for superior translation becomes the conoid ligament (68%).[21] The primary restraint to compression of the AC joint is the trapezoid ligament with both small and large displacements.[21]

When armed with this knowledge, surgeons can avoid potential complications in AC joint surgery. Concerns over stability may arise after distal clavicle resection. Corteen[22] investigated stability after resection of 1 cm of the distal clavicle. A 32% increase in posterior translation was seen with pure resection. Although capsular repair did not provide additional stability, capsular repair and coracoacromial ligament augmentation did result in decreased posterior translation.[22] Since instability after distal clavicle resection is believed to be a source of residual pain, protecting the soft tissue attachments should be a taken into account.

With forward elevation and abduction to 180°, there is approximately 5-8° of motion detected at the AC joint.[2] During full overhead elevation, the clavicle rotates between 40 and 50°, but this motion occurs via scapular rotation, rather than through the AC joint. This synchronous scapular-clavicular rotation during abduction and forward elevation was originally described by Codman, and is coordinated by the coraclavicular ligaments.[23] This is why even after AC joint fusion and coracoclavicular screw implantation, full forward elevation in abduction is still possible. However, this motion may also cause screws and hardware to migrate and break over time. The AC joint is not a fixed structure, and complications may occur with screw breakage, hardware migration, and loss of fixation, if this relationship is not appreciated.

Nonoperative Treatment

Although the focus of this chapter is to discuss complications associated with operative treatment of the acromioclavicular joint, it is important to realize that nonoperative treatment is not without complications as well.

Skin and wound complications can develop in patients treated nonoperatively. Abrasions or lacerations frequently accompany AC joint injuries and may develop local infection. Skin tenting associated with injury may lead to local skin necrosis. Previously, AC joint injuries have been treated with a Kenny-Howard device, but due to a 20% incidence of skin compromise,[1] they are no longer recommended.

Although the long-term sequelae of nonoperative treatment of AC joint injuries remains controversial, many authors have shown that rates of posttraumatic arthritis can be significant.[24-26] Cox reported a 36% rate of symptomatic arthritis after Grade I injuries, and a 48% rate after Grade II injuries.[26]

Distal clavicular osteolysis primarily presents as pain with abduction and flexion. While the etiology of distal clavicular osteolysis after AC joint injuries has been fully identified, it is not an uncommon outcome of AC joint injury.

Neurovascular complications can result from chronic instability after AC joint injuries treated nonoperatively. There are reports of symptoms consistent with brachial plexopathy after AC joint injury,[12,27] even up to 8 years after injury.[28]

Preoperative

Concominant injuries can be present and easily missed. Coracoid fractures may be overlooked,[12,29] and there are reports of pulmonary contusions and pneumothorax associated with AC joint injuries.[30] Skin injuries and abrasion may present a difficult scenario in operative treatment due to the need to alter incision sites. Allowing overlying abrasions and lacerations to heal prior to surgery can decrease the risk of subsequent skin breakdown and wound complications. However, skin tenting which is often seen with Type V injuries may need to be addressed early to limit skin necrosis and soft tissue compromise.[31]

Complications Associated with Commonly Utilized AC Joint Procedures

Coracoclavicular Ligament Repair: Described Technique and Complications

In 1941, Bosworth described a screw suspension procedure in which he percutaneously repaired the coracoclavicular ligament.[32] A subsequent report showed a 32% technical failure rate, however,[33] Several other methods of coracoclavicular ligament repair have been described, including screw fixation with acromioclavicular debridement and trapeziodeltoid repair,[34-36] wire or other materials looped around the clavicle and coracoid,[20,37-42] or reconstruction with the fascia lata.[43,44]

Several authors have recently reported results of coracoclavicular repair with use of polydioxanone (PDS) suture or cerclage.[45-51] Ghoring[46] compared AC joint dislocation treatments with PDS repair to tension band treatment and Wolter hook plate treatment and found early postoperative complications in 43% of patients treated with a tension band, 58% treated with a hook plate, and 17% treated with a PDS cord. Additionally, at an average of 35 months of follow-up, instability was seen in 32% with a tension band, 50% with plate fixation, and 24% with PDS cord treatment.[46] These results led the authors to recommend limiting surgery to young, athletic patients. Multiple surgeries have been described for AC injuries, and none has clearly emerged as the "gold-standard." Additional procedures will be described in historical context to the Bosworth technique.

Coracoacromial Ligament Transfer

Nevaiser[52] was the first to describe coracoacromial ligament transfer in 1968. While his initial description did not include coracoclavicular ligament repair, several authors have emphasized the importance of additional repair or reinforcement of the AC joint, noting that the coracoacromial ligament is usually too weak and too short for the treatment of AC dislocation.[53] Some advocate screw fixation in addition to coracoacromial ligament transfer.[54,55]

Distal Clavicle Resection and Coracoclavicular Ligament Reconstruction

There is controversy regarding distal clavicle excision in the setting of AC joint injuries. Although most agree that a high grade chronic AC injury (Type V) will not have the ability to develop AC arthrosis, some amount of distal clavicle resection is usually performed in conjunction with the stabilization procedure. The reason for this is to prevent the potential pain generator and complication that can arise from a reduction of a previously arthritic AC joint. Distal clavicle resection is usually performed for treatment of degenerative or osteolytic AC joint arthrosis, but may also be used as a salvage procedure for persistent pain after AC dislocation. In general, a high success rate can be expected. However, if fractures or instability are present, successful outcome may not be as likely. In Mumford's[56] original description of distal clavicle resection for persistent subluxation and degenerative changes, he emphasized the need for coracoclavicular ligament reconstruction when the distal clavicle was tender. It is generally accepted that distal clavicle resection should be accompanied by coracoclavicular ligament reconstruction with or without augmentation when the distal clavicle is unstable.

Modified Weaver Dunn with Augmentation

Weaver and Dunn[57] published their description of distal clavicle resection and coracoclavicular ligament reconstruction in 1972. They used the coracoacromial ligament for reconstruction. In this procedure, 7-8 mm is removed from the distal clavicle and 2-3 mm is removed from the medial edge of the acromion. A number 2 permanent suture is used to secure the coracoacromial ligament to the distal clavicle via drill holes. A gracilis or semitendinosis autograft is used in a figure of eight fashion to augment the reconstruction.

Distal Clavicle Resection Without Ligament Reconstruction

Blazar[58] has shown that visual analog pain scores correlate with the amount of translation of the distal clavicle resection. Although translation did not correlate with amount of apparent joint space after surgery, Klimkiewicz[17] has shown that sacrificing the superior and posterior capsular ligaments has significant effects on translation. This increased posterior translation can result in continued pain. Thus, it is important to perform distal clavicle resections that spare the posterior and superior capsular ligaments, especially when ligament reconstruction will not be performed. Complications arise from distal clavicular instability, especially when the distal clavicle is excised. Care should be taken to preserve as much of the capsule as possible. However, when performing open surgery (i.e., an AC reconstruction), the capsule should be preserved and repaired with nonabsorbable suture (#2 Ethibond, Ethicon, Somerville, NJ) after it has been subperiosteally dissected off the clavicle in a longitudinal fashion. The anterior and posterior limbs of the capsule are then imbricated after the AC procedure to provide a stable capsular repair.

Anatomical Coracocalvicular Ligament Reconstruction (ACCR) Technique and Complications

It has been shown that reconstruction of the clavicle with appropriate anatomical positioning of drill holes representing the conoid and trapezoid ligaments results in a stronger construct, especially in anterior[19,59] and posterior translation. Baker[59] demonstrated that as the drill hole in the clavicle moved more forward (anterior-superior to anterior-inferior drilling vector), the overall stability was improved, especially in the anterior direction. In essence, this approach to reconstruction of the AC joint was predicated on decreasing the postoperative complication of residual instability and loss of reduction. The technique, rationale, and surgical "bailouts" are described below.

Mazzocca et al.[19] investigated the effect of anatomical coracoclavicular ligament reconstruction (ACCR) in a cadaveric model by comparing it to a traditional Weaver-Dunn procedure or an arthroscopic reconstruction. They demonstrated that the Weaver-Dunn procedure had significantly greater laxity than an anatomical coracoclavicular reconstruction or arthroscopic reconstruction. Additionally, they showed that anterior and posterior translation were markedly improved with the anatomic techniques, even though superior displacement was not significantly different among the groups. The clinical and biomechanical success of using semitendinosis autografts or allografts allowed them to modify existing techniques in the literature and reconstruct the trapezoid and conoid ligaments in an "anatomic" position.

On the basis of past biomechanical studies, in addition to anatomical and clinical observations, an operative procedure was devised that would recreate both the conoid and trapezoid coracoclavicular ligaments individually as well as augment of any remaining superior and posterior acromioclavicular ligaments.

Approach (Fig. 14.7): In an osteological analysis of 118 clavicles, the mean length from the end of the clavicle, or the acromioclavicular joint, to the coracoclavicular ligaments was 46.3±5 mm; the distance between the trapezoid laterally and conoid medially was 21.4±4.2 mm. Thus, we center our incision roughly 3.5 cm from the acromioclavicular joint and make it curvilinear along Langer's lines toward the coracoid process. Control of the superficial skin bleeders down to the fascia of the deltoid is accomplished with a needle-tip bovie. Once the entire clavicle is palpated, full-thickness flaps are made from the midline of the clavicle both posteriorly and anteriorly, skeletonizing the clavicle. This is done in the area of the coracoclavicular ligament, making the osteological measurements listed above important.

There remains debate regarding the addition of a distal clavicle excision to an acromioclavicular joint reconstruction procedure. In the acute situation when the presence of acromioclavicular joint arthrosis is usually minimal, or in situations where stability is of paramount concern, the acromioclavicular reconstruction may be performed with retention of the distal clavicle. However, patients who have a chronic acromioclavicular joint injury, or preexisting acromioclavicular joint arthrosis may benefit from a distal clavicle excision. In these situations, approximately 10 mm of distal clavicle is removed with the use of a sagittal saw. The posterior edge of the clavicle is ensured to be smooth and free of abutment utilizing a sagittal saw and rasp.

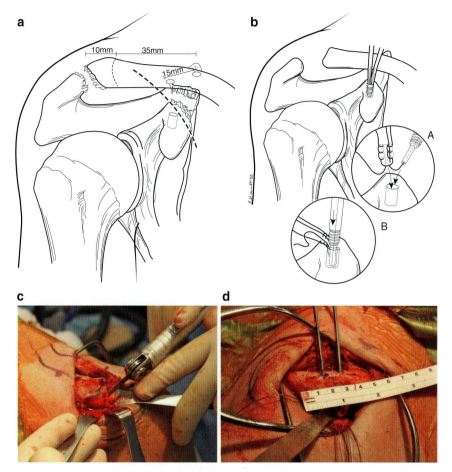

Fig. 14.7 Anatomic coracoclavicular reconstruction (ACCR) steps are shown. (**a**) Important anatomical landmarks, distances, and insertions of the trapezoid (lateral-most) and conoid (medial-most) ligaments on the distal clavicle. (**b**) A coracoid tunnel may be utilized in lieu of wrapping the autograft or allograft underneath the coracoid. (**c**) Utilizing a sagittal saw to remove approximately 8-10 mm of distal clavicle prior to fixing. Care is taken to preserve the joint capsule by elevating it off subperiosteally and protecting during the cut. (**d**) Measuring the two insertion points for the insertion of the conoid and trapezoid ligaments. Guide pins are placed in the locations for the ligament drill holes. (**e**) Schematic of passing the graft through the clavicle. (**f**) Graft passed through the two drill holes in the clavicle. (**g**) Schematic of one method to affix the graft in place - two tenodesis screws are placed in the clavicular drill holes and then the graft is tied to itself. (**h**) Postoperative AP radiograph demonstrating the two drill holes and reduction of the distal clavicle back to anatomic position

Complications and "bailouts" include:

- If too much of the distal clavicle was or is excised resulting in persistent instability despite reconstruction. Ensure adequate anterior to posterior repair of the deltotrapezial fascia with #2 nonabsorbable suture in a "pants over vest" fashion.

Graft Preparation: Depending upon surgeon preference, semitendinosis allograft or autograft or anterior tibialis allograft can be used for this procedure. Lee et al.[60,61] found no difference in peak load-to-failure between semitendinosis, toe extensors, and gracilis tendons for reconstruction of the acromioclavicular joint. In this technique, there are two options for handling the fixation to the coracoid process. One option involves a bone tunnel interference screw type fixation, and the other option involves looping the ligament around the coracoid process.

For interference screw fixation to the coracoid process, the graft is folded in its middle and a No. 2 Fiberwire (Arthrex, Inc., Naples, FL) or a No. 2 nonabsorbable suture is placed through the doubled-over

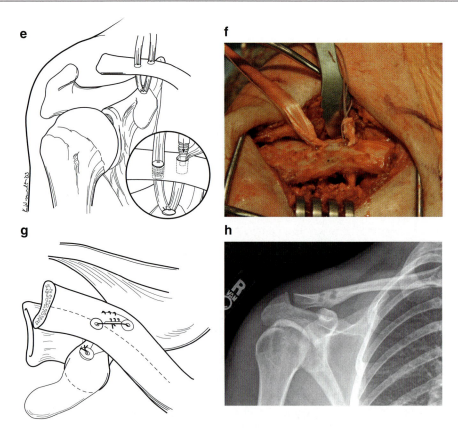

Fig. 14.7 (continued)

tendon graft in a Krakow type manner. One to two Krakow sutures are placed in the remaining two free ends of the graft. The graft is placed on the table in a moist sponge until the bone tunnels are prepared.

Complications and "bailouts" include:

- Intraoperative coracoid fracture. If this happens, the coracoid may be fixed with a 3.5 mm cortical screw that was temporarily fixed with k-wire(s). Additional complications include an inability to pass under the coracoid process the graft. Instrumentation such as a 90° right angle clamp, or commercially available 90° suture passers (akin to a Hewson suture passer) may be utilized to place passing sutures under the coracoid to transmit the graft.
- If graft passage under the coracoid is not possible, then a suture anchor (5.5 mm anchor, metal versus bio) or a Biotenodesis System with approximately a 5.0 mm screw (Arthrex, Naples, FL) are good solutions.

Bone Tunnel Preparation in the Coracoid: The diameter of the doubled-over portion of the graft is measured with a standard tendon-measuring device or using the handle of the Biotenodesis system (Arthrex, Inc., Naples, FL) to determine graft size. The appropriate cannulated reamer is chosen (usually, 6 or 7 mm). For fixation of graft to the base of the coracoid process, finger palpation of both lateral and medial portions of the coracoid process and drilling into the coracoid base under direct visualization with a cannulated reamer guide pin is completed. A coracoid drilling guide (Arthrex, Inc., Naples, FL) can also be used, which acts as a pipefitting device, fitting over the base of the coracoid process and angling the surgeon in the correct position. Once the guide pin has been inserted and confirmed by digital palpation not to be out of the coracoid process, the cannulated reamer of the specific graft size is used and the coracoid is reamed to a depth of 15-17 mm. Copious irrigation is used to remove any excess bone shavings from the reamings.

Complications and "bailouts" include:

- Drilling out the clavicle, or propagation of the bone tunnel. Accommodate with larger screw fixation or place around the clavicle and suture to remaining drill tunnel. "Cuff-links" have been used historically (plastic hole-savers placed into the drill holes) if too large or propagated.

- Improper coracoid graft position either under or superiorly fixated. Reposition and repass if under the coracoid through the inferior soft tissue and fascia. Avoid medial dissection to prevent musculocutaneous nerve injury. If improperly placed fixation device into the coracoid, bailout to passing underneath the coracoid.

Graft Fixation to Coracoid Process - Interference Fit Technique: The Biotenodesis driver is assembled and a 5.5×15 mm^2 bioabsorbable or PEEK Tenodesis screw is placed on the end. A Nitinol wire is placed through the center cannulation of the screwdriver complex and used to shuttle the suture from the graft through the driver. The long end of the Krakow suture attached to the graft should be placed through the cannulated portion of the Biotenodesis driver. The tenodesis driver is advanced to touch the tendon graft, and the entire tendon, driver, and screw complex is placed into the coracoid bone tunnel. The Krakow suture, usually measured to be about 15 mm in length running up and down the doubled portion of the tendon graft, should disappear from view when the tendon, driver, and screw complex is placed into the coracoid bone tunnel. A clamp is placed on the back portion of the teardrop handle of the driver to lock the suture in place. The screw is advanced over the driver-tendon complex, creating a secure interference screw fit. The clamp is released and the screwdriver complex is removed from the screw. Digital palpation confirms that the screw is flush with the bone tunnel, and by pulling on the two ends of the tendon it is confirmed that there is a secure fit. The sutures from the graft are tied together over the existing interference screw, giving both interference screw and suture anchor advantages.

Complications and "bailouts" include:

- Passage of autograft or allograft under the coracoid. Avoid medial dissection and injury to musculocutaneous nerve.
- Utilize fluoroscopy to confirm adequate reduction of the AC joint (Fig. 14.8)

Graft Fixation to Coracoid Process – Loop Technique: To avoid placing a bone tunnel in the coracoid process, the graft can be looped around its base. Looping the graft around the base of the coracoid process can be facilitated by the use of a curved aortic cross-clamp (Statinsky clamp) and a suture-passing device. At the same time that the graft is passed, a No.

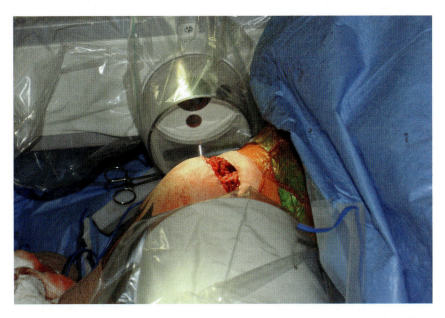

Fig. 14.8 Setup of how intraoperative fluoroscopy can be utilized during the case to ensure reduction of the distal clavicle

5 Fiberwire (Arthrex, Inc., Naples, FL) is also passed around the base of the coracoid. This will eventually become the nonbiologic fixation, reducing the clavicle to the scapula.

Bone Tunnels in the Clavicle: It is important to make the bone tunnels in as accurate a position as possible to recreate the coracoclavicular ligament. The complex osteological measurements provided are to aid the surgeon in finding the insertions of the conoid and the trapezoid and not meant as absolute numbers. A cannulated reamer guide pin is used for placement of the tunnels. The first tunnel, for the conoid process, is roughly 45 mm away from the distal end of the clavicle. The footprint of the conoid ligament is extremely posterior, along the entire posterior edge of the clavicle, and this is why making this bone tunnel as posterior as possible (i.e., in the posterior one-half of the clavicle) is extremely important. The guide pin is also angled approximately 45° from the direct perpendicular of the clavicle to recreate the oblique nature of the ligament. A 6 or 7 mm reamer is used to create the tunnel with careful attention confirming that the tunnel is as posterior as possible in the clavicle without "blowing out" the posterior cortical rim. Once this is confirmed, a 15-16 mm length bone tunnel is created.

The same procedure is repeated for the trapezoid ligament, which is a more anterior structure than the conoid and is usually placed in the center-point of the clavicle, approximately 15 mm away from the center portion of the previous tunnel. Two guide pins are used before reaming to confirm the accurate placement of the tunnels. After the tunnel reaming, copious irrigation follows to remove any bone fragments.

Complications and "bailouts" include:

– Blowing out the posterior or anterior cortical rim. Redrill in another location. However, this may not reproduce biomechanically the desired effect of the anatomic reconstruction. Alternatively, pass the graft over the top of the clavicle and affix to the remaining intact drill hole with sutures.

Interference Screw Fixation of Graft to Clavicle: One limb of the biologic graft is taken and placed through the posterior bone tunnel, recreating the conoid ligament. The other limb is passed through the anterior bone tunnel, recreating the trapezoid ligament. At the same time that the graft is brought through, each limb of a No. 5 Fiberwire (Arthrex, Inc., Naples, FL) should be brought through the respective bone tunnels as well. Upper displacement of the scapulohumeral complex by the assistant reduces the acromioclavicular joint. A large point-of-reduction forceps placed on the coracoid process and the clavicle can assist while securing the tendon grafts. The acromioclavicular joint should be over-reduced during initial fixation due to an inevitable amount of creep in the tendon graft. With complete upper displacement on the graft, ensuring its tautness, a 5.5×15 mm^2 bioabsorbable interference screw is placed in either the posterior or midline bone tunnel. The No. 5 Fiberwire (Arthrex, Inc., Naples, FL) is brought up through the cannulated process of this screw, and after assessment that this is done successfully, the second bioabsorbable interference screw is placed in the other unfilled bone tunnel. With both grafts secured using interference screw fixation, the No. 5 Fiberwire (Arthrex, Inc., Naples, FL) is tied over the top of the clavicle, becoming a nonbiologic fixation for the over-reduced acromioclavicular joint.

Complications and "bailouts" include:

– Avoid clamp placement medial to coracoid (musculocutaneous nerve injury)
– Improper reduction and excessive early strain on the repair. Assistant should help hold shoulder girdle and hold in place until fixation completed. Care should be taken to not allow shoulder to droop until sling is on the patient. Any compromise in repair should be retightened and fixed, potentially with larger interference screws.

Closure: One of the most important concepts with acromioclavicular or coracoclavicular joint reconstruction is the closure of the deltotrapezial fascial flaps from the dissection. A nonabsorbable suture, in a modified Mason-Allen type fashion is placed through the deltotrapezial fascia. Six or seven sutures are used, and the knots are tied on the posterior aspect of the trapezius. This closure of the deltotrapezial fascia should completely obscure the grafts as well as the clavicle. The subdermal skin is closed with 2-0 or 3-0 absorbable sutures, and the skin itself is closed with either a 2-0 running or interrupted nylon suture, everting the skin edges. A compression dressing is applied, and the patient is placed in a supportive sling with external rotation to 0° and an upward force on the arm.

Complications and "bailouts" include:

– If there is any concern regarding the fascial repair, the deltoid should be repaired through small drill holes in the anterior cortex of the clavicle. Some worry exists, though, that with two 6 mm bone tunnels in the clavicle, further smaller defects in the clavicle for deltoid fixation could lead to an iatrogenic fracture.

- Imbricate the deltotrapezial fascia by approximately 8-10 mm in a "pants-over-vest" fashion with #2 nonabsorbable suture in revision cases where the distal acromioclavicular joint capsule is likely compromised (Fig. 14.9).
- Distal clavicle options include bioabsorbable screws (Biotenodesis), metal, and PEEK (Fig. 14.10).

Surgery for Acriomioclavicular Joint Degenerative Pathology

Lemos and Tolo[61] have noted that very little is written about intraoperative complications of distal clavicle resection. They conclude that intraoperative complications in distal clavicle resection are rare.

Inadequate resection is the most common technical error in AC joint resection.[61] This is most often attributed to inadequate posterior resection secondary to poor visualization. At a minimum, 5 mm needs to be ressected for adequate decompression of arthritic AC joints.[62]

AC joint instability is also a potential complication of surgery. As noted earlier, sectioning the posterior and superior capsular ligaments can have deleterious effects on joint stability, which can lead to continued postoperative pain. Additionally, care must be taken to avoid dissecting the acromioclavicular ligaments, which can also cause postoperative instability. Distal clavicle excision of 5-8 mm has been recommended for this reason.[63] Cadaver models have not shown a difference in stability after distal clavicle resection when comparing open and arthroscopic techniques.[49]

Complications and bailouts:

- Excessive resection of the distal clavicle leads to residual instability. If recognized intraoperatively and if the lateral portion of the CC ligaments (trapezoid) are violated, then tenodese the trapezoid ligament

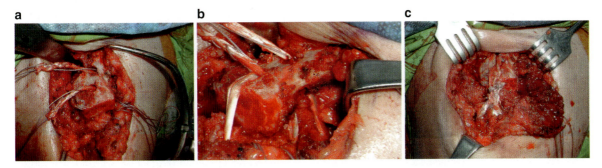

Fig. 14.9 A revision case in which the distal clavicle was unstable due to an incompetent acromioclavicular joint capsule. The graft is placed through the distal clavicular drill holes (**a**), affixed with tenodesis screws into the clavicle, and sutured into place. The graft is then routed to the acromion to reapproximate the joint capsule (**b**) and is secured (**c**)

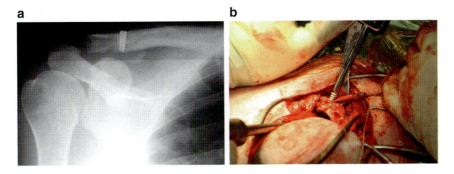

Fig. 14.10 Additional fixation options include metal screws (**a**) and PEEK (**b**) screws into the distal clavicle

into the remaining distal clavicle. Suture anchors (5.5 mm rotator cuff anchor) is adequate for tenodesis (Fig. 14.11).

Other General Complications

Hardware migration, the most serious complication of AC joint injury, is associated with surgical treatment of dislocations. Steinman pins, Hagie pins, and Kirschner wires have all been reported to migrate from the AC joint. There are reports of their migration to the lung,[64,65] the spinal cord,[66] and neck.[67] Grauthoff and Kalmmer reported five cases of migration into the aorta, subclavian artery, or lung.[68] Additionally, fixation can be associated with osteolysis.[69] Because of the high rate of migration, even with bending the end of the wire or using a tension band technique,[70] transfixion pins are not used if possible. The frequency of pin migration and seriousness of potential complications have prompted most surgeons to abandon their use, especially the use of smooth pins. Those who still use pins check their position with frequent radiographs and remove them after some interval of healing.

Failure of reconstruction is not uncommon in AC joint surgery. Tsou[33] reported technical complications in 32% of 53 AC joint dislocations treated with a Bosworth screw. These included screws missing the coracoid, screw failure, and subluxation after screw removal, as well as persistent drainage. A case of aseptic inflammatory loosening of a Gortex augmentation device leading to AC joint instability has also been reported.[71] Erosion of cerclage materials through the clavicle or coracoid has also been described.[39,72,73]

Infection of fixation or augmentation devices has also been reported. Neault et al.[74] reported on three cases in which the use of nonabsorbable tape or suture was related to postoperative infection. Colosimo[75] reported a case of aseptic foreign body reaction to Dacron graft. Reported rates of infection range from 0 to 9%, but seem to average around 6%.[47–49,76] Lemos and Tolo[63] recommend aggressive debridement with removal of all synthetic materials in such a case, antibiotic coverage should be initiated if infection is found, and reconstruction should be carried out in a staged fashion. If the failure is aseptic, the authors recommend a primary revision.[63]

Coracoclavicular ossification has also been reported, with an incidence of 50-85%.[63] Calcification of reconstructed ligaments does not appear to affect results.[48]

Loss of reduction of the AC joint is not uncommon. The weight of the arm and scapula places a tremendous static force on the coracoclavicular reconstruction. Younger patients have a tendency to discontinue efforts at supporting the arm for the first 6 weeks, which is necessary to protect the reconstruction. Efforts at augmentation of the repair and reconstruction have helped to reduce the incidence of complete failure, but partial loss of reduction remains common. In one report, Mayr[77] reported a lost reduction rate of 28%, with a less satisfactory outcome in these patients.

Erosion of cerclage material through the clavicle or coracoid is a well-documented complication.[39,72,73] A modification of the cerclage technique to place material through an osseous tunnel in the clavicle rather than completely around it decreases the severity of this complication because erosion does not create a complete discontinuity between the medial and lateral clavicle. Fracture of the coracoid may occur with placement of a coracoid screw.[78]

Osteolysis associated with acromioclavicular fixation has been reported.[69] Smith and Stewart[79] recommended resection of the distal clavicle at the time of surgical reduction to avoid this complication. The complication of late AC joint arthrosis is avoided and therefore distal clavicle resection has become an integral part of any acromioclavicular instability reconstruction.

Chronic pain after surgical treatment of acromioclavicular instability can be another challenging complication. Many possible causes need to be considered, including horizontal instability (anterior to posterior) of the clavicle, subacromial disease, and neurologic injury. Neurologic injury can occur with the initial trauma or with the surgical procedure. For example, suprascapular neuropathy may occur after distal clavicle resection and has been associated with resections of greater than 1 cm.[80]

Failed distal clavicle resection

The clinical evaluation of failed DCE is often subtle and difficult to evaluate. Nicholson GP (Presented AAOS, 1999) in an evaluation of 28 patients with unstable clavicles secondary to an aggressive DCE found a painful click/pinch at the posterior AC joint with forward elevation at and above 90°. He also found reproduction of pain with forced posterior clavicle

14 Avoiding and Managing Complications of Surgery of the Acromioclavicular Joint

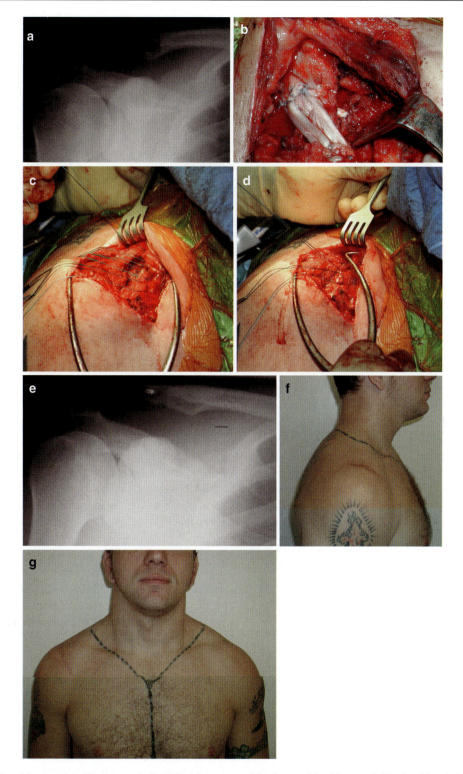

Fig. 14.11 A revision case in which too much distal clavicle was resected 2 years prior, leading to distal clavicle instability (**a**). In cases like this, the graft is brought out of drill holes lateral in the clavicle and then tied into the distal acromion (**b**). It is important to also obtain a tight closure of the deltotrapezial fascia with an imbrication of the tissues utilizing a series of #2 nonabsorbable sutures (**c** and **d**). The final radiograph (**e**) shows a metal button that can also be used to route sutures, and demonstrates an adequate reduction (**f** and **g**)

translation, trapezius spasm, and a manual AP translation of the distal clavicle of more than 1 cm.

There remains some controversy regarding the development of acromioclavicular joint symptoms following arthroscopic partial distal clavicle resections. Neer[81] recommended the removal of any osteophytes from the inferior aspect of the distal clavicle when performing open subacromial decompressions. He opined that these osteophytes could contribute to narrowing of the space available for the rotator cuff. With the development of arthroscopic techniques for subacromial decompression, some surgeons have suggested removing "osteophytes" from the inferior clavicle. However, after arthroscopic acromioplasty, part of the native distal clavicle is exposed and certainly some techniques have included removal of this inferior aspect of the clavicle in the "co-planing" procedure.

Fischer[82] reviewed 183 subacromial decompressions and divided them into three groups. The group in which the distal clavicle was not "co-planed" and the group that had a formal arthroscopic distal clavicle resection had no postoperative symptoms referable to the AC joint. However, the group that included a partial distal clavicle resection (co-planing) along with the subacromial decompression showed a high incidence of postoperative acromioclavicular joint symptoms (14 out of 36 or 39%). Because of these results an "all or none" philosophy has developed. In other words, the distal clavicle is left alone for routine subacromial decompression, or a formal distal clavicle resection is performed if the patient has significant acromioclavicular pathology.

Complications and "bailouts"

- Preoperative recognition of AC joint problems, or potential issues once reduced anatomically. Recognition that AC joint arthrosis may develop postinjury. Consideration of prophylactic AC joint resection at time of reconstruction surgery (Fig. 14.12).

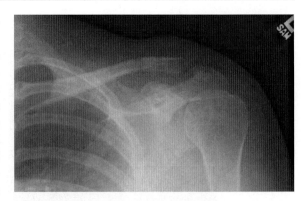

Fig. 14.12 Postoperative radiograph after anatomic coracoclavicular reconstruction with tibialis anterior allograft

injury and postsurgical films, and a thorough and accurate preoperative examination are essential prior to revision surgery. If failure of a previous surgery has occurred, the surgeon must account for the source of failure. As mentioned earlier, instability and posterior translation of the clavicle at the AC joint can be a cause of postoperative pain. Likely, revision surgery will require reconstruction that results in added stability with anatomic reconstruction of the distal clavicle.

If a coracoclavicular ligament repair or coracoacromial ligament transfer with or without augmentation was the index procedure, strong consideration should be given to anatomic coracoclavicular ligament reconstruction with deltotrapezial fascia repair. As mentioned earlier, anatomic coracoclavicular reconstruction has significantly less laxity compared with the Weaver-Dunn procedure.[19] It is important for the revision surgeon to be aware of any "burnt bridges" that may complicate revision surgery. If previous procedures used autograft augmentation, these harvest sites must be accounted for and planned around, and alternative autograft sites must be utilized. Semitendinosis, toe extensors, and gracilis tendons all have similar peak load-to-failure rates[60,61] and represent suitable sources. Allograft can provide an additional suitable biomechanical alternative.

Revision AC Repair/Reconstruction Surgery

Revision surgery for failed AC joint repairs and/or reconstructions remains a challenge. Central to any successful revision surgery is comprehensive appreciation of the previous surgery. Obtaining prior operative notes,

Arthroscopic repairs

Several technical reports[83–86] have described the ability to reconstruct an acromioclavicular joint dislocation arthroscopically, as first described by Wolf and Pennington.[86] The basic premise is that the procedure is performed through arthroscopic visualization in the subacromial space to facilitate viewing of graft and suture material into the clavicle. The purported advantages[83] are the ability to preserve the capsule of the distal clavicle (preserving the capsular ligaments), a staged procedure for screw removal is not required, and smaller, more cosmetic incisions. Overall, the procedure allows for a transcoracoid-transclavicular loop technique,[83,84] however, have yet to be clinically validated.

Complications and bailouts include:

- Failure to visualize structures and CC ligaments. The arthroscopic treatment of CC ligament injuries is challenging. Recommend step-wise approach to arthroscopic repairs. Start by doing half the case arthroscopically, then finish it open and then progress to full arthroscopic repairs once comfortable with anatomy.
- Easier to do acute (<3-4 weeks) repairs arthroscopically assisted. The Tight-Rope (Arthrex, Naples, FL), is a device designed for ease of arthroscopic application of CC repair and suture augmentation.

Postoperative Prescription, Outcomes Measurement, and Potential Complications

A variety of factors affect postoperative management of surgery involving the AC joint. If the procedure includes only a distal clavicle resection, then a short (1-3 days) period of immobilization is followed by range of motion activities. Strengthening begins at 4-6 weeks. Heavy weight training can begin at 3 months, but power athletes will often require 6-12 months to return to peak strength.

After a coracoclavicular ligament reconstruction, the arm is supported with an external device such as a sling and immobilizer. Gentle range of motion activities in the supine position can begin after 7-10 days. Range of motion with the arm unsupported in an upright position should be delayed until the reconstruction has had time to develop early biologic stability. For an acute repair, this takes 4-6 weeks. A chronic repair with severe soft tissue involvement, for example a Type V separation, may take up to 6-12 weeks before unsupported range of motion is allowed. An emphasis at this point should be placed on strengthening the scapular stabilizers. These muscles decrease the load on the joint by keeping the scapula in a relatively retracted position. Strengthening in an acute repair begins at 6-12 weeks, with weight training started at 3-4.5 months. Strengthening in a chronic repair is appropriately delayed. We utilize this protocol for the anatomic acromioclavicular reconstructions.

Historically, motion is limited until pins are removed at 6-8 weeks. After coracoclavicular screw fixation, range of motion begins when pain subsides. Bosworth[87] recommended no heavy activity for 8 weeks. Alldredge[88] recommended no immobilization, Bearden[20] a sling for 10-14 days, Jay[35] a sling for 4 weeks, and Gollwitzer[47] a Velpeau cast for 4 weeks. Recommendations regarding hardware removal have varied.[20,32,34,35,88,89] After coracoid transfer, Brunelli[90] recommended 90° of elbow flexion with gradual straightening starting on day 5 to reduce the AC joint, and protected activities for 6-8 weeks. Care should always be taken to avoid iatrogenic fractures (Fig. 14.13) due to excessively large drill holes, clavicular cortical blowout, or overly-aggressive rehabilitation.

Criteria for Return to Play/Activities

Power athletes and heavy physical demand workers are the longest to rehabilitate and generally take 9-12 months to reach peak strength, especially with pressing activities or lifting from the floor (i.e., dead lift). After an anatomic acromioclavicular reconstruction,

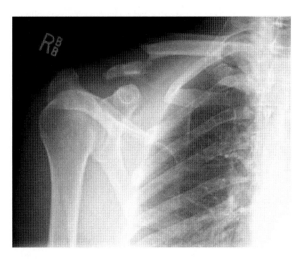

Fig. 14.13 A difficult situation in which the distal clavicle fractured through the medial anatomic reconstruction drill hole. This case was salvage with plate fixation and ligament reconstruction

return to contact sports is limited for a minimum of 6 months. Prior to this, the therapist should work with the athlete on sport-specific training exercises and also ensure that the Cybex upper extremity power testing is within 10-15% of the contralateral normal limb.

Conclusion

Successful outcomes in AC joint surgery are dependent on several factors. Surgeons must fully understand the common mechanisms of AC injury, recognize associated potential injuries, place the injury within a commonly used classification framework, obtain proper imaging, and have a full comprehension of potential surgical solutions. Even with all of this knowledge and planning, intraoperative and postoperative complications can occur. The surgeon that is prepared for potential confounders will be best suited to provide his or her patients with a painless, stable and functional acromioclavicular joint. Ideally, this chapter serves as a roadmap of contingency plans that will assist surgeons in achieving such outcomes for their patients.

References

1. Allman F (1967) Fractures and Ligamentous Injuries of the clavicle and its articulation. J Bone Joint Surg Am. 49:774-84
2. Rockwood C, Williams G, Young D (2004) Disorders of the Acromioclavicular Joint. In: Rockwood CJ, Matsen F (eds) The Shoulder. Vol 1. WB Saunders, Philadelphia, pp 521-95
3. Cave E (1961) Fractures and Other Injuries. Year Book Medical Publishers, Chicago
4. Lemos M (1998) The evaluation and treatment of the injured acromioclavicular joint in athletes. Am J Sports Med. 26:137-44
5. Garretson RIII, Williams G Jr (2003) Clinical evaluation of injuries to the acromioclavicular and sternoclavicular joints. Clin Sports Med. 22(2):239-54
6. Cadenat F (1917) The treatment of dislocations and fractures of the outer end of the clavicle. Int Clin. 1:145-69
7. Tossy J, Mead N, Sigmond H (1963) Acromioclavicular separations: Useful and practical classification for treatment. Clin Orthop. 38:111-19
8. Bossart P, Joyce S, Manaster B et al (1988) Lack of efficacy of "weighted" radiographs in diagnosing acute acromioclavicular separation. Ann Emerg Med. 17:47-51
9. Phillips A, Smart C, Groom A (1998) Acromioclavicular dislocation. Clin Orthop Rel Res. 353:10-17
10. Rudzki R, Matava J, Paletta A Jr (2003) Complications of treatment of acromioclavicular and sternoclavicular joint injuries. Clin Sports Med. 22(2):387-405
11. Larsen E, Bjerg-Nielsen A, Christensen P (1986) Conservative or surgical treatment of acromioclavicular dislocation. A prospective, controlled, randomized study. J Bone Joint Surg Am. 68:552-55
12. Nuber G, Bowen M (1997) Acromioclavicular joint injuries and distal clavicle fractures. J Am Acad Orthop Surg. 5:11-18
13. DePalma A, Callery G, Bennett G (1949) Variational anatomy and degenerative lesions of the shoulder joint. Instr Course Lect. 6:255-81
14. Petersson C (1983) Degeneration of the acromioclavicular joint: A morphological study. Acta Orthop Scand. 54:434-38
15. Salter E, Nasca R, Shelley B (1987) Anatomical observations on the acromioclavicular joint and supporting ligaments. Am J Sports Med. 15:199-206
16. Nicholson G (1999) Anterior and posterior instability of the distal clavicle after acromioclavicular resection: Clinical characteristics and results of operative stabilization. Orthop Trans. 22:1190-91
17. Klimkiewicz J, Williams G, Sher J et al (1999) The acromioclavicular capsule as a restraint to posterior translation of the clavicle: A biomechanical analysis. J Shoulder Elbow Surg. 8:119-24
18. Harris R, Vu D, Sonnabend D et al (Anatomic variance of the coracoclavicular ligaments) J Shoulder Elbow Surg. 10(6):585-8
19. Mazzocca D, Santangelo A, Johnson T et al (Feb 2006) A biomechanical evaluation of an anatomical coracoclavicular ligament reconstruction. Am J Sports Med. 34(2):236-46
20. Bearden J, Hughston J, Whatley G (1973) Acromioclavicular dislocation: Method of treatment. Am J Sports Med. 1:5-17
21. Fakuda K, Craig E, An K et al (1986) Biomechanical study of the ligament systems of the acromioclavicular joint. J Bone Joint Surg. 68A:434-39
22. Corteen D, Teitge R (Jan 2005) Stabilization of the clavicle after distal resection: A biomechanical study. Am J Sports Med. 33(1):61-7
23. Codman E, Codman E (1934) The Shoulder. Robert E. Krieger Publishing Company, Inc, Malabar, FL
24. Bergfeld J, Andrish J, Clancy W (1978) Evaluation of the acromioclavicular joint following first and second degree sprains. Am J Sports Med. 6:153-9
25. Cook D, Heiner J (1990) Acromioclavicular Joint Injuries. Orthop Rev. 19:510-16
26. Cox J (1981) The fate of the acromioclavicular joint in athletic injuries. Am J Sports Med. 9:50-3
27. Galatz L, Williams G Jr (2001) Acromioclavicular Joint Injuries. JB Lippincott, Philadelphia
28. Meislin R, Zuckerman J, Nainzadeh N (1992) Type III acromioclavicular joint separation associated with late brachial plexus neuropraxia. J Orthop Trauma. 6:370-2
29. Bernard T, Brunet M, Haddad R (1983) Fractured coracoid process in acromioclavicular dislocations: report of four cases and review of the literature. Clin Orthop. 175:227-32
30. Barber F (1987) Complete posterior acromioclavicular dislocation: A case report. Orthopaedics. 10:493-6
31. Guttman D, Paksima N, Zuckerman J (2000) Complications of treatment of complete acromioclavicular joint dislocations. AAOS, Rosemont, IL

32. Bosworth B (1941) Acromioclavicular separation: New method of repair. Surg Gynecol Obstet. 73:866-71
33. Tsou P (1989) Percutaneous cannulated screw coracoclavicular fixation for acute acromioclavicular dislocations. Clin Orthop. 243:112-21
34. Kennedy J (1968) Complete dislocation of the acromioclavicular joint: 14 years later. J Trauma. 8:311-18
35. Jay G, Monnet J (1969) The Bosworth Screw in Acute Dislocation of the Acromioclavicular Joint. Paper presented at: Clinical Conference; University of Oklahoma Medical Center.
36. Lowe G, Fogarty M (1977) Acute acromioclavicular joint dislocation: Results of operative treatment with the Bosworth screw. Aust NZ J Surg. 47(5):664-7
37. Albrecht F (1983) The Balser plate for acromioclavicular fixation. Chirurg. 53:732-4
38. Fleming R, Tomberg D, Kiernan H (1978) An operative repair of acromioclavicular separation. J Trauma. 18:709-12
39. Goldberg J, Viglione W, Cumming W et al (1987) Review of coracoclavicular ligament reconstruction using Dacron Graft material. Aust N Z J Surg. 57:441-5
40. Kappakas G, McMaster J (1978) Repair of acromioclavicular separation using a Dacron prosthesis graft. Clin Orthop. 131:247-51
41. Nelson C (1979) Repair of acromioclavicular separations with knitted Dacron graft. Clin Orthop. 143:289
42. Tagliabue D, Riva A (1981) Current approaches to the treatment of acromioclavicular joint separation in athletes. J Ital J Sports Traumatol. 3:15-24
43. Bunnell S (1928) Fascial graft for dislocation of the acromioclavicular joint. Surg Gynecol Obstet. 46:563-4
44. Lom P (67) Acromioclavicular disjunction: 1. Diagnosis and classification; 2. Surgical treatment-the author's modification. Rozhl Chir 67(4):253-70
45. Clayer M, Slavotinek J, Krishnan J (1997) The results of coraco-clavicular slings for acromioclavicular dislocation. Aust N Z J Surg. 67:343-6
46. Gohring H, Matusewicz A, Friedl W et al (1993) Results of treatment after different surgical procedures for management of acromioclavicular joint dislocation. Chirurg. 64:565-71
47. Gollwitzer M (1993) Surgical management of complete acromioclavicular joint dislocation (Tossy III) with PDS cord cerclage. Aktuelle Traumatologie 23(8):366-70
48. Hessmann M, Gotzen L, Gehling H (1995) Acromioclavicular reconstruction augmented with polydioxanonsulphate bands. Surgical technique and results. Am J Sports Med. 23:552-6
49. Matthews L, Parks B, Pavlovich L Jr et al (1999) Arthroscopic versus open distal clavicle resection: A biomechanical analysis on a cadaveric model. Arthroscopy 15(3):237-40
50. Morrison D, Lemos M (1995) Acromioclavicular separation. Reconstruction using synthetic loop augmentation. Am J Sports Med. 23:105-10
51. Pfahler M, Krodel A, Refior H (1994) Surgical treatment of acromioclavicular dislocation. Arch Ortho Traum Surg. 113(6):308-11
52. Neviaser J (1968) Acromioclavicular dislocation treated by transference of the coracoacromial ligament. A long-term follow-up in a series of 112 cases. Clin Orthop. 58:57-68
53. De la Caffiniere J, De la Caffiniere M, Lacaze F (1998) Treatment of acromioclavicular dislocations using coracoacromial ligament plasty. Revue de Chirurgie Orthopedique et Reparatrice de Appareil Moteur 84(1):9-16
54. Guy D, Wirth M, Griffin J et al (1998) Reconstruction of chronic and complete dislocations of the acromioclavicular joint. Clin Orthop. 347:138-49
55. Kumar S, Sethi A, Jain A (1995) Surgical treatment of complete acromioclavicular dislocation using the coracoacromial ligament and coracoclavicular fixation: report of a technique in 14 patients. J Orthop Trauma. 9:507-10
56. Mumford E (1941) Acromioclavicular dislocation- a new treatment. J Bone Joint Surg Am. 23:799-802
57. Weaver J, Dunn H (1972) Treatment of acromioclavicular injuries, especially complete acromioclavicular separation. J Bone Joint Surg Am. 54:1187-94
58. Blazar P, Iannotti J, Williams G (1998) Anteroposterior instability of the distal clavicle after distal clavicle resection. Clin Orthop Relat Res. March(348):114-20
59. Baker J, Nicandri G, Young D et al (Nov-Dec 2003) A cadaveric study examining acromioclavicular joint congruity after different methods of coracoclavicular loop repair. J Shoulder Elbow Surg. 12(6):595-8
60. Lee K, Debski R, Chen C et al (1997) Functional evaluation of the ligaments at the acromioclavicular joint during anteroposterior and superoinferior translation. Am J Sports Med. 25:858-62
61. Lee S, Nicholas S, Akizuki K et al (Sep-Oct 2003) Reconstruction of the coracoclavicular ligaments with tendon grafts: A comparative biomechanical study. Am J Sports Med. 31(5):648-55
62. Branch T, Burdette H, Shahriari A et al (1996) The role of acromioclavicular ligaments and the effect of distal clavicle resection. Am J Sports Med 24(3):293-6
63. Lemos M, Tolo E (Apr 2003) Complications of the treatment of the acromioclavicular and sternoclavicular joint injuries, including instability. Clin Sports Med. 22(2):371-85
64. Eaton R, Serletti J (1981) Computerized axial tomography - A method of localizing Steinmann pin migration. Orthopedics. 4:1357-60
65. Mazet R (1943) Migration of a Kirschner wire from the shoulder region into the lung: Report of two cases. J Bone and Joint Surg. 25A(2):477-83
66. Norrell H, Llewellyn R (1965) Migration of a threaded Steinmann pin from an acromioclavicular joint into the spinal canal: A case report. J Bone Joint Surg. 47A: 1024-6
67. Lindsey R, Gutowski W (1986) The migration of a broken pin following fixation of theacromioclavicular joint: A case report and review of the literature. Orthopedics. 9:413-16
68. Grauthoff V, Kalmmer H (1978) Complications due to migration of a Kirschner wire from the clavicle. Fortschr Rontgenstr. 128:591-4
69. Eskola A, Vainionpaa S, Korkala O (1987) Acute complete acromioclavicular dislocation. A prospective randomized trial of fixation with smooth or threaded Kirschner wires or cortical screw. Ann Chir Gynaecol. 76:323-6
70. Rockwood C Jr (1984) Injuries to the acromioclavicular joint. In: Rockwood C Jr, DP G (eds) Fractures in Adults, 2nd edn. JB Lippincott, Philadelphia, PA, pp 860-910
71. Jones H, Lemos M, Schepsis A (Mar-Apr 2001) Salvage of failed acromioclavicular joint reconstruction using autogenous semitendinosis tendon from the knee. Surgical technique and case report. Am J Sports Med. 29(2):234-7

72. Dahl E (1981) Follow-up after coracoclavicular ligament prosthesis for acromioclavicular joint dislocation (proceedings). Acta Chir Scand (Suppl.). 506:96
73. Dahl E (1982) Velour prosthesis in fractures and dislocations in the clavicular region. Chirurg. 53:120-2
74. Neault M, Nuber G, Marymont J (1996) Infections after surgical repair of acromioclavicular separations with nonabsorbable tape or suture. J Shoulder Elbow Surg. 5: 477-8
75. Colosimo A, Hummer C, Heidt R (1996) Aseptic foreign body reaction to Dacron graft material used for coracoclavicular ligament reconstruction after Type III acromioclavicular dislocation. Am J Sports Med. 24(4): 561-3
76. Winkler H, Schlamp D, Wentzensen A (1994) Treatment of acromioclavicular joint dislocation by tension band and ligament suture. Aktuelle Traumatologie 24(4):133-9
77. Mayr E, Braun W, Eber W et al (1999) Treatment of acromioclavicular joint separations. Central Kirschner wire and PDS augmentation. Unfallchirurg. 102:278-86
78. Monein M, Balduini F (1982) Coracoid fractures as a complication of surgical treatment by coracoclavicular tape fixation. Clin Orthop. 168:133-5
79. Smith M, Stewart M (1979) Acute acromioclaicular separations. A 20-year study. Am J Sports Med. 7:62-71
80. Mallon W, Bronec P, Spinner R et al (1996) Suprascapular neuropathy after distal clavicle excision. Clin Ortho Rel Res. 329:207-11
81. Neer C (1990) Shoulder Reconstruction. WB Saunders Company, Philadelphia
82. Fischer B, Gross R, McCarthy J et al (1999) Incidence of acromioclavicular joint complications after arthroscopic subacromial decompression. Arthroscopy 15(3):241-8
83. Baumgarten K, Altchek D, Cordasco F (2006) Arthroscopically assisted acromioclavicular joint reconstruction. Arthroscopy 22(2):228.e221-228.e226
84. Lafosse L, Baier G, Leuzinger J (Aug 2005) Arthroscopic treatment of acute and chronic acromioclavicular joint dislocation. Arthroscopy 21(8):1017
85. Rolla P, Surace M, Murena L (Jul 2004) Arthroscopic treatment of acute acromioclavicular joint dislocation. Arthroscopy 20(6):662-8
86. Wolf E, Pennington W (May 2001) Arthroscopic reconstruction for acromioclavicular joint dislocation. Arthroscopy 17(5):558-63
87. Bosworth B (1949) Complete acromioclavicular dislocation. N Engl J Med. 241:221-5
88. Alldredge R (1965) Surgical treatment of acromioclavicular dislocations (proceedings. J Bone Joint Surg. 47(A):1278
89. Weitzman H (1967) Treatment of acute acromioclavicular joint dislocation by a modified Bosworth method: Report on 24 cases. J Bone Joint Surg. 49(A):1167-78
90. Brunelli G, Brunelli F (1988) The treatment of acromioclavicular dislocation by transfer of the short head of biceps. Int Orthop. 12:105-08

Editors' Comments (AC)

If suture anchors are utilized on the coracoid process beware of suture anchor pullout or coracoid fracture. A 4.5 mm or 5.0 mm screw-in suture anchor can be used. Similarly, metal screw fixation can result in coracoid process fracture. Additional techniques for AC repair include the use of an endobutton with a closed loop that can be passed on the coracoid side and affixed on the clavicular side with a free endobutton passed underneath the free closed loop.

Prior to an arthroscopic AC repair, one should be thoroughly familiar with the approach to the coracoid through the rotator cuff interval. Best to practice on a cadaver in a learning center lab.

Chapter 15
Complications of Arthroscopic Shoulder Surgery: Miscellaneous Shoulder Conditions

Alexander Golant and Young W. Kwon

Introduction

Overall rate of complications after arthroscopic shoulder surgery was once believed to be quite low.[1–3] For instance, Ellman reported no major complications, one localized hematoma at a portal site, and three transient dysesthesias in the thumb (attributed to inadequate padding on the traction device) in his review of 50 consecutive subacromial decompressions.[4] Subsequently, a report from the Committee on Complications of the Arthroscopy Association of North America in the 1980s documented a wider range and scope of complications after arthroscopic shoulder surgery, and noted rates as low as 0.76% for subacromial space procedures and as high as 5.3% for arthroscopic anterior staple capsulorrhaphy.[5] Even for the "experienced" sureons, the committee noted a fairly high complication rate of 5.2% after arthroscopic shoulder surgery.[6] More recent retrospective review studies noted even higher complication rates, between 6.5 and 10.5%, with adhesive capsulitis being the most common complication.[7,8] In 2002, Weber and colleagues reviewed the available literature and found the overall complication rates after shoulder arthroscopy to be between 5.8 and 9.5%.[9] Thus, complications after arthroscopic shoulder surgery may be more common than once believed and warrant particular attention to increase awareness and to provide appropriate treatment.

A. Golant
Department of Orthopedic Surgery, NYU Hospital for Joint Diseases, New York, NY, 10003, USA
e-mail: golana1@med.nyu.edu

Y.W. Kwon (✉)
NYU Hospital for Joint Diseases, 301 E. 17th St., New York, NY 10003
email: young.kwon@nyumc.org

Adhesive Capsulitis

Adhesive capsulitis or "frozen shoulder" is a condition in which the glenohumeral joint exhibits inflammatory changes of the synovium followed by capsular thickening and contracture formation. As a result, patients have pain and loss of both active and passive shoulder motion. In contrast to several other shoulder conditions that are associated with shoulder stiffness in one particular plane of motion (e.g., rotator cuff impingement and loss of internal rotation), patients with adhesive capsulitis demonstrate loss of motion in all planes. To date, however, the actual pathophysiology of the disease is still not well understood.

Adhesive capsulitis can be divided into two general types. The primary, or idiopathic, type occurs without an identifiable cause, is often bilateral, and may be resistant to treatment. This disorder is more common and possibly more severe in patients with diabetes. In contrast, secondary or acquired, adhesive capsulitis develops after a recognizable inciting event, such as shoulder trauma or surgery.[10] For these patients, prolonged immobilization of the shoulder is believed to be the most common inciting factor.

All patients with adhesive capsulitis, both primary and secondary, should initially be managed with nonoperative modalities including regimented physical therapy program and appropriate anti-inflammatory medications. If inflammation of the joint persists, an intra-articular cortisone injection can also be considered. Finally, education regarding the disease process and its natural course may significantly improve patient's participation in their rehabilitation. A number of outcome studies on primary adhesive capsulitis have reported that nonoperative treatments are associated with a successful outcome in gross

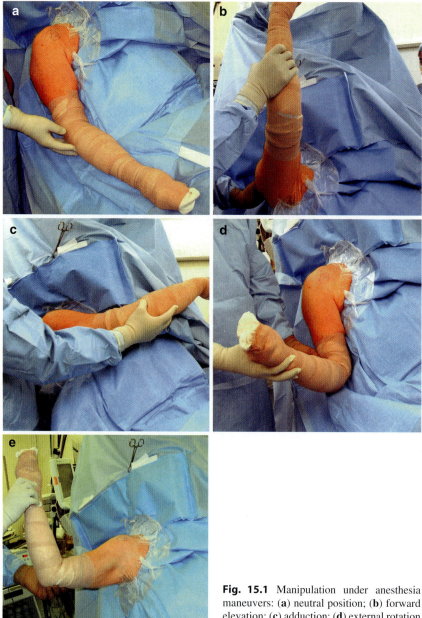

Fig. 15.1 Manipulation under anesthesia maneuvers: (**a**) neutral position; (**b**) forward elevation; (**c**) adduction; (**d**) external rotation in adduction; and (**e**) external rotation in abduction

majority of the patients and argue against aggressive initial management.[11–14] Although direct evidence on secondary adhesive capsulitis is lacking, most surgeons also proceed with nonoperative modalities for secondary adhesive capsulitis as well.

Surgical management should be considered for those patients who have failed nonoperative modalities for an extended period of time (typically, greater than 6 months) and still demonstrate significant disability from the disease. For these patients, several surgical options are available. One of the most commonly performed procedures is closed manipulation under anesthesia (MUA). The object of this procedure is to regain full shoulder motion through manual manipulation of the joint. This must be carried out in a careful and calculated manner. Specific maneuvers to regain flexion, adduction, abduction, and rotation at various angles of abduction should be performed sequentially. (Fig. 15.1) Any sudden or forceful maneuver may lead to reported complications including labral tears, instability, fractures, and nerve injuries. This is particularly important for high risk patients such as those with osteopenia or those who recently underwent a surgical repair of soft tissues.[10,15,16]

Another surgical option is an arthroscopic capsular release. In theory, this procedure provides a more controlled release of the capsule and minimizes the risks of the complications associated with the manipulation. Typically, a circumferential release of the glenohumeral capsule is usually required. In addition, for patients with prior shoulder surgeries, subacromial space should be inspected and debrided appropriately. If other intra-articular lesions are noted at the time of the arthroscopy, this pathology may also have to be addressed. Loew and colleagues, for example, reported that 12 of the 30 patients (40%) who underwent MUA and arthroscopy for adhesive capsulitis demonstrated additional intra-articular lesions. They included SLAP tears, partial rotator cuff tendon tears, anterior capsular avulsions, middle glenohumeral ligament tears, and osteochondral injury (Fig. 15.2).[17] Concomitant treatment of these lesions with the capsular release for adhesive capsulitis may pose a problem with the rehabilitation since temporary immobilization and gradual increase in motion is generally recommended after the treatment of these lesions. Therefore, each patient must be treated on an individual basis taking into consideration their primary source of pain as well as appropriate postoperative rehabilitation protocol that will not compromise the treatment of adhesive capsulitis.

Recently, a number of surgeons have argued for the combination of these two procedures. Some favor performing the manipulation first to loosen the scar tissues and to increase joint space for the arthroscopy. Then, the capsular release can be carried out accordingly. Others, including the senior author, tend to perform the arthroscopic capsular release first. The portions of the capsule that is difficult or dangerous to release arthroscopically (e.g., inferior capsule near the axillary nerve) are then released with the manipulation. There are practical and theoretical advantages for both of these approaches. For example, if arthroscopic release follows MUA, much of the adhesions are already disrupted as to allow easy introduction of arthroscopic instruments into the joint. On the other hand, however, arthroscopy after an MUA can be associated with significant intra-articular bleeding that may limit visualization and diagnostic abilities of arthroscopy. In addition, performing arthroscopic capsular release first will likely decrease the force required to manipulate the shoulder and may decrease the likelihood of iatrogenic injuries. In patients with advanced osteopenia from prolonged immobility, malnutrition, or rheumatologic diseases, this approach may be preferred. To date, however, neither approach has been clinically proven to be superior to the other.

Regardless of the surgical treatment, it should be stressed that adequate postoperative analgesia is paramount for a successful outcome. Sufficient pain relief should be obtained to in order to allow immediate postoperative motion exercises. In most surgical centers, this is typically obtained with an interscalene nerve block with long-acting agents.[18,19] Other options include indwelling intra-articular or subacromial catheters to deliver anesthetic agents.[20–23] Although there has been no direct comparison of these analgesia options, possible toxic effects of intra-articular anesthetic agents on the articular chondrocytes have raised concerns regarding the use of this modality.[24–26]

A relatively common complication after surgical treatment of adhesive capsulitis is recurrent stiffness. Patients at higher risk for recurrent stiffness include those who are diabetic, older, and with chronic medical illnesses.[27–30] For most patients, however, recurrent stiffness should be preventable Patients may be more likely to redevelop shoulder stiffness if the surgical release was inadequate. On the other hand, overly aggressive

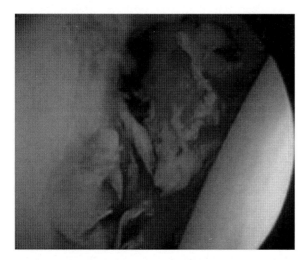

Fig. 15.2 Arthroscopic view of a capsulolabral tear with osteochondral involvement after manipulation under general anesthesia for adhesive capsulitis (reprinted from Loew et al.[17] copyright 2005, with permission from Elsevier)

manipulation or release of pericapsular tissues may result in postoperative instability. Therefore, care should be taken to adequately release the pathologically contracted glenohumeral capsule and the adhesions that restrain normal motion. After the procedure, full motion should be obtained without any evidence of instability. Finally, without appropriate postoperative rehabilitation, the released adhesions may reconsolidate, and the motion obtained during the surgery may be lost.

Infection

Deep infection after arthroscopy of the shoulder is a fairly rare complication with the reported rates between 0 and 3.6%.[4,7,31–33] Nevertheless, occurrence of a deep infection can significantly affect both the short- and long-term outcomes after shoulder arthroscopic surgeries. Administration of perioperative antibiotics and strict adherence to antiseptic surgical techniques should reduce the rate of postarthroscopic infection. For example, Herrera and colleagues initially reported a 1.9% incidence of deep infection after arthroscopically assisted mini-open rotator cuff repair in 360 patients. After introducing a second skin preparation and draping into their protocol, they noted that their rate of infection dropped to 0% after 200 similar procedures.[32]

Prompt identification of the infection is the key step in appropriate management of these patients. Systemic symptoms such as fevers, chills, or night sweats may be reported, but are infrequent. Rather, local signs such as pain, erythema, edema, and drainage are more common indications of infection. For example, the most common presentation of a deep infection after a rotator cuff repair surgery was persistent drainage from the wound.[34]

Once a deep infection is suspected, serologic markers such as a complete blood count (CBC) with differential, erythrocyte sedimentation rate (ESR), and C-reactive protein (CRP) can be measured. Without systemic symptoms, CBC is likely to remain within normal limits. In the setting of an acute postoperative period, ESR may also be elevated as well. Hence, CRP is likely to be the most reliable marker for an infection. In addition to these serologic markers, an aspiration may be carried out to confirm the infection and to identify the responsible organism. Previous studies have reported Staphylococcus and Propionibacterium to be the most common infecting organisms in postsurgical septic arthritis of the shoulder.[32,34,35]

If a deep infection is confirmed, surgical irrigation and debridement are required. This may be performed as an open procedure or through arthroscopic methods. Jeon et al. reported on successful management of septic arthritis of the native shoulder with a single arthroscopic debridement and antibiotic administration in 14 of 19 patients.[36] If arthroscopic procedure is performed, cultures should be sent at the beginning of surgery, preferably immediately after the insertion of the trocar for the arthroscope. After adequate visualization and inspection, all visibly affected and necrotic soft tissues should be debrided. In addition, copious amounts of saline should be used to irrigate the joint and the affected area. There is no evidence to suggest that adding antibiotics to the irrigating saline will improve the likelihood of eliminating the infection. However, if the infecting organism and its antibiotic sensitivities are identified, an appropriate antibiotic may provide additional means to eradicate the infection, and can be added to the saline at the discretion of a surgeon.

Depending on the clinical response after the first debridement procedure, a second debridement procedure may have to be performed. In patients with retained hardware such as suture anchors, all loose components should be removed at the time of the surgical debridement. For well-fixed hardware, retention of the hardware does not appear to preclude the successful eradication of the infection. A retrospective review of patients with early deep infection after open or arthroscopically assisted mini-open rotator cuff repair demonstrated that infection was successfully eradicated in six shoulders with at least one retained implant. The authors also noted, however, that the average number of surgical debridements and the duration of antibiotic administration required to eradicate infection in these patients were slightly higher compared to those with no retained implants.[34]

Once the surgical debridement is completed, administration of intravenous antibiotics is generally recommended. The duration of the therapy will depend on the degree of infection and the causative organism, and may last up to 6 weeks. For most patients, a consult from an infectious disease specialist is also recommended. If the infection is under control, appropriate rehabilitation may also be initiated during this period.

Nerve Injuries

Among the most serious complications after arthroscopic shoulder surgery are nerve injuries. Although relatively infrequent, these injuries can have significant impact on patient outcomes and satisfaction. Hence, precautions should be taken to avoid injuries to the nearby nerves during all steps of the procedure.

Improper arm position, excessive traction, and overdistension of the glenohumeral joint have all been postulated to play a role in increasing the risk of neuropraxias after shoulder arthroscopy.[31,37] A study using electrodiagnostic modalities to assess nerve function during shoulder arthroscopy found musculocutaneous nerve to be most susceptible to injury.[38] Other reports in the literature have also noted possible dangers to the axillary, ulnar, medial antebrachial cutaneous nerves, as well as the brachial plexus.[37] Due to these findings, some authors advocate the use of the "beach chair" position during shoulder arthroscopy. If lateral decubitus position is to be used, it is advisable to avoid excessive arm abduction and extension.[31] Minimal amount of weight should be used for joint distraction and the length of time in traction must be minimized. Specifically, Pitman and colleagues recommended using no more than 5 lbs of traction perpendicular to the arm (classically known as "Position 2") and less than 12 lbs of longitudinal traction in "Position 1".[38] The traction rope should not be attached to a fixed point, and appropriate padding of the wrist and forearm should be used to prevent distal neuropraxias.[4,37]

A significant portion of the nerve injuries during shoulder arthroscopy is believed to occur during placement of the portals. Segmuller and colleagues, for example, reported a 7% rate of cutaneous nerve neuropathies after shoulder arthroscopy, with nearly half of these lesions remaining symptomatic at 8 months after surgery. They noted that majority of these injuries were about the portal sites and attributed them to the blunt trauma during the introduction of the trocar.[39] Similarly, the anterior portals must be placed well lateral to the coracoid process in order to avoid injury to the musculocutaneous nerve.[40]

Due to its proximity to the joint, one of the most commonly injured structure is the axillary nerve. Injury to the axillary nerve has been associated with excessive traction in the lateral position, improper portal placement, fluid extravasation from the glenohumeral joint, use of electrocautery near the axillary pouch, and overly aggressive manipulation.[37] Establishment of the anterior portals, especially the so-called "5-o'clock portal," should be performed carefully as it has been demonstrated to be within 13 mm to the axillary nerve.[41] However, standard portal placement is generally associated with a relatively low risk of axillary nerve injury.[42] Similarly, when performed appropriately, MUA for adhesive capsulitis is relatively unlikely to injure the axillary nerve with only anecdotal reports of postoperative neuropraxia.

Higher risk of axillary nerve injury after shoulder arthroscopy has been documented with the use of radiofrequency or electrocautery probes in the inferior aspect of the glenohumeral joint just superior to the inferior capsule and the nerve. One study, for example, noted an axillary nerve injury in 21% of the patients treated with arthroscopic thermal capsulorrhaphy.[43] Several cadaveric studies found that the axillary nerve is located closer to the humeral head than to the glenoid underneath the inferior capsule, and recommended approaching the inferior capsule near the glenoid with the arm in an abducted and externally rotated position in order to decrease the risk of nerve damage (Fig. 15.3).[44–47]

If a nerve palsy is documented, most authors recommend observation as initial treatment since spontaneous recovery is likely. In general, sensory neuropathy is more likely to spontaneously resolve than a motor or a combined neuropathy.[48] If no recovery is noted within 3–4 weeks, electrodiagnostic studies should be considered to assess the degree of the injury and to establish a baseline for future study comparison. For those rare patients whose axillary nerve injury persists without electrodiagnostic evidence of recovery after 6 months, an open exploration may be considered.

Conclusion

With the recent advancements in arthroscopy, a variety of shoulder disorders are now treated almost exclusively with an arthroscopic surgery. The use of shoulder arthroscopy is likely to gain even more popularity as the next generation of surgeons pioneer new surgical technologies and expertise. Although most of these procedures can be performed safely with a low rate of morbidity, it should be noted that complications will continue to occur, even in the hands of the most expert arthroscopists.

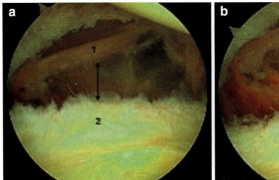

Fig. 15.3 Arthroscopic view of cadaver shoulder through the anterior portal. (**a**) In neutral (adducted arm) position the axillary nerve lies close to the glenoid margin; (**b**) Abduction of the arm moves the axillary nerve further away from the glenoid. (1 – axillary nerve; 2 – inferior edge of the glenoid) (reprinted from Yoo et al.[47] copyright 2007, with permission from Elsevier)

Hence, careful techniques should be utilized to minimize these risks and increased attention should be provided to identify these complications.

References

1. Andrews J, Broussard T, Carson W (1985) Arthroscopy of the shoulder in the management of partial tears of the rotator cuff: a preliminary report. Arthroscopy 1:117-22
2. Cofield R (1983) Arthroscopy of the shoulder. Mayo Clin Proc 58:501-8
3. Wiley A, Older M (1980) Shoulder arthroscopy. Investigations with a fibrooptic instrument. Am J Sports Med 8:31-8
4. Ellman H (1987) Arthroscopic subacromial decompression: analysis of one- to three-year results. Arthroscopy 3:173-81
5. AANA (1986) Complications in arthroscopy: the knee and other joints. Committee on Complications of the Arthroscopy Association of North America. Arthroscopy 2:253-8
6. Small N (1988) Complications in arthroscopic surgery performed by experienced arthroscopists. Arthroscopy 4: 215-21
7. Brislin K, Field L, Savoie FIII (2007) Complications after arthroscopic rotator cuff repair. Arthroscopy 23:124-8
8. Curtis A, Synder S, Del Pizzo W et al (1992) Complications of shoulder arthroscopy. Arthroscopy 8:395
9. Weber S, Abrams J, Nottage W (2002) Complications associated with arthroscopic shoulder surgery. Arthroscopy 18: 88-95
10. Warner JJ (1997) Frozen shoulder: Diagnosis and management. J Am Acad Orthop Surg 5:130-40
11. Diercks R, Stevens M (2004) Gentle thawing of the frozen shoulder: a prospective study of supervised neglect versus intensive physical therapy in seventy-seven patients with frozen shoulder syndrome followed up for two years. J Shoulder Elbow Surg 13:499-502
12. Griggs S, Ahn A, Green A (2000) Idiopathic adhesive capsulitis. A prospective functional outcome study of nonoperative treatment. J Bone Joint Surg Am 82-A:1398-407
13. Kivimaki J, Pohjolainen T, Malmivaara A et al (2007) Manipulation under anesthesia with home exercises versus home exercises alone in the treatment of frozen shoulder: a randomized, controlled trial with 125 patients. J Shoulder Elbow Surg 16:722-6
14. Levine W, Kashyap C, Bak S et al (2007) Nonoperative management of idiopathic adhesive capsulitis. J Shoulder Elbow Surg 16:569-73
15. Neviaser R, Neviaser T (1987) The frozen shoulder. Diagnosis and management. Clin Orthop Relat Res Oct(223):59-64
16. Harryman DII (1993) Shoulders: frozen and stiff. Instr Course Lect 42:247-57
17. Loew M, Heichel T, Lehner B (2005) Intraarticular lesions in primary frozen shoulder after manipulation under general anesthesia. J Shoulder Elbow Surg 14:16-21
18. Brown A, Weiss R, Greenberg C et al (1993) Interscalene block for shoulder arthroscopy: comparison with general anesthesia. Arthroscopy 9:295-300
19. Kinnard P, Truchon R, St-Pierre A et al (1994) Interscalene block for pain relief after shoulder surgery. A prospective randomized study. Clin Orthop Relat Res Jul(304):22-4
20. Axelsson K, Gupta A, Johanzon E et al (2008) Intraarticular administration of ketorolac, morphine, and ropivacaine combined with intraarticular patient-controlled regional analgesia for pain relief after shoulder surgery: a randomized, double-blind study. Anesth Analg 106:328-33 table of contents
21. Yamaguchi K, Sethi N, Bauer G (2002) Postoperative pain control following arthroscopic release of adhesive capsulitis: a short-term retrospective review study of the use of an intra-articular pain catheter. Arthroscopy 18:359-65
22. Webb D, Guttmann D, Cawley P et al (2007) Continuous infusion of a local anesthetic versus interscalene block for postoperative pain control after arthroscopic shoulder surgery. Arthroscopy 23:1006-11
23. Savoie F, Field L, Jenkins R et al (2000) The pain control infusion pump for postoperative pain control in shoulder surgery. Arthroscopy 16:339-42
24. Gomoll A, Kang R, Williams J et al (2006) Chondrolysis after continuous intra-articular bupivacaine infusion: an experimental model investigating chondrotoxicity in the rabbit shoulder. Arthroscopy 22:813-9

25. Hansen B, Beck C, Beck E et al (2007) Postarthroscopic glenohumeral chondrolysis. Am J Sports Med 35:1628-34
26. Dogan N, Erdem A, Erman Z et al (2004) The effects of bupivacaine and neostigmine on articular cartilage and synovium in the rabbit knee joint. J Int Med Res 32:513-9
27. Arkkila P, Kantola I, Viikari JS et al (1996) Shoulder capsulitis in type I and II diabetic patients: association with diabetic complications and related diseases. Ann Rheum Dis 55:907-14
28. Rauoof M, Lone N, Bhat B et al (2004) Etiological factors and clinical profile of adhesive capsulitis in patients seen at the rheumatology clinic of a tertiary care hospital in India. Saudi Med J 25:359-62
29. Pal B, Anderson J, Dick W et al (1986) Limitation of joint mobility and shoulder capsulitis in insulin- and non-insulin-dependent diabetes mellitus. Br J Rheumatol 25:147-51
30. Massoud S, Pearse E, Levy O et al (2002) Operative management of the frozen shoulder in patients with diabetes. J Shoulder Elbow Surg 11:609-13
31. Bigliani L, Flatow E, Deliz E (1991) Complications of shoulder arthroscopy. Orthop Rev 20:743-51
32. Herrera M, Bauer G, Reynolds F et al (2002) Infection after mini-open rotator cuff repair. J Shoulder Elbow Surg 11:605-8
33. Ogilvie-Harris D, Wiley A (1986) Arthroscopic surgery of the shoulder. A general appraisal. J Bone Joint Surg Br 68:201-7
34. Kwon Y, Kalainov D, Rose H et al (2005) Management of early deep infection after rotator cuff repair surgery. J Shoulder Elbow Surg 14:1-5
35. Athwal G, Sperling J, Rispoli D et al (2007) Deep infection after rotator cuff repair. J Shoulder Elbow Surg 16:306-11
36. Jeon I, Choi C, Seo J et al (2006) Arthroscopic management of septic arthritis of the shoulder joint. J Bone Joint Surg Am 88:1802-6
37. Stanish W, Peterson D (1995) Shoulder arthroscopy and nerve injury: pitfalls and prevention. Arthroscopy 11:458-66
38. Pitman M, Nainzadeh N, Ergas E et al (1988) The use of somatosensory evoked potentials for detection of neuropraxia during shoulder arthroscopy. Arthroscopy 4:250-5
39. Segmuller H, Alfred S, Zilio G et al (1995) Cutaneous nerve lesions of the shoulder and arm after arthroscopic shoulder surgery. J Shoulder Elbow Surg 4:254-8
40. Flatow E, Bigliani L, April E (1989) An anatomic study of the musculocutaneous nerve and its relationship to the coracoid process. Clin Orthop Relat Res Jul(244):166-71
41. Meyer M, Graveleau N, Hardy P et al (2007) Anatomic risks of shoulder arthroscopy portals: anatomic cadaveric study of 12 portals. Arthroscopy 23:529-36
42. Lo IK, Lind C, Burkhart S (2004) Glenohumeral arthroscopy portals established using an outside-in technique: neurovascular anatomy at risk. Arthroscopy 20:596-602
43. Miniaci A, McBirnie J (2003) Thermal capsular shrinkage for treatment of multidirectional instability of the shoulder. J Bone Joint Surg Am 85-A:2283-7
44. Uno A, Bain G, Mehta J (1999) Arthroscopic relationship of the axillary nerve to the shoulder joint capsule: an anatomic study. J Shoulder Elbow Surg 8:226-30
45. Price M, Tillett E, Acland R et al (2004) Determining the relationship of the axillary nerve to the shoulder joint capsule from an arthroscopic perspective. J Bone Joint Surg Am 86-A:2135-42
46. Jerosch J, Filler T, Peuker E (2002) Which joint position puts the axillary nerve at lowest risk when performing arthroscopic capsular release in patients with adhesive capsulitis of the shoulder? Knee Surg Sports Traumatol Arthrosc 10:126-9
47. Yoo J, Kim J, Ahn J et al (2007) Arthroscopic perspective of the axillary nerve in relation to the glenoid and arm position: a cadaveric study. Arthroscopy 23(12):1271-7
48. Wong K, Williams G (2001) Complications of thermal capsulorrhaphy of the shoulder. J Bone Joint Surg Am 83-A(Suppl 2 Pt 2):151-5

Editors' Comments: Miscellaneous Shoulder Conditions

Adhesive Capsulitis

Although forward elevation can often be improved with manipulation alone, full external and particularly internal rotation is much more difficult to achieve without surgical release of the capsule. In addition, in postsurgical adhesive capsulitis, particularly after a repair, controlled release is greatly preferable to blind manipulation, to avoid disrupting the repaired tissue. In addition, in postsurgical adhesive capsulitis, adhesions are also often found in the subacromial space and subscapularis bursa which are most amenable to direct surgical release.

We recommend direct release of the inferior capsule as well as anterior and inferior capsule. This can be facilitated by the use of an accessory posterior inferior portal while viewing from the standard posterior portal. Capsule is released with an electrocautery device facing the glenoid just off the labral surface. The axillary nerve is >1.5 cm away from the inferior glenoid margin, and should be safe as long as the release is performed adjacent to the inferior labrum and inferior glenoid margin. A complete release has been obtained when muscle fibers are visible through the release. The rotator interval and coracohumeral ligament will also usually need to be released to obtain full external rotation. It is also important to release adhesions around the rotator cuff including those in the subscapularis bursa. In rare cases, usually after open shoulder surgery, some of the adhesions are extramuscular and will not be accessible arthroscopically. If impaired motion persists intraoperatively after adequate arthroscopic releases, the surgeon may want to consider open extramuscular releases. Beware of patients who have had previous radiation about the shoulder, since their scarring is quite extensive, thus making full motion as a final outcome extremely difficult even with open releases.

Patients who develop postoperative adhesions often are timid with their subsequent physical therapy and have some psychological barriers to believing they will ever get their motion back. We have found benefit to photographing the patients arm in full range of motion after the surgery, which we show to the patients postoperatively as encouragement, and will occasionally even leave the patients arm in full foward flexion until they are awake in the recovery room and can visualize the success of the procedure.

Some surgeons use CPM machines postrelease, but we have found these cumbersome and unpredictable We prefer to start the patient on physical therapy post-op day #1, 3–5 times a week. If adhesions seem to be recurring at 6 weeks, we will schedule a repeat manipulation at this point, before the adhesions become thick enough to require additional surgical release. We place all patients on a nonsteroidal for at least 1 month post-op, and will also use Medrol dose packs on occasion.

The best way to treat postoperative adhesions is to avoid them. We being pendulum exercises day one post-op for all shoulder surgery patients, and emphasize external rotation to avoid scarring of the anterior capsule and coracohumeral ligament. We also utilize an abduction/external rotation pillow along with a sling to avoid capsular scarring. Patients are advised to take pain medication 1 h prior to their physical therapy sessions which begin 7 days post-op. Proper physical therapy is also essential in avoiding other complications. If patients do not receive glenohumeral joint mobilization, they will often compensate with scapulothoracic motion. To the inexperienced therapist, the patient will appear to be meeting range of motion milestones, but in fact they are getting a stiff glenohumeral joint, and straining their AC joints due to transference of force to this joint and then to the scapula to obtain arm elevation. This is a common cause for secondary AC joint pain following previous unrelated shoulder surgery. To truly test your patients recovery of motion, stabilize their scapula with your hand, or have them stand leaning backward against a wall to stabilize their scapula and then have them raise their arm. This will accurately test glenohumeral motion.

Nerve Injury

The exact etiology of reported neuropraxias after shoulder arthroscopy is not clear. In our experience, the most likely culprit is from the distal holding devices. We avoid use of rigid gauntlets which can easily compress superficial nerves, and take care not to wrap the distal traction devices too tightly. Traction up to 15 lbs appears to be well tolerated, and we have not had a neuropraxia in thousands of cases using this technique. However, it should be noted that most cases are under an hour or hour and a half and in general excessively long surgical times even with lighter traction should be avoided. Interscalene anesthesia blocks can also cause neuropraxia, and should be carefully considered as a cause when evaluating the etiology of a postoperative complication. When performing shoulder instability surgery, care must be taken when utilizing suture hooks in the inferior pouch, since the axially nerve can be injured if an overly aggressive bite of tissue is taken. Avoid going too deep, or more than 1 cm inferior to the inferior labrum.

Others

Always place a gauze or ABD pad under the patient's axilla postoperatively, especially in warm humid climates. This will avoid secondary fungal infections which will slow recovery and lead to a very unhappy patient.

Encourage elbow wrist and hand motion immediately postoperatively. This will help avoid distal edema and secondary joint stiffness.

Encourage patients to sleep in a lounge chair or use multiple pillows so that they are in a beach chair position while sleeping for several weeks after reconstructive shoulder surgery. This will prevent them rolling onto the surgical site and potentially disrupting your repair.

Index

A
Abduction stress testing, 98
Abrams, J.S., 175
ACCR. *See* Anatomical coracoclavicular ligament reconstruction
ACDs. *See* Articular cartilage defects
ACI. *See* Autologous chondrocyte implantation
ACL. *See* Anterior cruciate ligament
Acromioclavicular (AC) joint surgery
    athletes, 261–262
    complications
        ACCR technique, 252–257
        augmentation, 251–252
        coracoacromial ligament transfer and repair, 251
        distal clavicle resection, coracoclavicular ligament, 251–252
    degenerative pathology
        complications, 258
        distal clavicle resection, 257–259
        failed distal clavicle resection, 258, 260
    distal clavicle fracture, 261
    functional anatomy
        static and dynamic stabilizers, 249
        vertical stability, 250
    injury diagnosis and pathophysiology
        classification, 246–247
        imaging, 247–249
        mechanism, 246
        treatment, 249
    nonoperative treatment, 250
    preoperative, 251
    radiographic evaluation, 247
    revision/reconstruction
        arthroscopic, 260–261
        postoperative management, 261
    revision repair/reconstruction, 260
    type V separation, 248
Ahlback, 169
Alhalki, M., 30
Alldredge, R., 261
Amendola, A., 115
AMG. *See* Anterior midglenoid
Amis, A.A., 152
Anatomical coracoclavicular ligament reconstruction (ACCR) technique
    clavicle
        bone tunnels, 256
        graft interference screw fixation, 256
        osteological analysis, 252–253
    closure
        complications and bailouts, 256–257
        of deltotrapezial fascial flaps, 256
    complications and bailouts, 253
    coracoid, bone tunnel preparation
        cannulated reamer, 252
        complications and bailouts, 254–255
    coracoid process graft fixation
        interference fit technique, 255
        loop technique, 255–256
    effect in cadaveric model, 252
    graft preparation
        complications and bailouts, 254
        coracoid process screw fixation, 253–254
Andrews, J., 189
Andrish, J., 140–141
Anterior cruciate ligament (ACL), 3, 11, 14, 16, 20–21, 25, 34, 97
    bucket-handle meniscal tears, 23
    intraoperative factors, reconstruction
        anterior tibial tunnel, 58–59
        anteromedial portal, 59–60
        cross pin break, 64
        devices breakages, 62–63
        divergent fixation, 64–65
        dropped graft, 56–57
        femoral back wall, 60–61
        gastrocnemius, 55–56
        graft amputation, 55
        grafting technique, 55
        graft passage, 61
        graft–tunnel length mismatch, 61–62
        knee hyperflexion, 59–60
        loose fixation, 63
        no touch technique, 57–58
        PCL damages, 65–66
        push-pull drill technique, 59–60
        risks, graft handling, 58
        tibial footprint, 59
        traction sutures break, 62–63
        trapezoidal-shaped graft, 56
        tunnel malposition, 57–59

Anterior cruciate ligament (ACL) (cont.)
    postoperative factors, reconstruction
        femoral tunnel placement, 70
        fractures, 67–69
        infection, 66–67
        PL tibial tunnel, 70–71
        scarring/keloid formation, 69–71
        stiffness, 66–68
        tensioning devices, 68
        tibial tunnel placement, 70
        widening, tibial tunnel, 69
    reconstruction, 23, 27–28, 31–33
        back up tibial fixation, 72–73
        complications, 129
        description, 53
        graft loosening prevention, 73
        patella bone plug harvest, 72
        preoperative factors, 53–54
        risk, functional anatomy, 54
        surgeries, 130
        tibial slope, 129–130
    tibial insertion, 27
Anterior midglenoid (AMG), 210, 213
    cannula and crochet hook, 199
    portal and crochet hook, 200
Anterior superior portal (ASP), 196
Anterolateral (AL) bundle, 75–77, 79–85
Anteromedial rotatory instability (AMRI), 97
Arnoczky, S., 2
Arthrofibrosis, 165–172
Arthroscopic biceps tenodesis
    anatomy, 208
    description, 207
    interference screw fixation, 216
    pain, clinical source, 208
    SCOI subpectoral technique
        final fixation and closure, 219–220
        humeral drilling and tendon passing, 219
        identification and release, 217
        incision and tendon preparation, 217–219
        proximal drill hole, 220
        repositioning, 217
    in shoulder function, 208
    soft tissue suture fixation
        anterior cannula, 210
        glenohumeral joint, 209
        high-strength braided suture, 211
    suture anchor fixation
        SCOI, 212–216
        subacromial, 211–212
    techniques, 209
    tendons, 208–209
Arthroscopic knee surgery
    arthrofibrosis
        diagnosis of, 165
        flexion contractures, 166
        ligament reconstruction, 165–166
        motion loss, inflammation and symptoms, 167
        open treatment, 168165
        postoperative rehabilitation protocols, 168–169
        prevention, 171
        risk factors, 166
        surgical indications, 167–168
        treatment, 165, 171–172
        varieties, 166–167
    broken instrumentation, 171
    osteonecrosis
        and arthroscopic meniscectomy, 169–170
        bone marrow edema syndrome, 170
        staging systems, 170
    portals, 171
    postoperative infection
        joint infection classic signs, 169
        sterile technique and prophylactic antibiotics, 169
Arthroscopic rotator cuff repair
    adhesed excavation, 240–241
    compaction bone grafting, 241–242
    failure, 239–240
    functional anatomy
        coracoid process, 226
        suprascapular nerve, 226–227
    impaction grafting technique, 243
    intraoperative complications
        anchor pull out, 232–233
        arthroscopic view, 232
        cuff tissue, 236–237
        knot tying, 237–238
        outfoldings/dog-ears, 237
        suture, 234–236
        turbulence control, 233
        unloading anchor, 233–234
        visualization, 231–232
    positioning, 227–228
    postoperative complications
        infection, 238–239
        stiffness, 238
    principles, 228
    residual metal anchors, 241–242
    revision, 240
    steps
        bony bed preparation, 230
        repair constructs, 231
        rotator cuff tear, 228
        suture-anchor insertion and management, 230
        suture passing and tying knots, 230–231
        tear mobility determination, 228–229
Arthroscopic shoulder surgery
    adhesive capsulitis
        capsular release, 267
        capsulolabral tear, 267
        complication, 267–268
        MUA maneuvers, 266
        postoperative adhesions, 270–271
        types, 265
    infection
        serologic markers, 268
        surgical irrigation and debridement, 268
    nerve injuries
        cadaver shoulder, 270
        distal holding devices, 271
        5-o'clock portal, 269

Arthroscopic suture anchor fixation
    SCOI
        anchor placement, 213–214
        biceps release and, 215–216
        biceps tendon hitch, 212–215
        rotator interval and bone preparation, 212
    subacromial, 211–212
Articular cartilage defects (ACDs)
    rational and systematic care, 42
    treatment plans, 41
Athwal, G., 239
Autologous chondrocyte implantation (ACI), 22, 23
    factors and tools, 38
    key components, 46–47
    objective assessments, 38
    partial detachment, 48
    procedure, 43, 46
    sandwich technique, 47
    treatments, 47–48
Ayeni, O, 53

B
Bahk, M.S., 189, 207
Baker, J., 252
Barber-Westin, S., 109
Bearden, J., 261
Beck, P., 149
Belfie, D., 109
Bellemans, J., 135
Bert, J., 169
Biceps tendon hitch
    AMG cannula, 214–215
    epidural needle, 212–213
    Mehalik hitch, 215
    SCC cannula, 213
Bishop, J., 226
Blazar, P., 252
Bone block technique, 31
Bone marrow edema syndrome
    patterns and stages, 170
    symptoms, 170–171
Bone plug technique, 29–31
Bosworth, B., 251, 258, 261
Brahme, S., 170
Brislin, K., 225, 238
Brunelli, G., 261
Bugbee, W., 46
Bunnell stitch, 5, 6, 85
Burkhart, S., 229
Burks, R., 183
Burmester curve
    ligament insertions, 96
    MCL attachment, 96–97
    sMCL, 97
Burns, J.P., 207

C
Cadenat, F., 246
Cartilage restoration surgery
    complications
        ACD, patient preoperative assessment, 38–39
        ACI, 46–48
        arthroscopic assessment, 39
        chondropenia, 39–41
        DVT and pulmonary embolism, 43–44
        marrow stimulation techniques, 44–45
        osteochondral allograft transplantation, 45–46
        osteochondral autograft transplantation, 45
        treatment algorithms, 41–42
    description, 37–38
    index procedure, 48
    infections, 43
    rehabilitation, 42–43
    transfer techniques, 48–49
Caton–Deschamps measurement techniques, 134
Chondropenia severity score (CSS), 40–41
Chondropenic pathway, treatment algorithms
    clinical failure, 41
    femoral and trochlear defects, 41
    intraoperative complications, 42
Codman, E., 250
Cole, B., 33
Collateral ligament surgery, knee
    LCL injuries
        anatomy and biomechanics, 107–108
        examination, 108
        graft breaks, 112
        postoperative care, 111
        treatments, 109–111
    MCL injuries
        ACL reconstruction, 112
        anatomy, 92–95
        biomechanics, 95–96
        Burmester curve, 96–97
        classification and examination, 97
        femoral origin screw and post fail, 111–112
        first line of defense *vs.* primary restraint, 97
        grade III *vs.* ACL combined treatment, 100–101
        isolated tears, treatment, 99–100
        physical examination, 98–99
        and POL proximal avulsion, 102
        surgical treatment, 101–106
        vertical tear, 102
        Y-shaped tear, 102–103
        zigzag and diagonal tears, 103
    motion problems avoidance, 111
Colosimo, A., 258
Compression-rotation test, 192
Concomitant injuries, 3
Continuous passive motion (CPM), 43, 91, 101
Cooper, D., 190
Coracoclavicular (CC) ligament, 249
Corteen, D., 250
Cosgarea, A., 135, 159
Cox, J., 250
CPM. *See* Continuous passive motion
Crank test, 192
CSS. *See* Chondropenia severity score
Cummins, C.A., 240
Curl, W., 37

D
Deep venous thrombosis (DVT), 43–44
Dehaven, K., 169
DePalma, A., 249
Distal clavicular ligaments, anatomy, 247
Distal femoral osteotomy (DFO), 116, 120
Dodds, J., 167
Dovetail/slot technique
    LM and MM transplants, 28–29
        press-fit, 25
        trough preparation, 28
Dudich, 6
Dunn, H., 251–252, 260
DVT. *See* Deep venous thrombosis
Dye, S., 133, 160

E
Eager, M., 135, 159
Electromyography (EMG), 208
Ellsasser, J., 100
Elman, M.V., 133
Excessive lateral pressure syndrome (ELPS), 137

F
Fanelli, G., 75
Farr, J., 33, 152
FasT-fix™, 6–7
Fast fix device, 16
Fischer, B., 260
Fithian, D., 137, 154
Fithian's technique, 154
Franceschi, F., 239
Freedman, E., 166
8 French pediatric feeding tube, 82–83
Frozen shoulder, 265
Fulkerson, J., 134, 140, 155, 160

G
Galatz, L., 226
Gardiner, J., 95
Grauthoff, V., 258
Giffin, J.R., 115
Goble, E., 33
Godfrey test, 77
Golant, A., 265
Gollehon, D., 107
Gollwitzer, M., 261
Grafting technique, 55
Grood, E., 95, 107

H
HAGL lesions, 186
Halbrecht, J., 144–145
Harner, C.D., 30, 75
Hauser procedure, 148, 150, 155
Hemarthrosis, 138–139, 145
Henry, J., 149
Herrera, M., 239, 268

Heterotopic ossification, 168
High tibial osteotomy (HTO)
    closing and opening wedge, 119–120
    infection, 117
    reconstruction, 129
    salvage operation, 117
Howell, S., 30
HTO. *See* High tibial osteotomy
Hughston, J., 97–99, 108, 140
Human leukocyte antigen (HLA), 38
Hunter, W., 37

I
Iliotibial band (ITB), 107
Indelicato, P., 100, 101
Inside-out meniscal repair techniques
    lateral approach, 12
    medial approach, 11
Interference fit technique, 255
International Cartilage Repair Society (ICRS), 38, 39
Intra-articular fracture, knee osteotomies
    HTO, 123
    microsagittal saw, 122
    opening and closing wedge, 122–123

J
Jarvinen, M., 100
Jay, G., 261
Jeon, I., 268
Johnson, D., 53
Johnston, J.A., 37–50
Jones, R., 19, 100
Judd, D., 169
Jump test, 140

K
Kannus, P., 100
Kaplan-Meier survival analysis, 22
Kibler's anterior slide test, 192
Kim's biceps load tests, 192
Kim, T., 168
Kalmmer, H., 258
Klimkiewicz, J.J., 20, 252
Kline, A., 136
Kolowich test, 138
Koshino, 170
Kuroda, R., 144
Kurzweil, P.R., 1
Kwon, Y.W., 239, 265

L
LaPrade, R., 102
Larson, R., 109
Lateral collateral ligament (LCL) injuries
    anatomy and biomechanics
        knee lateral side, 107–108
        tissue isometric behavior analysis, 108
    examination, 108

graft breaks, 112
postoperative care, 111
surgical treatment
achilles tendon allograft, 110
acute avulsions, 109
reconstruction technique, 109–110
Lateral patellar instability
CT tracking study, 143
derotational osteotomy, 142
4+ lateral glide, 141
MPFL reconstruction, 144
Q-angle and TT-TG, 141–142
LeClere, L., 245
Lee, K., 253
Lee, S., 253
Lemos, M., 257–258
Loew, M., 267
Lo, I.K.Y., 225, 226
Loop technique, 255–256
Lotke, P., 170

M

Magnetic resonance imaging (MRI)
diagnostic techniques, 38
matrix-specific, 39
tools, 38
Mandelbaum, B.R., 37–50
Manipulation under anesthesia (MUA), 266–267, 269
Mansat, P., 225
Mariani, E., 208
Marrow stimulation techniques
chronic lesions, 45
intralesional osteophyte, 44–45
mesenchymal stem cells, 44
Marshall, J., 92
Marti, C., 116
Marumoto, J., 138
Mayr, E., 258
Mazzocca, A.A., 245
Mazzocca, D., 245, 252
McFarland, E., 238
MDI. See Multidirectional instability
Mechanoreceptors, 2
Medial collateral ligament (MCL) injuries, 4, 5, 17, 166
capsuloligamentous structures, 92
chronic instability
medial laxity, 106
reconstruction, 107
classifications, 97
femoral origin screw and post fail, 111–112
grade III vs. ACL combined treatment, 100–101
isolated tears treatment
grade I and II, 99
grade III tears, 99–100
physical examination
grade I and II, 98
grade III, 98–99
grade IV, 99
sMCL stability, 98
and POL proximal avulsion, 102
postoperative care, 106–107

semimembranosus corner, vertical tear, 102
sMCL, 93–95
surgical treatment
dMCL repair, 103–104
general principals, 101–102
grade IV, 102
slocum test, 103–104
sMCL interstitial tear, 104, 106
Y-shaped tear, 102–103
zigzag and diagonal tears, 103
Medial patellofemoral ligament (MPFL), 141–143, 161
arthroscopic reefing
Halbrecht technique, 144–145
open reefing, 145–146
suture breakage, 145
tissue advancement, 144
open reefing
anteriorization, 149–150
bone graft technique, 150
complications, 146
groove deepening procedure, 149
opening wedge osteotomy, 148
osteochondral fracture, 147
tug test, 146
X-ray, 147–148
reconstruction
biotenodesis, 152
Fithian's technique, 154
overtensioning, 151
semitendinosis autograft, 151–152
soft tissue restrain, 150
two incisions, 153
Meislin, R., 165
Mendez, K., 91
Meniscofemoral ligaments (MFLs), 76, 80
Meniscus repair
complex, 17
complications, 14–15
fast fix device, 16
fibrin clot, 16
functional anatomy
microvascular, 2
ultrastructure of, 2–3
indications, bucket-handle medial meniscus, 3
intraoperative details
diagnostic arthroscopy, 4
enhancement agents, 5
fixation devices, 5–10
inside-out repair techniques, 10–13
outside-in repair technique, 13
setting up, 3–4
site preparation, 4–5
postoperative pain control protocol and rehabilitation, 14, 16
unstable bucket handle tears, 16
zone-specific
cannulae, 16–17
inside-out repairs, fluid management, 17
Meniscus transplantation
allograft, 34
bone plug technique
MCL and, 29–31
notchplasty, 30

Meniscus transplantation (cont.)
    clinical results, 32–34
    complications, 21
    functional anatomy
        horn insertion, 20–21
        medial meniscus transmission, 21
        two tunnel technique, 20
    graft fixation
        bone and augmenting, 31–32
        suture balancing, 31
    graft passage and seating, 29–31
    graft preparation
        bone plugs and, 26
        dovetail technique, 27
    graft-specific considerations
        meniscal dimensions, 25
        sizing, 24
    intraoperative considerations
        arthroscopy and remnant meniscectomy, 25–26
        rim preparation, 26
    operative instrumentation, 25
    postoperative considerations, 32
    preoperative considerations
        patient-specific factors, 22
        pitfalls, 22–24
    revision surgery, 32, 33
    tunnel establishment
        anterior and posterior, 27–28
        dovetail/slot technique, 28–29
Menschik, A., 96
Menscius Mender II™, 13
MFLs. See Meniscofemoral ligaments
Milachowski, K., 32
Morgan, C., 191–193
MPFL. See Medial patellofemoral ligament
MRI. See Magnetic resonance imaging
Muller, W., 93, 97, 102, 104, 105
Multidirectional instability (MDI), 186
Multiligamentous injuries, 165
Mumford, E., 251
Muscolo, D., 170
Myositis ossificans, 168

N
Neault, M., 258
Neer, C., 260
Nevaiser, 251
Nguyen, T.B., 1
Nicholson, G., 258
No touch technique, 57–58
Noyes, F., 33, 88, 109, 110, 165, 167

O
O'Brien's test, 192, 193
Osteochondral allograft transplantation
    complications, 46
    components of, 45–46
    treatments, 45
Osteochondral autograft transplantation, 45
Osteotomies, knee
    complications, 116
        AP radiographs, 117–119
        compartment syndrome, 126
        fixation failure, 127–128
        fracture–unstable hinge, 120–122
        hardware, 127, 129
        HTO and ACL reconstruction, 129–131
        infection, 126–127
        intra-articular fracture, 122–123
        nerve injury, 126
        patella baja, 120
        sagittal slope alteration, 123–125
        stiffness, 129
        undercorrection and overcorrection, 117–120
        union/malunion, 127
        vascular injury, 125–126
    description, 115–117
    risk, functional anatomy, 117
    treatments, 116

P
Pagnani, M., 190
Paletta, G., 30–31
Panossian, V., 190
Partial thickness articular sided repairs (PASTA), 242
Patella surgery
    anterior knee pain, 133–134
    arthroscopic medial reefing, 144–146
    Caton–Deschamps measurement techniques, 134
    functional anatomy
        drilling, 137
        tubercle osteotomies, 136
    intraoperative complications
        cold therapy, 139
        hemarthrosis, 138
        ligament reconstruction, 141
        medial patellar subluxation, 140
        saber device, 139
        tendon graft, 140
        vastus lateralis, 138–139
    lateral patellar instability, 141–144
    lateral retinacular release
        contraindications, 137–138
        ELPS and, 137
        limited vs. extensive fashion, 138
        recurrent patellar instability, 137
        X-ray and Kolowich test, 138
    MRI vs. CT, 161
    open reefing, 146–150
    patellofemoral joint, 133
    proximal patellar realignments, 144
    revision surgery, 160–161
    synovectomy, 161–162
    tibial tubercle osteotomy
        anteriorization and medialization, 155
        2 drill bit technique, 158
        free-hand osteotomy, 157
        postoperative complication, 158–160

Q-angle, 156
tracker guide, 156–157
trochlear dysplasia, 135
TT–TG distance measurement, 136
weight-bearing, 135
Paulos, L., 91, 166, 167
PCL. *See* Posterior cruciate ligament
Pennington, W., 260
Petersson, C., 249
Pinch-tuck technique, 6
Pitman, M., 269
Pizzo, D., 166
Platelet-Rich Fibrin Matrix™ (PRFM), 5, 6
Platelet-rich plasma (PRP), 5
Pohl, A., 228
POL. *See* Posterior oblique ligament
Popliteofibular ligament (PFL), 107
Posterior cruciate ligament (PCL) reconstruction
   AL and PM bundle, 76
   AL tibial tunnel, 80
   anesthesia, 76
   arthroscopic debridement, 80
   curette and rasp, 81
   diagnostic arthroscopy
      compartment syndrome, 78
      meniscal injuries, 79
      tibial origin, debridement, 79
   drilling/reaming, 83
   fluoroscopy
      AL guidewire and tunnel, 82
      intraoperative, 81
   graft passage and fixation
      bolster placement, 84–85
      tibialis anterior allograft and metal skid, 84
      ticron suture, 83
   graft selection and fixation
      allograft *vs.* autograft, 85
      autograft, 84
   injuries, 75
   intraoperative complications
      prevention, 85–86
      recognizing and dealing, 86–87
   patient positioning, 78
   postoperative
      complications, 87–88
      immediate care, 89
   preoperative evaluation
      external rotation test, 77
      surgical site marking, 76
   revision surgery, 88–89
   surface anatomy and skin marking, 77–78
Posterior oblique ligament (POL)
   attachment sites, 93
   and capsule detachment, 100
   functions, 95
   and MCL
      primary repair, 101–102
      proximal avulsion, 102
   origination, 92
   and SMCL, 94
   valgus stress, 98

Posterior sag test, 77
Posterolateral rotatory instability (PLRI), 109
Price, M., 226
Prophylactic preoperative antibiotics, 3
Provencher, M.T., 245
Prues-Latour, V., 170
Push-pull drill technique, 59–60

R
Ramappa, A., 155
Rapid-Loc™ system
   advantage, 7
   needle insertion, 9
Ricchetti, E., 137
Rockwood, C., 246
Rodosky, M., 190
Romeo, A.A., 245
Rudzki, J.R., 19
Ryu, R., 33

S
Salter, E., 249
Sanchis-Alfonso, V., 134, 139
Santori, N., 170
Schepsis, A.A., 133
Schottle's point, 152
Schweitzer, M., 170
SCOI repair technique
   biceps tendon, 196
   single anchor with double suture
      anchor placement, 197–198
      closure, 201
      labrum fixation, 199–201
      labrum, glenoid and cyst decompression, 197
      portals establishment, 196
      suture management, 199
SCOI subpectoral technique
   arthroscopic identification and release, 217
   final fixation and closure, 219–220
   humeral drilling and tendon passing, 219
   incision and tendon preparation
      biceps tendon, 218
      pectoralis major muscle, 217–218
   repositioning, 217
Scoop, J.M., 37–50
Segmuller, H., 269
Seroyer, S.T., 75
Setteceri, 239
Shaffer, B., 19
Shaikh, N., 171
Shapiro, M., 166
Shelbourne, K., 166
Shoulder labral repair
   arthroscopic revision surgery
      bone-grafting procedure, 184–185
      glenoid preparation, 185
   complication techniques
      arthroscopy *vs.* open repair, 178
      Hill-Sachs lesion, 177

Shoulder labral repair (*cont.*)
  load-and-shift exam, 178–179
  patient positioning, 177–178
  suture anchors, 178
 description, 175–176
 intraoperative complications
  anterior fovea, 180
  Bankart lesion, 179
  bone graft, 183
  capsular mobilization, 179–180
  chondral injuries, 181
  diagnostic arthroscopy, 179
  glenoid rim fractures, 181
  Hill-Sachs lesion, 179–180
  inferior capsular repair, 179–180
  knot-tying, 182
  metallic glenoid anchor, 181
  open surgical repairs, 182
  suture anchors, 180–181
  suture problems, 181–182
 postoperative complications
  anchor insertion and loosening, 183
  chondrolysis, 183
  glenohumeral joints, 184
 risk, functional anatomy, 176–177
 surgical procedures, 176
Shoulder Rescue Plug® system, 202
Shoulder superior labrum (SLAP) repair
 biomechanics
  arthroscopic, 190–191
  biceps and glenoid-labral anchor, 190
 classification, 191–192
 diagnosis
  physical, 192–193
  traumatic origin, 192
 fixation techniques, 195–196
 functional anatomy
  biceps and glenoid variation, 190
  sublabral recess, 189–190
 imaging
  Buford complex and MRI coronal, 195
  ganglion and spinoglenoid cysts, 194
  MRI, 193
  pathological signal, 193–194
  type III SLAP lesion, 194
  type II SLAP lesion, 193
 immobilization, 201
 intraoperative complications and revision surgery
  anchors, axillary radiograph, 201–202
  arthroscopic grasper, 202
 lesion types, 191
 postoperative considerations and rehabilitation, 203
 SCOI repair technique
  biceps tendon, 196
  single anchor with double suture, 196–201
 single portal, 202

  tear, arthroscopic diagnosis, 194
  type III and IVs with bucket handle component., 202–203
  type II lesions, 194–195
Shoulder traction and rotation (STaR), 217
Shuttle relay suture passer, 199
Sidles, J., 107
Slocum, D., 101, 103
Slocum test, 101, 103
Smith, M., 258
Snyder, S.J., 189, 191, 192, 207
Spalteholz technique, 2
Speed's test, 192, 193
Spielmann, A., 240
Staphylococcus sp., 169
STaR. *See* Shoulder traction and rotation
Steiner, T., 147
Stetson, W., 135, 159
Stewart, M., 258
Stone, K., 22, 25
Strauss, E.J., 165
Streptococcus sp., 169
Superficial medial collateral ligament (SMCL), 94

T
Teitge, R., 140, 142, 161
Tolo, E., 257–258
Tossy, J., 246
Total knee arthroplasty (TKA), 116
Trantalis, J., 225
Tsou, P., 258
Tug test, 146
Two tunnel technique, 20

V
Vasconcellos, D.A., 115
Vascular synovial tissue, 2
Verdonk, P., 33

W
Warren, L., 92
Warren, R., 2
Weaver-Dunn procedure, 252
Weaver, J., 251–252, 260
Weber, S., 225
Westerheide, K., 194
White, L., 170
Witonski, 134
Wolf, E., 260

Z
Zimmer, S., 133

Printed in the United States of America